WORK, HEALTH AND '.. _____ __
THE CONSTRUCTION INDUSTRY

This book covers a wide range of topics relating to the health and wellbeing of the construction workforce. Based on more than two decades of work examining various aspects of workers' health and wellbeing, the book addresses a key topic in construction management: how the design of work environments, construction processes and organisation of work impact upon construction workers' physical and psychological health.

Occupational health is a significant problem for the construction industry. However, the subject of health does not receive as much attention in occupational health and safety research or practice as the subject of safety. Traditional management approaches (focused on the prevention of accidents and injuries) are arguably ill-suited to addressing issues of workers' health and wellbeing. This book seeks to explain how workers' health and wellbeing are impacted by working in the construction industry, and suggest ways in which organisations (and decision makers within them) can positively shape workplaces and practices in ways that better support construction workers to maintain healthy and productive working lives.

Including chapter summaries and discussion questions to encourage student readers to reflect on and formulate their own viewpoints about the issues raised in each chapter, the book has the potential to be used as a textbook in undergraduate or postgraduate occupational health and safety, or construction management courses dealing with occupational health and safety. It could also be used as supplementary recommended reading in undergraduate or postgraduate programmes in architecture, engineering or management.

Helen Lingard is RMIT Distinguished Professor and Director of The Centre for Construction Work Health and Safety Research at RMIT University, Melbourne, Australia. Helen has been an active researcher in the field of construction work health and safety for more than 20 years. Helen has authored or co-authored three other books published by Taylor & Francis.

Michelle Turner is an Associate Professor at the School of Property, Construction and Project Management, is a member of The Centre for Construction Work Health and Safety Research at RMIT University, Melbourne, Australia, and co-leads the Health and Wellbeing stream with Distinguished Professor Helen Lingard. Michelle has more than fifteen years of experience working with the construction industry in her capacity as a health, wellbeing and resilience researcher.

WORK, HEALTH AND WELLBEING IN THE CONSTRUCTION INDUSTRY

Helen Lingard and Michelle Turner

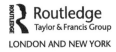
Routledge
Taylor & Francis Group

LONDON AND NEW YORK

Designed cover image: © Getty Images

First published 2023
by Routledge
4 Park Square, Milton Park, Abingdon, Oxon OX14 4RN

and by Routledge
605 Third Avenue, New York, NY 10158

Routledge is an imprint of the Taylor & Francis Group, an informa business

British Library Cataloguing-in-Publication Data
A catalogue record for this book is available from the British Library

Library of Congress Cataloging-in-Publication Data
Names: Lingard, Helen, author. | Turner, Michelle, author.
Title: Work, health and wellbeing in the construction industry /
Helen Lingard, Michelle Turner.
Description: Abingdon, Oxon ; New York, NY : Routledge, 2023. |
Includes bibliographical references and index. | Identifiers: LCCN 2022050655 |
ISBN 9780367410087 (hardback) | ISBN 9780367410094 (paperback) |
ISBN 9780367814236 (ebook)
Subjects: LCSH: Building–Safety measures. | Construction industry–Employees–Health
and hygiene. | Construction industry–Health aspects.
Classification: LCC TH443 .L5624 2023 |
DDC 690.068–dc23/eng/20230103
LC record available at https://lccn.loc.gov/2022050655

ISBN: 978-0-367-41008-7 (hbk)
ISBN: 978-0-367-41009-4 (pbk)
ISBN: 978-0-367-81423-6 (ebk)

DOI: 10.1201/9780367814236

Typeset in Bembo
by Newgen Publishing UK

CONTENTS

Preface   *xi*

1 Introduction: The health imperative   1

   1.1   Introduction 1

   1.2   The global burden of work-related disease and injury 1

   1.3   Workers' health in the construction industry 2

   1.4   Social determinants of health 4

   1.5   Motivation for managing workers' health 9

       1.5.1   Moral/ethical considerations 10

       1.5.2   The business case 10

       1.5.3   Legal requirements 11

   1.6   What constitutes a healthy workplace? 12

   1.7   The way work is done in construction 17

   1.8   Gender, work and health 18

   1.9   The rest of this book 19

   1.10 Discussion and review questions 22

   References 22

2 Attending to the "H" in OH&S   27

   2.1   Introduction 27

   2.2   Who should be responsible for managing workers' health? 28

   2.3   Managing occupational health is more complicated than
       managing safety 30

   2.4   Deciding on appropriate risk controls for occupational health
       hazards 32

   2.5   Occupational cancer 34

2.6   Exposure to respirable silica 37

2.7   Occupational hearing loss 41

2.8   Other factors contributing to occupational hearing loss 47

2.9   Products causing occupational skin disease 47

2.10 Musculoskeletal disorders 49

2.11 Conclusion 51

2.12 Discussion and review questions 52

2.13 Acknowledgements 52

References 52

3 Work-related factors impacting construction workers'
   psychological health   60

3.1   Introduction 60

3.2   The relationship between job quality and psychological health 61

3.3   Theories linking work with psychological health 62

3.4   Work-related stress in construction work 64

3.5   Psychosocial hazards and the management of risk 67

3.6   ISO 45003 71

3.7   Workplace mental health programmes 78

3.8   Conclusion 82

3.9   Discussion and review questions 83

3.10 Acknowledgements 83

References 83

4 Working time, health and wellbeing   88

4.1   Introduction 88

4.2   Time in project-based construction work 88

4.3   Long work hours, health and wellbeing 89

4.4   Long hours of work in construction 90

4.5   The balance between work and non-work life 91

4.6   The gendered nature of work hours and health 91

4.7   Other facets of working time with relevance to health 93

4.8   Taxonomy of work schedules: Long hours, overtime and
        work schedule control 97

4.9   Working time modifications and reductions 98

4.10 Working-time modifications in the Australian construction
        industry 99

4.11 Recovery and the right to disconnect 104

4.12 Conclusion 106

4.13 Discussion and review questions 107

4.14 Acknowledgements 107

References 107

5 Women's health in construction   113
    5.1   Introduction 113
    5.2   Health inequality: A societal issue 113
    5.3   Gender as a social determinant of health 116
    5.4   Health and minority status 122
    5.5   Discrimination–health relationship 125
    5.6   Bullying in the workplace 127
    5.7   Perpetuating work hazards for women 127
    5.8   Neurosexism 130
    5.9   #MeToo in construction 130
    5.10   Workplaces designed for women 132
           5.10.1 Ergonomic design of tools and equipment 132
           5.10.2 Personal protective equipment (PPE) 133
           5.10.3 Reproductive hazards 135
           5.10.4 Sanitary facilities 135
    5.11   Conclusion 136
    5.12   Discussion and review questions 136
    References 137

6 Employee resilience   145
    6.1   Introduction 145
    6.2   What is resilience? 145
    6.3   Team resilience 148
    6.4   Employee resilience 150
    6.5   Protective factors, assets and resources 153
    6.6   Occupational approach to resilience 155
    6.7   Employee resilience in construction 156
    6.8   Navigating difficult work environments 157
    6.9   Resilience training in the workplace 160
    6.10   Conclusion 161
    6.11   Discussion and review questions 163
    References 163

7 Health issues in the construction industry in developing
    countries: The case of Sub-Saharan Africa   169
    7.1   Introduction 169
    7.2   Occupational wellbeing 169
    7.3   The Sub-Saharan region 171
    7.4   Development issues 172
    7.5   The construction industry 173
           7.5.1   Construction industry economic issues 173
           7.5.2   Construction industry social issues 175

7.6 Occupational health and wellbeing in the construction industry in Southern Africa 176
    7.6.1 COVID-19 176
    7.6.2 Malaria 177
    7.6.3 Tuberculosis 178
7.7 HIV/AIDS and the construction industry 178
    7.7.1 Disease anatomy and treatment 178
    7.7.2 HIV/AIDS in Sub-Saharan Africa – an overview 180
    7.7.3 HIV/AIDS in South Africa – an overview 182
    7.7.4 HIV/AIDS and the South African construction industry 184
7.8 Industry health testing in South Africa 188
7.9 Family and lifestyle issues 189
7.10 Organisational support for workers 189
7.11 Conclusion 190
7.12 Discussion and review questions 190
References 191

8 Young construction workers' health and wellbeing   194
8.1 Introduction 194
8.2 The apprenticeship model 195
8.3 Young workers' safety experiences at work 197
    8.3.1 Non-fatal injury incidence 197
    8.3.2 Fatal injury incidence 198
8.4 Why young workers are a high-risk group for workplace safety incidents 198
8.5 Young construction workers' health-related behaviour 204
8.6 Young workers' mental health experiences 205
8.7 Social support and mental health and wellbeing 209
8.8 Protecting and promoting the health and wellbeing of young workers 213
8.9 Conclusion 214
8.10 Discussion and review questions 216
8.11 Acknowledgements 216
References 216

9 Healthy ageing at work   222
9.1 Introduction 222
9.2 The ageing population 222
9.3 The ageing process 223
9.4 Age and work ability 227
9.5 Are health risk factors individual or environmental? 228
9.6 Older construction workers' physical work health experiences 229

9.7 The workplace safety of older construction workers 231

9.8 Older workers' experience of psychosocial health risk factors 232

9.9 A lifespan perspective 238

9.10 The social context of work 240

9.11 Effective age management 241

9.12 Interventions designed to protect and promote the health and wellbeing of older workers 242

9.13 Conclusion 245

9.14 Discussion and review questions 245

9.15 Acknowledgements 246

References 246

10 Building a sense of place   252

10.1 Introduction 252

10.2 What is sense of place (SoP)? 252

10.3 Developing a sense of place in a dynamic workplace 253

10.4 Positive approach to mentally healthy workplaces 254

    10.4.1 Prevention and promotion 254

    10.4.2 Positive psychology in the workplace 255

    10.4.3 Positive psychology interventions 256

10.5 Sense of place conceptual model 258

    10.5.1 Social support 258

    10.5.2 Community 259

    10.5.3 Life balance 260

    10.5.4 Engagement 260

    10.5.5 Respect/civility 261

    10.5.6 Employee resilience 262

10.6 Sense of place tool 262

10.7 Link between sense of place and mental wellbeing 263

10.8 Conclusion 267

10.9 Discussion and review questions 267

10.10 Acknowledgements 268

References 268

11 Thinking about the future   273

11.1 An unexpected turn 273

11.2 Lessons learned about working from home during the COVID-19 pandemic 277

11.3 Future issues in work and health 279

11.4 Climate change and workers' health 280

11.5 New models of work and health 284

11.6 Technology 290

11.7 Conclusion 292
11.8 Discussion and review questions 292
References 292

Index *298*

PREFACE

In writing this book we sought to tie together a body of work undertaken over a period spanning 20 years. Some of this work has been undertaken individually but much of it we have conducted jointly. We felt it was timely and important to collate this work as construction workers' health is increasingly recognised as a neglected aspect of management practice in the construction industry (particularly when compared to the management of occupational safety). Construction workers are exposed to a wide variety of health risks in their daily work, including a vast array of chemical, physical and psychosocial hazards. Again, compared with safety hazards, many health hazards experienced by construction workers are not well understood or effectively controlled. Construction workers are also a high-risk group for suicide, with shocking statistics around this being reported in many countries of the world. There is a growing emphasis on the broader concept of workers' wellbeing, of which health is a part. This reflects a desire to ensure that workers are able to live and work in ways that enable them to remain physically, mentally, emotionally and socially well. Thinking about the long hours and weekend work that typically prevents project-based construction workers from engaging satisfactorily in life outside work, construction workers' wellbeing may seem to be an improbable prospect.

We wanted this book to challenge readers to think more deeply about the factors contributing to poor health in the construction workforce. In particular, we drew on the social determinants and social ecological models of health to position construction workers' health within the broader industrial systems within which construction projects are planned, procured and delivered.

As we have written this book, our understanding of the relationship between occupational and public health domains has evolved. This was, in part, due to the COVID-19 pandemic that placed workers' health in sharp relief. During the pandemic, the management of workers' health became critical for many construction organisations as the case for business continuity was predicated on the industry's ability to control the risk of COVID transmission. The stress caused by the global pandemic, lockdowns and other containment measures also highlighted the importance of supporting workers' mental health during this time.

As John F. Kennedy famously observed, crises bring with them both danger and opportunity. It is possible that the COVID-19 pandemic has irreversibly shifted the focus of construction industry participants to pay more attention to the protection and promotion of construction workers' health in the future. We sincerely hope this is the case. However, it is also apparent that changing the industry's culture and deeply entrenched practices is needed to effect sustainable improvements.

No single organisation or entity is likely to be able to change the challenge of long work hours, for example, because these are driven by deep-rooted characteristics of the competitive tendering and procurement processes. Greater collaboration between client organisations, construction firms and unions is likely to be needed to resolve some of the long-standing (and well-documented) characteristics of construction jobs that affect workers' health and wellbeing. It is also important that researchers continue to address ways to improve the health and wellbeing of construction workers. Rigorous intervention studies are particularly necessary as much research to date has focused on diagnosing the problems rather than evaluating ways to resolve them. Multidisciplinary work is also much needed in the context of increasingly complex challenges with the potential to cause harm (e.g., climate change).

We see this book as the starting point for an industry-academic conversation about what is needed to produce measurable improvements in construction workers' health and wellbeing in the coming years.

1

INTRODUCTION

The health imperative

1.1 Introduction

There has been a great deal of focus and many resources allocated to understanding and preventing injury in the construction industry (the "S" in OH&S) but limited attention has been given to workers' health. This book seeks to consolidate what we know about construction workers' health, offers guidance and suggestions to organisations on how they can protect and support the health of construction workers, and identifies some important areas for future research. This book may also be used by construction management and occupational health and safety (OH&S) educators to inform curriculum. Importantly, this book seeks to shift the emphasis away from a sole focus on health as an individual responsibility and takes a broader approach to understanding the characteristics of work and the workplace which can affect workers' health. Critically, we acknowledge that the construction industry's workforce is diverse and heterogeneous, including different groups of workers who perform a wide variety of work tasks across a range of work locations under different organisational and environmental conditions. This diversity has a bearing on health risks and outcomes. However, in this book we suggest that taking a systems approach to construction workers' health can assist in identifying causes of ill-health and guide the controls necessary to protect and promote the health of all workers, irrespective of role, age, or gender.

1.2 The global burden of work-related disease and injury

The United Nations 2030 Agenda of Sustainable Development Goals (SDGs) was adopted by all United Nations Member States in 2015. In order to achieve these goals, specifically SDG3 (Ensure healthy lives and promote well-being for all at all ages) and SDG8 (sustained, inclusive and sustainable economic growth, full

DOI: 10.1201/9780367814236-1

and productive employment and decent work), there is a need to reduce exposure to occupational health risks and promote health and wellbeing through the provision of well-designed and decent work.

The results of a global monitoring study undertaken on behalf of the World Health Organization and the International Labour Organization found that work-related diseases and injuries were responsible for 1.9 million deaths in 2016 and 89.7 million disability-adjusted life years (DALYs)[1] (WHO/ILO, 2021). Non-communicable diseases accounted for a much larger proportion of deaths (80.7%) than injuries (19.3%). The proportion of disease-related DALYs was also substantially greater (70.5%) than injury-related DALYs (29.5%).

These figures are a stark reminder that occupational health and safety programmes need to focus on the reduction of work-related risks to health as a matter of priority and urgency. The WHO/ILO Global Monitoring Report found that the most frequent causes of work-related deaths attributable to disease were chronic obstructive pulmonary disease (450,381 deaths); stroke (398,306 deaths) and ischaemic heart disease (346,618 deaths). The analysis considered 19 occupational risk factors, including workplace exposure to air pollution, asthmagens, carcinogens, ergonomic risk factors, and noise. Importantly, the 2021 report included exposure to long work hours for the first time. Long work hours were defined as working more than 55 hours each week. Long work hours was the occupational risk factor with the largest number of attributable deaths (744,924) followed by occupational particulate matter, gases and fumes (450,381 deaths). Importantly, deaths from heart disease and stroke associated with exposure to long work hours increased by 41 and 19 per cent respectively between 2000 and 2016, leading the WHO/ILO to identify long work hours as an increasingly important psychosocial occupational risk factor (WHO/ILO, 2021).

The WHO/ILO Global Monitoring Report also suggests preventive actions for each identified risk factor; for example, agreement on healthy maximum limits on working time is suggested to address the risk of exposure to long work hours. Given the prevalence of long work hours in project-based work, the health impacts of long hours of work in the construction industry are specifically addressed in Chapter 4 of this book.

1.3 Workers' health in the construction industry

Construction workers are reported to be relatively unhealthy when compared to the general population. This is sometimes attributed to lifestyle behaviour. For example, the *Australian National Health Survey 2017–2018* found that, compared to workers in other industries, construction workers have higher rates of smoking and alcohol consumption. Further, poor nutrition and levels of overweight and obesity remain high among construction workers. This is a problem for the industry because construction, perhaps more than other industries, relies on fit and healthy workers to perform work tasks that are often physically demanding (Sherratt, 2018). Consequently, construction organisations have sought to introduce health promotion programmes focused on improving a variety of lifestyle behaviours (see, for example, Lingard & Turner, 2015). What these programmes often fail to address is the fact that occupational causes of unhealthy lifestyle behaviours are not addressed by behaviour-focused health promotion programmes. That is people who are exposed to hazardous conditions, physically demanding tasks, high stress levels and long work hours are more likely to smoke and consume too much alcohol and less likely to exercise and eat well (WorkSafe Queensland, 2021).

Construction workers are exposed to a wide variety of occupational health hazards and have a higher incidence of work-related illness including contact dermatitis, all types of skin neoplasma, non-malignant pleural disease, mesothelioma, lung cancer, pneumoconiosis and musculoskeletal disorders compared to workers in other industries (Stocks et al., 2010; Snashall, 2005; Stocks et al., 2011). According to the UK Health and Safety Executive (HSE, 2021), construction has the largest incidence of cancer of any industry sector, accounting for 40 per cent of occupational cancer deaths and cancer registrations. The HSE also estimates that over 5,000 occupational cancer cases and approximately 3,700 deaths each year can be attributed to past exposures in the construction industry. Asbestos (70%), silica (17%), working as a painter and exposure to diesel engine exhaust (6–7% each) were the most prevalent exposures associated with occupational cancer cases in the construction industry (HSE, 2021). Further, lung disease and breathing problems are linked to exposures to dusts, fumes, vapours or gases in the air, while dermatitis is associated with handling many commonly used (but hazardous) construction materials. Construction workers are also exposed to physical occupational hazards, including exposure to noise, hand-arm and whole-body vibration. Construction is a high-risk industry for musculoskeletal disorders (MSDs) (Hartmann & Fleischer, 2005; Latza, et al., 2000). For example, in the USA, 40 per cent of construction workers over the age of 50 are reported to experience chronic back pain (Dong et al., 2012). As a result of exposures to hazardous work conditions, many construction workers experience work disability necessitating early retirement (Brenner & Ahern, 2000; Welch, 2009; Oude Hengel et al., 2012; Arndt et al., 2005).

It has been widely observed that, while considerable attention has been paid to the identification and management of risks to construction workers' immediate safety, far less attention has been paid to the systematic management of workers' health (Jones et al., 2019). The critical need to focus on reducing occupational health risks and some of the challenges associated with doing so are further discussed in Chapter 2 of this book.

Construction workers are also susceptible to mental ill health. The incidence of psychological distress among construction workers is reported to be twice the level of the general male population (Borsting Jacobsen et al., 2013). Petersen and Zwerling (1998) similarly report that construction workers experience a significantly higher incidence of emotional/psychiatric disorders than other manual/non-managerial workers. Suicide rates in the industry are reported to be high in the United Kingdom, Australia and the USA (Meltzer et al., 2008; Centers for Disease Control and Prevention, 2018; Milner et al., 2013). In the context of an already substantial suicide problem, King and Lamontagne (2021) argue that the COVID-19 pandemic has created the "perfect storm" for suicide rates among construction workers to rise steeply. Most at risk are unskilled workers who are often young and who experience lower levels of job security and control than skilled workers (King & Lamontagne, 2021).

1.4 Social determinants of health

It is widely accepted that social – as distinct from biological and genetic – factors have a significant impact on health outcomes. Social determinants of health include "the conditions in which people are born, live, work, and age, and the health systems they can access, which are in turn shaped by a wider set of forces: economics, social, environmental policies, and politics" (Allen et al., 2014, p.392).

The "Dahlgren and Whitehead model" (Figure 1.1) is widely used to depict determinants of population health. Although first developed in 1991, Dahlgren and Whitehead (1991, 2021) observe that the model has proven so popular because it encourages professionals and policymakers (beyond those directly engaged in healthcare or health services) to consider how their activities affect health and what they can do in their sectors and local environments to influence the health of the groups potentially affected by their activities. The model also supports the development of a holistic understanding of health and promotes multisectoral action. While disease-focused models of health can result in fragmented initiatives in which strategies for the prevention of a disease are developed independently of one another, the social determinants model encourages a more comprehensive strategy focused on determinants of health that may contribute to many diseases (Dahlgren & Whitehead, 2021).

Inequality in health (e.g., differences by socioeconomic characteristics, such as education and income) has been reported in many countries, with the worst health experienced by those in the lowest socioeconomic groupings (Denton & Walters, 1999; Braveman & Gottlieb, 2014). However, Dahlgren and Whitehead (2021) also observe that their model does not (nor was it intended to) explain the causes of health inequalities within a particular country or context. In order to understand health inequality, Dahlgren and Whitehead (2021) argue there is a need to examine the ways that the various social determinants create social gradients in health. In particular, the ways that social determinants of health can create inequality have been identified as differences in power and resources, differences in exposure, differences in vulnerability and differences in the consequences of being sick (Diderichson et al., 2001).

Case example 1.1 considers health inequality in the construction workforce which emerged during the COVID-19 pandemic and identifies some of the mechanisms contributing to health inequality for a particular cohort of workers.

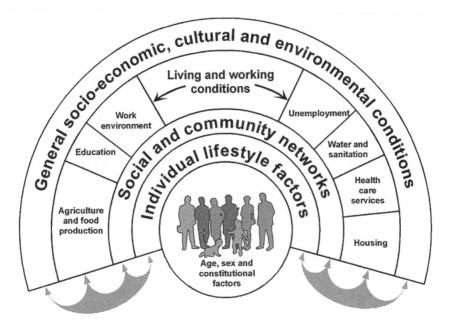

FIGURE 1.1 Model of social determinants of health

Source: Dahlgren & Whitehead, 2021, p.22.

CASE EXAMPLE 1.1 MECHANISMS CONTRIBUTING TO HEALTH INEQUALITY IN THE COVID-19 PANDEMIC

While the COVID-19 pandemic affected the whole workforce in the construction industry, there is emerging evidence to suggest that it had a greater impact on some groups of workers who were more vulnerable than others. The vulnerability was likely to escalate the health, safety and wellbeing risks posed by COVID-19 among these worker groups, leading to health inequalities in the construction workforce (Brown et al., 2020).

In the United Kingdom socioeconomic inequalities between people who were able to work from home (to protect themselves against exposure to COVID-19) and those who could not were observed (Marmot et al., 2020). In particular, 70 per cent of workers in occupations requiring higher qualifications reported they were working from home during a reference week in April 2020 compared with 19 per cent of those in skilled trade occupations and only 5 per cent of process, plant and machine operatives (Marmot et al., 2020). This suggests that people in occupations requiring higher qualifications were afforded greater protection from COVID-19. However, while occupation was an important risk factor for COVID-19 infection and death, the effect of occupational exposure was amplified when people were living in a more deprived area, in poor quality or overcrowded housing, and where they had a pre-existing underlying health condition. People from a black, Asian or minority ethnic background were also more susceptible (Marmot et al., 2020). The vulnerability of migrant construction workers became even more obvious during the COVID-19 pandemic. For example, in Singapore, migrant workers were housed in congested dormitories isolated from the rest of the population and had less access to masks (Koh, 2020; Geddie & Aravindan, 2020), making infection risk among migrant workers significantly higher than the rest of the population.

Recognising that individuals' opportunities and choices in relation to health-related behaviours can be influenced by the contexts in which they work highlights the opportunity for organisations to promote health and/or remove barriers that might prevent people from engaging in healthy behaviours (Braveman et al., 2011). Systematic reviews have identified workplace interventions as having a positive impact in improving health and reducing health inequality (Bambra et al., 2010). However, primary interventions that focus on changing job conditions or work characteristics (rather than changing workers' lifestyle behaviour) are most beneficial. For example, interventions designed to increase workers' participation and control over their conditions of work, changing the organisation of shift patterns and addressing specific occupational hazards were all found to have positive impacts on workers' health (Bambra et al., 2010). Allen et al. (2014) similarly report that poor quality employment and jobs with low levels of reward and control have a damaging effect on mental health. By promoting greater job control and decreased demand, employers can reduce stress, anxiety and depression and increase self-esteem, job satisfaction and productivity (Allen et al., 2014).

As previously noted, many workplace health promotion programmes aim to modify individuals' lifestyle behaviours, such as smoking, alcohol consumption, exercise and diet (Bambra et al., 2010). Examples in construction include programmes that have: encouraged exercise to address shoulder pain (Ludewig & Borstad, 2003) and improve aerobic capacity (Gram et al., 2012); sought to help workers to reduce their weight and risk of cardiovascular disease (Groeneveld et al., 2010); and to encourage smoking cessation and the consumption of fruit and vegetables (Sorensen et al., 2007). However, the extent to which these programmes are genuinely informed by workers' participation and choice has been questioned (Sherratt, 2015).

Research also confirms that fundamental structures of social inequality are more influential in determining a person's health than behavioural factors (Denton & Walters, 1999). In particular, structural sources of inequality may actually underpin unhealthy lifestyle behaviours. Consequently, Dahlgren and

Whitehead (2021) argue that "vertical links" are needed in the determinants of health model depicted in Figure 1.1 to show how social, economic and cultural factors are linked to lifestyle behaviours. In reality, what appear to be lifestyle "choices" may be substantially constrained by structural factors, including work and family responsibilities, occupational status and income adequacy. These structural socioeconomic factors can impact health directly as well as indirectly, through their influence on health-related behaviours (Denton & Walters, 1999).

Zoller (2003) argues that the lifestyle focus of many workplace health promotion programmes de-emphasises social factors that shape the way people behave. The emphasis on living a healthy lifestyle thus shifts the focus away from the underlying (and often very deeply entrenched) causes of workplace-generated disease and frames health as a matter of individual choice. Sherratt (2018) similarly argues that the positioning of worker health as a personal lifestyle choice does not reflect the way that work practices in the construction industry induce high levels of stress that contribute substantially to unhealthy lifestyle behaviours.

To illustrate this point, the role of long work hours and time poverty in shaping construction workers' response to a lifestyle-focused workplace health programme is described in case example 1.2, as follows:

CASE EXAMPLE 1.2 TIME POVERTY AS A STRUCTURAL IMPEDIMENT TO HEALTH BEHAVIOUR CHANGE IN THE CONSTRUCTION INDUSTRY

A health promotion programme targeting the behaviour of construction workers at two worksites in the Queensland construction industry was evaluated by the authors. At these sites, initiatives were introduced including:

- a smoking cessation campaign,
- health-based information sessions and healthy food tasting sessions,
- a change of food options sold in the site canteen,
- a waistline measurement activity,
- yoga/stretching sessions, and
- discounted gym memberships.

Workers worked six days per week, and often had to travel long distances for work. During the summer months, the site operated from 6am, and during winter from 6.30am. Finishing time varied according to overtime worked. Participants indicated they were frequently unable to find the time to prepare and eat healthy food or engage in physical exercise. During the programme the authors used diary-based methods to record workers' health behaviour. The results produced no evidence of significant or sustained behaviour change (Lingard & Turner, 2015).

Site workers' comments revealed that a shortage of time acts as a major structural impediment to leading a healthy lifestyle. One described their day as follows: "[I] *leave home at 4.45am because I kick off in the mornings. By the time you come home, feed the dog, clean the house, wash your clothes, eat, that's it.*" Another worker commented: "*I don't have time to go for a walk. When I lived in town (closer to work) I'd get up at 4.30am and walk for an hour. Now if I did that I'd get up at 2.30am (because of extra travel time). I just wouldn't have any time to sleep.*" Another commented: "*Time is the biggest barrier. If you don't have the time, you don't have the time. If you want to do something extra in your day, you will be doing it before you go to work in the dark. By the time you get home, you are exhausted and just want to sit down, you don't want to do anything.*"

A shortage of time was identified as a factor contributing directly to lifestyle and poor health: "*You get into a cycle. There's not enough time. It's hard to step back and make a change in your lifestyle. You get into a pattern of eat, smoke, drink, sleep. Then you wake up and do it all again. Before you know it you have put on 20 kilos.*"

Adapted from Lingard & Turner, 2015, 2017

However, workplace health promotion programmes are rarely subjected to critical examination. One of the challenges lies in the fact that the boundary between factors that influence health at work and outside work is blurred. In this way, health is arguably far more complex an issue to deal with than workplace safety. Assessing the work-relatedness of illness and disease is not always simple. Similarly, concerns have been raised as to whether it is appropriate for organisations to try to control or manage workers' health beyond the workplace (and, if so, to what extent?).

Some studies have examined the operation of workplace wellness programmes in relation to their underlying rationale and motivation, as well as potentially negative impacts. These more critical perspectives are important to acknowledge and consider in relation to how construction organisations can better address issues of worker health and wellbeing.

For example, Sherratt (2015) argues that the implementation of workplace health promotion interventions may be motivated more by corporate interests than by a philanthropic interest in workers' health. This view is shared by Holmqvist (2009) who suggests that a desire to manage uncertainty in the organisation's operational environments underpins many corporate health promotion activities. Conrad and Walsh (1992) similarly view workplace health/wellness programmes as a means through which business tries to shape the values, attitudes and behaviour of workers for the purpose of improving productivity and performance.

Value statements used to promote workplace health initiatives often reflect a managerial ethic of production efficiency and performance (Johannson &

Edwards, 2021). Sherratt (2015) points out how a significant UK industry policy document (The Responsibility Deal Construction Pledge) emphasises the number of days lost due to sickness in its appeal to construction employers to "step up" and do something about workers' health. She argues that this constructs worker health as "simply the ability to be present and participate in work" (Sherratt, 2015, p.448).

Workplace health/wellness programmes have also been criticised for defining health in specific and often quite narrow ways. The social construction of what a "healthy" body looks like is largely based on notions of physical fitness and performance linked to behaviours characterised by abstinence, self-control, hard work and competitiveness (Zoller, 2003). In painting a narrow and homogeneous interpretation of what it means (and looks like) to be healthy, workplace health promotion programmes can also stigmatise workers who do not conform to organisationally created norms and values (Johannson & Edwards, 2021). This can marginalise certain groups in the workforce, e.g., those whose bodies for reasons of gender, class, caring responsibilities, disability, maternity, etc., do not conform to the idealised notion of what a healthy (and therefore competent) worker looks like (Holmqvist, 2009).

1.5 Motivation for managing workers' health

The World Health Organization (2019) identifies an inextricable link between employment and health and observes the important contribution to be made by workplaces in the pursuit of global Sustainable Development Goals (SDGs) and reduction of health inequalities. In particular, Goal 3 "Ensure healthy lives and promote well-being for all at all ages" and Goal 8 "By 2030 have sustained, inclusive and sustainable economic growth, full and productive employment and decent work for all" focus attention on workers' health and the provision of good quality jobs. However, other SDGs also apply to the protection of workers' health, for example, SDG 10: "Reduced inequalities" and SDG 16: "Peace, justice and strong institutions." Moreover, in June 2022, delegates attending the International Labour Conference (ILC) adopted a resolution to add the principle of a safe and healthy working environment to the International Labour Organization's (ILO) Fundamental Principles and Rights at Work. Thus, occupational health and safety was added to the previously agreed four principles:

- freedom of association and the effective recognition of the right to collective bargaining;
- the elimination of all forms of forced or compulsory labour;
- the effective abolition of child labour; and
- the elimination of discrimination in respect of employment and occupation (ILO, 2022).

Smallwood and Lingard (2009) argue that the motivation for organisations to protect and promote workers' health (and also safety) is multi-faceted and can include legal considerations, moral/religious beliefs, ethical considerations; humanitarian concerns and a respect for people; a desire for sustainability; compliance with national and international standards; a desire to reduce the costs of workers' compensation, absenteeism and turnover; the desire to reduce organisational risk; adherence with total quality management principles; support of local industry, corporate image and reputation considerations and the pursuit of better practice. The World Health Organization (2010a) similarly suggests three primary reasons for organisations' willingness to exert effort and expend resources to protect and promote workers' health.

1.5.1   Moral/ethical considerations

The "golden rule" establishing a moral level of care for other people is common to most of the world's major religions, philosophies and value systems (Eckhardt, 2001). Thus, it is morally wrong to treat people in certain ways (Rowan, 2000) and the avoidance of inflicting harm on others is a basic ethical/moral principle (WHO, 2010a). Organisational activities (for example, exposure to workplace hazards as a result of the way that work is designed and performed) can have consequences for workers' physical and mental health. The moral nature of organisational decision-making is amplified because workers are often dependent upon jobs for their livelihood, may have little knowledge of the health hazards to which they are exposed, and have little control over conditions of work. Consequently, there have been calls for organisational decision-making to be guided by ethical codes and guidelines (Greenwood, 2002). However, the World Health Organization (2010a) argues that moral codes adopted by many societies and cultures are often limited in their application to "personal" decisions and actions and are seldom considered in relation to the operation of business. As previously noted, the right to a healthy and safe work environment, identified as a fundamental human right at the XVIII World Congress on Safety and Health at Work held in Seoul, Korea (WHO, 2010a), has now also been included in the International Labour Organization's (ILO) Fundamental Principles and Rights at Work (ILO, 2022). Thus, the right to a healthy and safe workplace is universally held by workers, and employers therefore have a concomitant duty to provide a healthy and safe work environment.

1.5.2   The business case

The economic impacts of workers' poor health and potential benefits to be gained from protecting and promoting workers' health are often cited as the incentive for organisations to invest in workplace health programmes. For private businesses this motivation aligns with the view that the principal responsibility of business is to make a profit. Success in non-profit and public sector organisations involves the achievement of an established purpose. The ability to meet organisational goals is dependent upon workers in private as well as non-profit and public organisations. Unhealthy (and unsafe) work environments have been linked to increased operating costs, decreased productivity, decreased quality of products and services leading to customer dissatisfaction, fines and even potentially imprisonment (WHO, 2010a). These factors are preceded by higher levels of absenteeism, presenteeism, rising health insurance costs and workers' compensation claims, industrial disputes and employee turnover (WHO, 2010a). The "business case" is widely accepted as a driver for organisational initiatives to protect and promote workers' health. Indeed, commentators identify the need to evaluate the impacts of workplace health programmes using a variety of health and economic measures to properly understand the business outcomes of these programmes (Adams, 2019). The return on investment of workplace wellness programmes has received considerable attention in the business/management literature, with analysts claiming an impressive ratio of total benefits achieved for every monetary unit spent on a programme (Berry et al., 2010; Baicker et al., 2010). However, it is also recognised that some health-related phenomena (for example, presenteeism) are difficult to monetise and may not be reliably captured in organisationally generated datasets (McLellan, 2017). Despite multiple accounts of favourable cost-benefit ratios, a systematic review of workplace wellness programmes conducted in Europe (and evaluated in rigorous randomised controlled trials) showed the economic impacts to be mostly negative, i.e., the costs of implementation outweighed the monetised benefits (Martinez-Lemos, 2015). A similar review of studies undertaken in the USA also failed to find evidence of a positive return on investment in the short term (Baid et al., 2021). The expectation of a favourable ratio of costs to financial benefits may not, therefore, act as a motivator for the implementation of workplace wellness initiatives where clear and measurable cost benefits are not evident. In such circumstances questions arise as to whether or not employers are willing to pay for workers' improved health, the extent to which they are willing to do so and what types of mechanisms may be needed to encourage organisations to more fully address issues of workers' health (Martinez-Lemos, 2015).

1.5.3   Legal requirements

Most countries have enacted some form of legislation requiring employers to take measures to protect their workers from workplace hazards that could cause illness or injury. In some countries, these laws are sophisticated and impose duties on other parties whose activities could be harmful to workers who may not be their direct employees (for example, designers, manufacturers, importers and suppliers of plant or substances, as well as owners and managers of facilities/workplaces and designers of structures). In many instances, laws specifically focus on the elimination or reduction of risks. For example, in Australia, the Model Work Health and Safety Act (which was established as the basis for creating national consistency between Australia's states and territories, each of which has its own occupational health and safety legislation) states that the duty to "ensure health and safety requires the person:

a) to eliminate risks to health and safety, so far as is reasonably practicable; and
b) if it is not reasonably practicable to eliminate risks to health and safety, to minimise those risks so far as is reasonably practicable" (Safe Work Australia, 2019, p.15).

The Model Act is also supplemented with a raft of more detailed and prescriptive requirements in the Model Work Health and Safety Regulations. Many of these regulations refer specifically to occupational health-related hazards/risks, including managing risks in relation to noise, hazardous manual tasks, hazardous chemicals, lead and asbestos. The regulations include detailed health monitoring requirements for workers exposed to lead, asbestos and certain specified hazardous chemicals, as well as audiometric testing for people exposed to high levels of noise. Detailed requirements are specified for risk controls that must be implemented in certain situations, specific personal protective equipment requirements and facilities that need to be provided for changing, washing, laundering or disposing of contaminated personal protective equipment following exposure to hazardous environments and substances (Safe Work Australia, 2021).

Given the existence of occupational health and safety legislation in most countries, employers may be motivated to take steps to reduce risks of work-related illness and protect workers' health in order to avoid fines or imprisonment in the case of serious breaches. However, the WHO (2010a) observes that occupational health and safety legislation varies significantly from country to country so coverage will be inconsistent. The extent to which employers are focused on preventing harm to workers' health may also depend upon the efficacy of enforcement activity in a particular jurisdiction. Further, Sherratt (2018) observed that UK construction contractors' emphasis on public health issues, such as diet and exercise, detracted from their willingness to invest in programmes focused on the reduction of widely recognised occupational health risks. This is reflected in a quotation attributed to a senior occupational health and safety manager in the industry that "it's no good giving people fruit and porridge as they come through the turnstile if we're then giving them exposure to dust and carcinogens..." (CIOB, 2016, cited in Jones et al., 2019, p.546).

Given the serious and potentially irreversible effects of work exposures on health, the World Health Organization (2010a) advocates for the precautionary principle to be applied. That is: employers and workers should not delay implementing interventions to address workplace conditions and promote health simply because intervention effectiveness has not yet been rigorously evaluated and its efficacy demonstrated (p.43).

1.6 What constitutes a healthy workplace?

The World Health Organization has defined health broadly as "a state of complete physical, mental and social well-being, and not merely the absence of disease" (WHO, 2010b, p.15). In most countries, employers have responsibilities under occupational health and safety legislation for the prevention of work-related illness and injury. However, workplaces are increasingly viewed as an appropriate setting within which health promotion can occur.

The WHO defines a healthy workplace as "one in which workers and managers collaborate to use a continual improvement process to protect and promote the health, safety and well-being of all workers and the sustainability of the workplace by considering the following, based on identified needs:

- health and safety concerns in the physical work environment;
- health, safety and well-being concerns in the psychosocial work environment, including organization of work and workplace culture;
- personal health resources in the workplace; and
- ways of participating in the community to improve the health of workers, their families and other members of the community" (WHO, 2010b, p.6).

This definition reflects the importance of collaboration between managers and workers in relation to preventing illness and promoting health and of being inclusive in providing support to all workers.

To support the practical development of healthy workplaces, the WHO (2010a) developed a healthy workplace model, depicted in Figure 1.2. This model shows four avenues through which employers (in collaboration with workers) can influence the health of their workers, including the physical work environment, the psychosocial work environment, workers' personal health resources and the involvement of an enterprise within the broader community in which it operates.

The definitions of each of these avenues is included in Table 1.1 below:

The WHO healthy workplace model also incorporates an organisational implementation process (based on existing "continual improvement" models) through which workplace health programmes can be initiated, collaboratively designed, planned, resourced, implemented, evaluated and improved (Figure 1.2).

At the heart of the WHO model lie some fundamental principles that are likely to be critical to the success of a workplace health initiative. These are:

- the engagement of leaders within the organisation to ensure workplace health initiatives are integrated into an organisation's business strategy, goals and values, and senior management commitment that is communicated clearly and consistently to all within the organisation; and
- the meaningful and active involvement of workers and/or their representatives across the entire implementation process. Workers' opinions should be sought at each step in the implementation process and their ideas listened to and used to inform decision-making.

Another model of worker health, the Total Worker Health model, was developed by the National Institute for Occupational Safety and Health (NIOSH) in the United States and aims to integrate occupational safety and health protection

TABLE 1.1 Avenues of workplace influence on worker health

Avenue	Definition
Physical work environment	"The part of the workplace facility that can be detected by human or electronic senses, including the structure, air, machines, furniture, products, chemicals, materials and processes that are present or that occur in the workplace, and which can affect the physical or mental safety, health and well-being of workers. If the worker performs his or her tasks outdoors or in a vehicle, then that location is the physical work environment." (WHO, 2010a, pp.77–78)
Psychosocial work environment	"Includes the organization of work and the organizational culture; the attitudes, values, beliefs and practices that are demonstrated on a daily basis in the enterprise /organization, and which affect the mental and physical well-being of employees. These are sometimes generally referred to as workplace stressors, which may cause emotional or mental stress to workers." (WHO, 2010a, p.79)
Personal health resources	"The supportive environment, health services, information, resources, opportunities and flexibility an enterprise provides to workers to support or motivate their efforts to improve or maintain healthy personal lifestyle practices, as well as to monitor and support their ongoing physical and mental health." (WHO, 2010a, p.80)
Enterprise community involvement	"The activities, expertise, and other resources an enterprise engages in or provides to the social and physical community or communities in which it operates; and which affect the physical and mental health, safety and well-being of workers and their families. It includes activities, expertise and resources provided to the immediate local environment, but also the broader global environment." (WHO, 2010a, p.81)

Source: After WHO, 2010a.

with workplace efforts to promote worker health and wellbeing (Schill & Chosewood, 2013). NIOSH describes a Total Worker Health approach as the "policies, programs, and practices that integrate protection from work-related safety and health hazards with promotion of injury- and illness-prevention efforts to advance worker well-being" (Lee et al., 2016, p.1). Total Worker Health has five defining elements, many of which are consistent with models of workers' health that take an integrated approach:

1. Demonstrate leadership commitment to worker safety and health at all levels of the organisation.
2. Design work to eliminate or reduce safety and health hazards and promote worker wellbeing.
3. Promote and support worker engagement throughout program design and implementation.

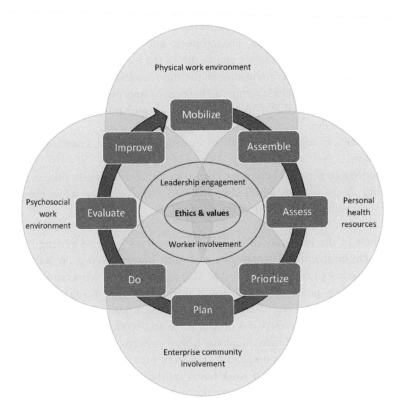

FIGURE 1.2 Healthy workplace model
Source: (WHO, 2010a, p.8).

4. Ensure confidentiality and privacy of workers.
5. Integrate relevant systems to advance worker wellbeing (Lee et al., 2016, p.3).

The five defining elements are positioned as guiding principles for organisations seeking to develop workplace policies, programmes, and practices that contribute to worker safety, health and wellbeing (Tamers et al., 2019).

To strengthen the link between traditional OH&S approaches and Total Worker Health, the Office for Total Worker Health published the "Hierarchy of Controls Applied to NIOSH Total Worker Health," adapted from the hierarchy of controls framework traditionally used in OH&S (Lee et al., 2016). The controls and strategies are arranged in descending order of likely effectiveness and protectiveness (NIOSH, 2017):

• **Eliminate** workplace conditions that cause or contribute to worker illness and injury, or otherwise negatively impact wellbeing. For example, remove harmful supervisory practices throughout the management chain.

- **Substitute** unsafe, unhealthy working conditions or practices with safer, health-enhancing policies, programmes, and management practices that improve the culture of safety and health in the workplace.
- **Redesign** the work environment for improved safety, health, and wellbeing. Examples include removing barriers to improving wellbeing, enhancing access to employer-sponsored benefits, and providing more flexible work schedules.
- **Educate** on safety and health to enhance individual knowledge for all workers.
- **Encourage** personal behaviour change to improve safety, health, and wellbeing. Assist workers with individual risks and challenges, while providing support in making healthier choices.

As implicit in the hierarchy of control, the emphasis is on addressing system-level or environmental determinants of health before relying on individual-level approaches (Tamers et al., 2019). The central role of working conditions in shaping safety, health and wellbeing is shown in Figure 1.3 (Sorensen et al., 2021). Recently, the Total Worker Health approach was expanded to include the broader forces that affect the organisation and workers' health, and this is reflected in Figure 1.3. Employment and labour patterns are particularly relevant to construction workers, as employment is often precarious, providing little job security, and long and irregular work hours are the norm. It is common practice that trade and semiskilled workers are subcontracted by the primary contractor to undertake a specific and time-limited task, and it is possible that workers can work across multiple sites for different contractors and therefore experience multiple health and safety practices. Such employment and labour patterns are

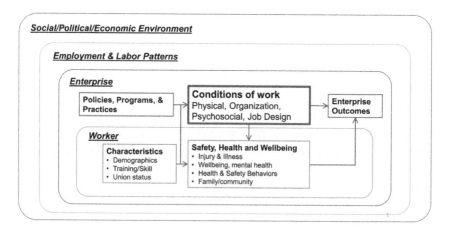

FIGURE 1.3 Systems level conceptual model of work, safety, health and wellbeing
Source: (Sorensen et al., 2021, p.3).

known to be associated with poor health outcomes (Sorensen et al., 2021). Social, political and economic environments include structural forces that influence employment and labour patterns, shape working conditions at the organisation (enterprise) level, and affect worker safety and health. For example, governments vary widely in their approach to protecting workers' safety and health and this is reflected in policy and regulatory requirements.

1.7   The way work is done in construction

The construction industry presents some particular challenges in relation to the protection and promotion of workers' health. The delivery of a construction project is characterised by complex inter-organisational relationships and long (and often complicated) supply chains (Dubois & Gadde, 2000; Hartemann & Caerteling, 2010). The allocation of risk in a construction project is stipulated in contracts, which have become highly diversified to respond to the variety of procurement options and situations. Unfortunately, rather than foster a genuinely collaborative approach, competitive tendering and commercial arrangements can create structural (cost and time) impediments to the protection and promotion of workers' health. Some of these structural impediments are discussed in Chapter 4 in relation to long work hours and health.

Further, most physical construction work is performed by workers who are engaged by subcontractors, are self-employed or are engaged via labour hire agencies. Research suggests that different forms of precarious and/or indirect employment create particular challenges for workers' health. For example, subcontracted workers are reported to be significantly more affected by work-related disease than direct employees (Min et al., 2013). Similarly, the health and safety of agency workers are negatively affected due to pressures, disorganisation and regulatory failure reflected in Table 1.2.

TABLE 1.2 Risk factors associated with precarious employment

Economic and Reward Pressures	Disorganisation	Regulatory Failure
Insecure jobs (fear of losing job)	Short tenure, inexperience	Poor knowledge of legal rights, obligations
Contingent, irregular payment	Poor induction, training and supervision	Limited access to OH&S, workers' compensation rights
Long or irregular work hours	Ineffective procedures and communication	Fractured or disputed legal obligations
Multiple jobholding	Ineffective OH&S management systems/ inability to organise	Non-compliance and regulatory oversight (stretched resources)

Source: Underhill & Quinlan, 2011.

The transient nature of employment in the construction industry has been identified as a challenge for implementing health assessments, arranging follow-ups as workers move from project to project and managing systematic health surveillance programmes (Jones et al., 2019). Sherratt (2018) points out that, even when construction organisations commit to ambitious targets for health education, training, screening, etc., in reality, many health initiatives are limited to directly employed workers or those who remain at a worksite long enough to partake. Consequently, health protection and promotion in the construction industry are likely to require initiatives that extend beyond the boundaries of a single organisation and operate at an industry or sector level.

1.8 Gender, work and health

The World Health Organization (2011) also recommends a gender-based approach or analysis (GBA) be applied to the design, implementation, monitoring and evaluation of workplace health-related policies, programmes and practices (p.21). The WHO argues that women and men experience work health and safety in different ways and are affected differently by risk exposures and health problems. Women are very under-represented in the construction industry in many countries and, consequently, relatively little is known about the risk exposures and health experiences of women in this sector. Many studies of workplace health "control" for gender in statistical analysis, thereby masking potentially important differences between men and women workers' experiences (Messing & Östlin, 2006). Owing to the fact that women are not well-represented in the construction workforce, it is difficult to collect sufficient population-level data to properly understand their health experiences and more research in this area is needed. Notwithstanding this, even when doing the same job, women and men can experience and be affected by working conditions differently. In particular, equipment, tools and clothing designed for men may not be suitable for women, given differences in average body size and dimensions (WHO, 2011). Women and men also differ in terms of their domestic and unpaid work responsibilities, including providing care for children and the elderly and undertaking household work. This can place women under particular strain as unpaid work combined with participation in paid work can contribute to stress, fatigue and depression (WHO, 2011). Hochschild famously described how women effectively work a "second shift" when they return home from work each day (Hochschild & Machung, 1989).

Moreover, women in traditionally male-dominated industries, such as construction, are more frequently exposed to gender-based violence (including sexual harassment) at work. For example, the Australian Human Rights Commission (2020) reports that male-dominated workplace cultures have a higher prevalence of sexual harassment due to the unequal gender ratio (a higher proportion of men than women in the workplace). Construction was singled out as a high-risk industry for gender-based violence against women. Gender-based violence is a serious occupational health issue (WorkSafe Victoria, 2020) and research highlights the urgency of ensuring that construction workplaces are both psychologically and physically safe for women (Turner et al., 2021).

A gender-based approach to understanding and responding to the needs of women workers can help to ensure workplace health policies, programmes and practices support equity in health and gender within a work environment and can ensure that, in male-dominated industries like construction, the specific health risks and experiences of women workers are effectively addressed (WHO, 2011). We explore the health issues related to women in construction in Chapter 5.

1.9   The rest of this book

This book draws on research work that has been undertaken over a ten-year period. During this period, construction industry stakeholders, including client organisations, employers and trade unions, have grown increasingly aware of the impact of the construction industry's employment practices and working conditions on workers' health. The emphasis has shifted from an exclusive focus on the management of occupational health and safety risks to a recognition that organisations can and should also implement programmes to promote the health and wellbeing of their workforce. It is now widely understood that employment in the construction industry affects the health and wellbeing of workers whether they occupy manual/non-managerial or managerial/professional roles. Yet the work health challenges of the construction industry cannot be resolved by behavioural solutions alone. Recognising the social determinants of health and addressing the systemic environmental factors that affect the health of construction workers is critical. This will require careful consideration of entrenched industry structures and modification to long-standing working conditions and practices.

The remaining chapters of the book recognise that social determinants of health are at play in the construction industry and explore the manner in which these operate. Where possible, health promotion interventions are described and evidence as to their effectiveness presented.

The chapters are organised in the following structure:

Chapter 2 considers the "H" in OH&S. It commences with a discussion of who should be responsible for managing workers' health in an industry in which work is decentralised, the workforce is peripatetic and workers are exposed to a wide range of work-related health hazards. The chapter then goes on to explore why managing occupational health is more complicated than managing safety but emphasises that implementing the most effective control measures for occupational health hazards is critical. Following this is an overview of some of the common hazards and related health issues that are found in construction, including occupational cancer, respirable silica, occupational hearing loss, and musculoskeletal disorders.

Chapter 3 examines the work-related factors which can affect construction workers' psychological health. The key theories linking work with psychological health are outlined, followed by a description of the relationship between conditions of work and work-related stress among construction industry workers. The chapter then provides an overview of psychological hazards and the types of workplace mental health programmes implemented to address these hazards. These programmes are considered in relation to the extent to which they address systemic and environmental issues or whether they primarily focus on individuals' behaviour and ability to cope with work-related stressors. An overview of ISO 45003 (Occupational health and safety management – Psychological health and safety at work) is provided which considers the management of psychosocial risks and promotion of wellbeing at work as part of an organisation's occupational health and safety management system.

Chapter 4 examines different approaches to working time and its effects on the health and wellbeing of workers. The chapter considers how time is understood in project-based construction work, and the connection between long work hours and health and wellbeing is outlined. Challenges experienced in balancing time spent at work and non-work related activities are explored, and consideration is given to the role played by gender in shaping work–life interactions and experiences. The chapter outlines the relationships between long work hours, overtime, and the way that work is scheduled, including modifications and reductions in the "working week," and outlines what alternatives are possible for project-based construction workers. The right to disconnect from the pressures and activity of work after leaving the worksite is discussed, as are the new-found flexible working arrangements that have been adopted by necessity during the COVID-19 pandemic. The chapter ends with a consideration of the systemic factors contributing to long and rigid hours in construction and identifies the need for a whole-of-industry approach to addressing these factors.

Chapter 5 focuses on the occupational health of women working in construction. The health inequality of women from a societal perspective is outlined, and consideration is given to how this is reflected in occupational health research. We consider gender as a social determinant of health, and how the health of women is impacted by their status as a numerical minority group in the male-dominated construction industry. The chapter outlines the characteristics of work and the workplace and how they can be detrimental for the physical and mental health of women. We explore the discrimination-health relationship and in what manner this manifests for women in construction. The psychosocial risk factor of bullying is considered, and the ways in which gendered work hazards are perpetuated in the construction industry are outlined and their impacts on health are identified. We finish the chapter by determining how construction workplaces designed for men can have a detrimental impact on the health of women, and argue that sex (biological differences) and gender (social roles) must be considered in the design of work which seeks to reduce or remove harmful work hazards.

Chapter 6 explores the role of employee resilience and its relationship to wellbeing. Resilience is defined in multiple ways and we review the various definitions of resilience and consider how this translates into definitions of team resilience and employee resilience. Given the definitional and empirical limitations of team resilience, the chapter goes on to focus on the antecedents and outcomes of employee resilience. Protective factors emerging from the individual and organisation which support employee resilience are outlined. The interactionist approach to resilience is considered, and this is important as it positions the organisation as an important contributor to employee resilience. Criteria guiding resilience-building programmes in the workplace are outlined. The chapter also considers how organisations can support the resilience of their employees and outlines various interventions which have been trialled and met with mixed results.

Chapter 7 reviews construction workers' health and wellbeing in the Sub-Saharan African region. The chapter describes how economic and social issues affect the characteristics and working environment of the construction industry in the Sub-Saharan African region. Diseases and infections prevalent in the community are outlined, together with a description of how these affect the construction workforce. The chapter also describes the regulations and practices relating to industry health testing in South Africa. Family and lifestyle issues and their impact on health and wellbeing are described. The chapter finishes with a consideration of organisational supports which are available to construction workers in the Sub-Saharan African region.

Chapter 8 provides an overview of the occupational hazards young construction workers are exposed to when working onsite. Consideration is given to why the health of young workers is more adversely affected than that of older workers. Research on the work experience of apprentices is described, and the mental health implications are considered. Why young workers hesitate to speak up about unsafe work practices is explored, as are psychologically damaging incidences of humour, banter and teasing. The importance of social support from supervisors for young construction workers is examined. The chapter finishes by outlining programmes which seek to protect and promote the health and wellbeing of young workers. Finally, the importance of focusing on the work and social environment of young workers rather than focusing solely on the individual is examined.

Chapter 9 addresses the health and wellbeing of manual/non-managerial construction workers as they age. The chapter starts by considering global trends of the ageing workforce and more specifically the construction workforce. The ageing process and its impact on construction workers' workability is then examined. The interplay between occupational risk factors and individuals' health-related behaviours and how they shape work disability outcomes are explored. The chapter then considers the impacts of exposure to occupational health risks, workplace fatalities and severe injuries, and psychosocial risk factors and how these are associated with older workers. A lifespan perspective is used to examine the sequence of interactions between individual (biological and psychological) and contextual (social and environmental) determinants of development to understand older workers' work and health-related experiences. The chapter finishes with an overview of effective age management and outlines interventions designed to protect and promote the health and wellbeing of older workers.

Chapter 10 presents and discusses a new theoretically based model developed for supporting a mentally healthy workforce. This model is based on the sense of place concept and is aligned with a positive psychology approach which focuses on creating a work environment in which workers can flourish. The six elements of the sense of place model are examined to explore their relationship with workers' mental wellbeing. The six elements of the model comprise social support, community, life balance, engagement, respect, and resilience. The chapter finishes by presenting results of a pilot study which tested the reliability, validity and usefulness of the sense of place model in a construction project workplace.

Chapter 11 draws out the conclusions of the book. The chapter starts with a description of the unexpected turn of a global pandemic and consideration of how this affected workers' health and wellbeing in construction. Lessons learned from working from home during the COVID-19 pandemic are examined, followed by a discussion of future issues in work and health. Following this, the implications of climate change for construction workers' health and new models of work and health are explored. Finally, the use of technology in construction and its impact on workers' health are considered.

1.10   Discussion and review questions

1. Why is the social determinants of health model an important perspective to use when considering workers' health?
2. What are the main motivations for managing workers' health?
3. Whose responsibility is it to ensure that workers have and are able to sustain a positive state of physical and mental health?

Note

1 One DALY represents the loss of the equivalent of one year of full health. DALYs for a disease or health condition are the sum of the years of life lost due to premature mortality (YLLs) and the years lived with a disability (YLDs) due to prevalent cases of the disease or health condition in a population. www.who.int/data/gho/indicator-metad ata-registry/imr-details/158, accessed 4 October 2021.

References

Adams, J. M. (2019). The value of worker well-being. *Public Health Reports*, 134(6), 583–586.

Allen, J., Balfour, R., Bell, R., & Marmot, M. (2014). Social determinants of mental health. *International Review of Psychiatry*, 26(4), 392–407.

Arndt, V., Rothenbacher, D., Daniel, U., Zschenderlein, B., Schuberth, S., & Brenner, H. (2005) Construction work and risk of occupational disability: a ten year follow up of 14,474 male workers. *Occupational and Environmental Medicine*, 62(8), 559–66.

Australian Human Rights Commission. (2020). Respect@Work: National Inquiry into Sexual Harassment in Australian Workplaces. Australian Human Rights Commission.

Baicker, K., Cutler, D., & Song, Z. (2010). Workplace wellness programs can generate savings. *Health Affairs*, 29, 304–311.

Baid, D., Hayles, E., & Finkelstein, E. A. (2021). Return on investment of workplace wellness programs for chronic disease prevention: a systematic review. *American Journal of Preventive Medicine*, 61(2), 256–266.

Bambra, C., Gibson, M., Sowden, A., Wright, K., Whitehead, M., & Petticrew, M. (2010). Tackling the wider social determinants of health and health inequalities: evidence from systematic reviews. *Journal of Epidemiology & Community Health*, 64(4), 284–291.

Berry, L. L., Mirabito, A. M., & Baun, W. B. (2010). What's the hard return on employee wellness programs. *Harvard Business Review*, 88(12), 104–112.

Borsting Jacobsen, H., Caban-Martinez, A., Onyebeke, L., Sorensen, G., Dennerlein, J. T., & Endresen Reme, S. (2013) Construction workers struggle with a high prevalence of mental distress and this is associated with their pain and injuries. *Journal of Occupational and Environmental Medicine*, 55(10), 1197–204.

Braveman, P., & Gottlieb, L. (2014). The social determinants of health: it's time to consider the causes of the causes. *Public Health Reports*, 129(1_suppl2), 19–31.

Braveman, P., Egerter, S., & Williams, D. R. (2011). The social determinants of health: coming of age. *Annual Review of Public Health*, 32, 381–398.

Brenner, H., & Ahern, W. (2000) Sickness absence and early retirement on health grounds in the construction industry in Ireland. *Occupational and Environmental Medicine*, 57(9), 615–20.

Brown, S., Brooks, R. D., & Dong, X. S. (2020). *Coronavirus and Health Disparities in Construction Data Bulletin*. Center for Construction Research and Training. Accessed 1 September 2022 from: www.cpwr.com/update_newsletter/new-data-bulletin-examines-the-coronavirus-and-health-disparities-among-construction-workers/.

Centers for Disease Control and Prevention (2018). *Suicide Rates by Major Occupational Group – 17 States, 2012 and 2015*. Accessed 14 October 2021. www.cdc.gov/mmwr/volumes/67/wr/mm6745a1.htm?s_cid=mm6745a1_w

Conrad, P., & Walsh, D. C. (1992). The new corporate health ethic: lifestyle and the social control of work. *International Journal of Health Services*, 22(1), 89–111.

Dahlgren, G., & Whitehead, M. (1991). *Policies and strategies to promote social equity in health. Background document to WHO-Strategy paper for Europe* (No. 2007: 14). Institute for Futures Studies.

Dahlgren, G., & Whitehead, M. (2021). The Dahlgren-Whitehead model of health determinants: 30 years on and still chasing rainbows. *Public Health*, 199, 20–24.

Denton, M., & Walters, V. (1999). Gender differences in structural and behavioral determinants of health: an analysis of the social production of health. *Social Science & Medicine*, 48(9), 1221–1235.

Diderichsen, F., Evans, T., & Whitehead, M. (2001). The social basis of disparities in health. In T. Evans, M. Whitehead, F. Diderichsen, A. Bhuiya, and M. Wirth (Eds.), *Challenging Inequities in Health: From Ethics to Action*. Oxford Academic (pp.12–23).

Dong, X. S., Wang, X., Fujimoto, A., and Dobbin, R. (2012), Chronic back pain among older construction workers in the United States: a longitudinal study. *International Journal of Occupational and Environmental Health*, 18(2), 99–109.

Dubois, A., & Gadde, L. E. (2000). Supply strategy and network effects – purchasing behaviour in the construction industry. *European Journal of Purchasing & Supply Management*, 6(3–4), 207–215.

Eckhardt, R. E. (2001). The moral duty to provide for workplace safety. *Professional Safety*, 46(8), 36–38.

Geddie, J. & Aravindan, A. (2020). *In Singapore, Migrant Coronavirus Cases Highlight Containment Weak Link*. Accessed 1 December 2020 from: www.reuters.com/article/us-health-coronavirus-singapore-migrants-idUSKCN21X19G

Gram, B., Holtermann, A., Søgaard, K., & Sjøgaard, G. (2012). Effect of individualized worksite exercise training on aerobic capacity and muscle strength among construction workers – a randomized controlled intervention study. *Scandinavian Journal of Work, Environment & Health*, 38(5), 467–475.

Greenwood, M. R. (2002), Ethics and HRM: A Review and conceptual analysis, *Journal of Business Ethics*, 36, 261–278.

Groeneveld, I. F., Proper, K. I., Van der Beek, A. J., & Van Mechelen, W. (2010). Sustained body weight reduction by an individual-based lifestyle intervention for workers in the construction industry at risk for cardiovascular disease: results of a randomized controlled trial. *Preventive Medicine*, 51(3–4), 240–246.

Hartmann, A., & Caerteling, J. (2010). Subcontractor procurement in construction: The interplay of price and trust. *Supply Chain Management: An International Journal*, 15(5), 354–362.

Hartmann, B. & Fleischer, A. G. (2005). Physical load exposure at construction sites. *Scandinavian Journal of Work, Environment and Health*, 31 (Supplement 2), 88–95.

Health and Safety Executive (2021). Construction Health Risks: Key Points. Accessed 14 October 2021from: www.hse.gov.uk/construction/healthrisks/key-points.htm

Hochschild, A. R., & Machung, A. (1989). *The Second Shift: Working Parents and the Revolution at Home*. Viking.

Holmqvist, M. (2009). Corporate social responsibility as corporate social control: The case of work-site health promotion. *Scandinavian Journal of Management*, 25(1), 68–72.

International Labour Organization (2022). International Labour Conference adds safety and health to Fundamental Principles and Rights at Work, www.ilo.org/global/about-the-ilo/newsroom/news/WCMS_848132/lang--en/index.htm, accessed 27 September 2022.

Johansson, J., & Edwards, M. (2021). Exploring caring leadership through a feminist ethic of care: The case of a sporty CEO. *Leadership*, 17(3), 318–335.

Jones, W., Gibb, A., Haslam, R., & Dainty, A. (2019). Work-related ill-health in construction: the importance of scope, ownership and understanding. *Safety Science*, 120, 538–550.

King, T. L., & Lamontagne, A. D. (2021). COVID-19 and suicide risk in the construction sector: preparing for a perfect storm. *Scandinavian Journal of Public Health*, 49(7), 774–778.

Koh, D. (2020). Migrant workers and COVID-19. *Occupational and Environmental Medicine*, 77(9), 634–636.

Latza, U., Karmaus, W., Stürmer, T., Steiner, M., Neth, A., & Rehder, U. (2000). Cohort study of occupational risk factors of low back pain in construction workers. *Occupational and Environmental Medicine*, 57(1), 28–34.

Lee, M. P., Hudson, H., Richards, R., Chang, C. C., Chosewood, L. C., & Schill, A. L. (2016). *Fundamentals of Total Worker Health Approaches: Essential Elements for Advancing Worker Safety, Health, and Well-Being*. U.S. Department of Health and Human Services,

Centers for Disease Control and Prevention, National Institute for Occupational Safety and Health.

Lingard, H., & Turner, M. (2015). Improving the health of male, blue collar construction workers: a social ecological perspective. *Construction Management and Economics*, 33(1), 18–34.

Lingard, H., & Turner, M. (2017). Promoting construction workers' health: a multi-level system perspective. *Construction Management and Economics*, 35(5), 239–253.

Ludewig, P. M., & Borstad, J. D. (2003). Effects of a home exercise programme on shoulder pain and functional status in construction workers. *Occupational and Environmental Medicine*, 60(11), 841–849.

Marmot, M., Allen, J., Goldblatt, P., Herd, E., & Morrison, J. (2020). *Build Back Fairer: The Covid-19 Marmot Review*. Institute of Health Equity. Accessed 5 October 2021 from: www.instituteofhealthequity.org/about-our-work/latest-updates-from-the-institute/build-back-fairer

Martínez-Lemos, R. I. (2015). Economic impact of corporate wellness programs in Europe: A literature review. *Journal of Occupational Health*, 57(3), 201–211.

McLellan, R. K. (2017). Work, health, and worker well-being: Roles and opportunities for employers. *Health Affairs*, 36(2), 206–213.

Meltzer, H., Griffiths, C., Brock, A., Rooney, C., & Jenkins, R. (2008). Patterns of suicide by occupation in England and Wales: 2001–2005. *British Journal of Psychiatry*, 193(1), 73–76.

Messing K., & Östlin P. (2006). *Gender Equality, Work and Health: A Review of the Evidence*. World Health Organization.

Milner, A., Spittal, M. J., Pirkis, J., & LaMontagne, A. D. (2013). Suicide by occupation: Systematic review and meta-analysis. *British Journal of Psychiatry*, 203(6), 409–416.

Min, K. B., Park, S. G., Song, J. S., Yi, K. H., Jang, T. W., & Min, J. Y. (2013). Subcontractors and increased risk for work-related diseases and absenteeism. *American Journal of Industrial Medicine*, 56(11), 1296–1306.

National Institute for Occupational Safety and Health (NIOSH) (2017). *The Hierarchy of Controls Applied to Total Worker Health*. Accessed 5 November 2021: www.cdc.gov/niosh/twh/letsgetstarted.html

Oude Hengel, K. M., Blatter, B. M., Joling, C. I., van der Beek, A. J., & Bongers, P. M. (2012) Effectiveness of an intervention at construction worksites on work engagement, social support, physical workload and the need for recovery: Results from a cluster randomized controlled trial. *BMC Public Health*, 12, 1–10.

Peterson, J. S., & Zwerling, C. (1998). Comparison of health outcomes among older construction and blue-collar employees in the United States. *American Journal of Industrial Medicine*, 34(3), 280–287.

Rowan, J. J. (2000), The moral foundation of employee rights. *Journal of Business Ethics*, 25, 355–361.

Safe Work Australia (2019). *Model Work Health and Safety Bill*. Safe Work Australia.

Safe Work Australia (2021). *Model Work Health and Safety Regulations*. Safe Work Australia.

Schill, A. L., & Chosewood, L. C. (2013). The NIOSH Total Worker Health program: an overview. *Journal of Occupational and Environmental Medicine*, 55(12 Suppl), S8–11.

Sherratt, F. (2015). Legitimizing public health control on sites? A critical discourse analysis of the Responsibility Deal Construction Pledge. *Construction Management and Economics*, 33(5–6), 444–452.

Sherratt, F. (2018). Shaping the discourse of worker health in the UK construction industry. *Construction Management and Economics*, 36(3), 141–152.

Smallwood, J., & Lingard, H. (2009) Occupational health and safety and corporate social responsibility. In M. Murray and A. Dainty (Eds.), *Corporate Social Responsibility in the Construction Industry*. Spon Press (pp.261–286).

Snashall, D. (2005) Occupational health in the construction industry. *Scandinavian Journal of Work, Environment & Health*, 31(Suppl. 2), 5–10.

Sorensen, G., Barbeau, E. M., Stoddard, A. M., Hunt, M. K., Goldman, R., Smith, A.,... & Wallace, L. (2007). Tools for health: the efficacy of a tailored intervention targeted for construction laborers. *Cancer Causes & Control*, 18(1), 51–59.

Sorensen, G., Dennerlein, J. T., Peters, S. E., Sabbath, E. L., Kelly, E. L., & Wagner, G. R. (2021). The future of research on work, safety, health and wellbeing: A guiding conceptual framework. *Social Science & Medicine*, 269, 1–9.

Stocks, S. J., McNamee, R., Carder, M., and Agius, R. M. (2010) The incidence of medically reported work-related ill health in the UK construction industry. *Occupational and Environmental Medicine*, 67(8), 574–576.

Stocks, S. J., Turner, S., McNamee, R., Carder, M., Hussey, L., and Agius, R. M. (2011) Occupational and work-related ill-health in UK construction workers. *Occupational Medicine*, 61(6), 407–15.

Tamers, S. L., Chosewood, L. C., Childress, A., Hudson, H., Nigam, J., & Chang, C. C. (2019). Total worker health 2014–2018: The novel approach to worker safety, health, and well-being evolves. *International Journal of Environmental Research and Public Health*, 16(3), 321, 1–19.

Turner, M., Holdsworth, S., Scott-Young, C. M., & Sandri, K. (2021). Resilience in a hostile workplace: The experience of women onsite in construction. *Construction Management and Economics,* 39(10), 839–852.

Underhill, E., & Quinlan, M. (2011). How precarious employment affects health and safety at work: the case of temporary agency workers. *Relations Industrielles/Industrial Relations*, 66(3), 397–421.

Welch, L. S. (2009) Improving work ability in construction workers – let's get to work. *Scandinavian Journal of Work, Environment & Health*, 35(5), 321–324.

WorkSafe Queensland (2021). *National Health Survey Construction Industry Data Released*. Accessed 14 October 2021 from: www.worksafe.qld.gov.au/news-and-events/news letters/esafe-newsletters/esafe-editions/esafe-construction/november-2019/national-health-survey-construction-industry-data-released

WorkSafe Victoria (2020). *Work-Related Gendered Violence Including Sexual Harassment. A Guide for Employers on Preventing and Responding to Work-Related Gendered Violence and Work-Related Sexual Harassment*. Accessed 13 October 2021from: www.worksafe.vic. gov.au/resources/work-related-gendered-violence-sexual-harassment,

World Health Organization (2010a). *Healthy Workplaces: A Model for Action: For Employers, Workers, Policymakers and Practitioners*. World Health Organization.

World Health Organization (2010b*)*. *A Conceptual Framework for Action on the Social Determinants of Health*. World Health Organization.

World Health Organization (2011). *Building healthy and equitable workplaces for women and men: A Resource for Employers and Worker Representatives*. World Health Organization.

World Health Organization (2019). *Health, decent work and the economy*. World Health Organization. Regional Office for Europe. Copenhagen.

World Health Organization/International Labour Organization (2021). *WHO/ILO Joint Estimates of the Work-related Burden of Disease and Injury, 2000–2016: Global Monitoring Report*.

Zoller, H. M. (2003). Working out: Managerialism in workplace health promotion. *Management Communication Quarterly*, 17(2), 171–205.

2

ATTENDING TO THE "H" IN OH&S

I still think there is a bit of a view that health is secondary to safety, which is obviously what we're trying to eliminate. I think if we see good performance in the health bit, it's normally quite a good indicator that an area is taking everything very seriously.

Health and Safety Director

2.1 Introduction

In this chapter we provide a brief overview of the challenges inherent in managing occupational health in the construction industry and some of the major occupational health risk factors to which construction workers are exposed. We highlight the importance of applying the hierarchy of control to ensure that occupational health risks are controlled as effectively as possible, by targeting health hazards at source and preventing (or at least substantially reducing) exposures. Examples are provided of initiatives that have effectively reduced exposures to occupational health risks in the sector. Some of these initiatives involve changes to national and international regulatory frameworks governing the manufacture, importation and supply of products and materials, others involve the adoption and use of new tools and technologies within particular organisations or projects. While the chapter cannot cover all occupational health issues relevant to construction work, the discussion and examples we offer are intended to provide evidence of the need to do more to manage occupational health (as well as safety) in the construction sector. The chapter also provides insights into actions that can be taken at government, industry, organisation and project levels to reduce the construction industry's unacceptably high incidence of work-related disease.

DOI: 10.1201/9780367814236-2

2.2 Who should be responsible for managing workers' health?

While everybody can and should take responsibility for looking after their own health in relation to the things over which they have control, workers are often exposed to conditions that can adversely affect their health, and over which they have little or no control. Occupational health and safety legislation exists to ensure that organisations and individuals who manage worksites, and other parties such as organisations and individuals who design, manufacture and supply plant, equipment and substances take reasonable steps to control risks of harm to workers' health, as well as to their safety.

The point of departure for this chapter is the position that it is unhelpful that occupational health has been subsumed into the catch-all, singular concept of "OH&S." We argue that occupational health is distinct from safety, requiring specific and focused attention and effort in both its regulation and management. However, the identification and control of hazards that present the potential for acute injury (with immediate effects) have tended to take precedence over the management of health risks, the effects of which are often delayed, less well understood, and difficult to envisage. This situation has led to calls for occupational health to be given a higher priority, and recognised as being of equal importance to occupational safety in the construction industry (Jones et al., 2019).

While adverse safety events tend to have immediate effects and occur almost exclusively within the physical workplace, occupational illnesses often develop over a long time period and can also be influenced by individual characteristics and behaviours and environmental factors outside the workplace. Sherratt (2016) argues these differences have reduced the degree of organisational attention that is paid to the elimination or reduction of significant occupational health risks, while placing an unrealistically high degree of emphasis on individual workers' responsibility for managing their own health. This is evident in the emphasis on wellbeing programmes that focus on improving workers' "lifestyle" behaviours, for example providing fruit in workplaces to encourage healthy eating, providing fitness programmes, smoking cessation programmes, etc. While well-intentioned, these programmes do not reduce the risk associated with exposure to many known and serious occupational health risks present in many workplaces. The systematic identification, assessment and control of occupational health risk must be primarily an organisational/managerial responsibility, rather than the responsibility of individual workers.

Construction workers are a high-risk group for poor health that is caused by or made worse by their employment. In the United Kingdom in 2020, 81,000 construction workers were reported to be suffering from work-related ill health (including new or long-standing illnesses) (HSE, 2020a). Musculoskeletal disorders accounted for 57 per cent of these illnesses, followed by stress, depression and anxiety (26 per cent). Reflecting the diversity of exposure to health risks,

17 per cent of reported occupational illnesses in UK-based construction workers were classified as "other illnesses" and included occupational asthma, chronic obstructive pulmonary disease (COPD), contact dermatitis, occupational cancer, occupational deafness and hand-arm vibration (HSE, 2020a). In the USA, the risk of chronic occupational illness over a 45-year working life in construction is 2–6 times greater for construction workers than non-construction workers (Ringen et al., 2014). Ringen et al. (2014) estimate that, in their working lives, 16 per cent of construction workers developed COPD, 11 per cent experienced chest x-ray abnormality, and 74 per cent developed hearing loss.

Understanding the prevalence of occupational illness in the construction industry can be challenging due to the diverse nature of the industry's workforce and the vast array of work-related health hazards to which construction workers are exposed. In European countries, large-scale national health surveillance schemes have been implemented which allow a detailed examination of trends in the annual incidence of occupational disease (defined as "clinically established diseases mainly caused by work" (van der Molen et al., 2016, p.350)). For example, in the Dutch construction industry, van der Molen et al. (2016) report that approximately 13 per cent of construction workers have an occupational disease that has been reported and diagnosed by an occupational physician. Noise-induced hearing loss accounted for two-thirds of these diagnoses, while musculoskeletal disorders were the second most frequently occurring occupational disease. Over a five-year period between 2010 and 2014, the incidence of noise-induced hearing loss increased significantly by 7 per cent and contact dermatitis increased by 19 per cent (van der Molen et al., 2016).

Snashall (2005) argues that, because of the wide variety of activities and tasks involved in construction work, almost every known occupational illness has been reported in the construction workforce. Also, the health risk exposure of construction workers varies considerably depending on their trade. Some health issues are more prevalent in particular trades due to the exposures associated with their work. For example, plasterers, bricklayers and masons are at high risk of contact dermatitis (HSE, 2020a), while tunnellers are exposed to a variety of airborne substances that reduce lung function (Ulvestad et al., 2015). Historically, painters have been at risk of neuropsychiatric disorders arising from exposure to organic solvents (Kaukiainen et al., 2004). However, the increasing use of water-based rather than solvent-based paint that has occurred since the 1970s has reduced the occurrence of chronic toxic encephalopathy or so-called "painters' syndrome" (Decopaint, 2000; Järvholm & Burdorf, 2017).

The substantial variation in hazard exposures and occupational health effects experienced by construction workers requires a nuanced understanding of the risk profile of the workforce in an organisation or project, recognising this may vary between project stages as particular construction activities commence and finish. The ageing construction workforce in many countries is also likely to increase the risk of occupational disease as workers experience higher cumulative exposures over their working lives.

Aside from the human impacts and losses borne by workers and their families who experience a debilitating illness or death arising from a work-related disease, the economic costs of occupational disease are substantial. For example, UK data indicates that occupational illness in the construction industry resulted in more than 1.5 million lost working days each year between 2017/18 and 2019/20. This is compared with 500,000 workdays lost as a result of workplace injury (HSE, 2020a). The UK's Health and Safety Executive also estimates that, in 2018/19, new cases of work-related ill health cost society around £10.6 billion, compared with £5.59 billion for workplace injury (HSE, 2020a).

2.3 Managing occupational health is more complicated than managing safety

Many of the occupational risk factors and resulting diseases experienced by construction workers have been well understood for some time and effective risk controls have been identified. This raises the important question as to why construction workers are still exposed to hazardous work conditions that affect their health to the extent that they do. A variety of reasons has been provided as to why, historically at least, occupational health risks have not been as well managed as occupational safety risks. Some of the challenges are described briefly below.

The long latency period of many diseases (for example, cancers arising as a result of asbestos exposure or neurological damage associated with hand-arm vibration), in which illness may not be experienced until many years after exposure, is sometimes identified as a barrier to effective prevention. An extended time lag between exposure and illness can make attribution of responsibility for harmful exposure to individual employers difficult in an industry like construction in which workers move frequently between projects and may change employers multiple times in their working lives. For example, Dement et al. (2005) suggest that the peripatetic nature of the construction industry's workforce combined with the cost of investment in prevention has contributed to a failure of employers to implement effective and known controls for the risk of noise-induced hearing loss in the US construction industry. Importantly, even if it is difficult to identify employer responsibility for historical exposure leading to illness, this should not preclude the implementation of appropriate measures to eliminate and reduce potentially harmful exposures in the present. As knowledge about the links between workplace exposure and occupational illnesses grows, it is incumbent upon employers and others with responsibility for workplace health and safety to ensure that health risks are identified, understood and effectively controlled to reduce the burden of illness in the future. This may require more significant regulatory intervention to ensure that organisations invest appropriately in the prevention of occupational ill health.

Further, the effects of occupational exposures on ill health can be obscured because of the cumulative and combined effect of exposures at work and outside work. For example, construction workers are a high-risk group for COPD (progressive and irreversible limitation in airflow in the lungs, including chronic bronchitis and emphysema) (Murgia & Gambelunghe, 2021). The primary cause of COPD is smoking, but COPD is also caused by exposures to welding fumes, silica, man-made vitreous fibres, and other chemicals such as isocyanates, cadmium, vanadium and polycyclic 1 aromatic hydrocarbons and wood dust (HSE, 2020b). The extent to which COPD is linked to occupational exposures in construction workers reportedly depends upon whether they are smokers or not. In a study of Swedish construction workers exposed to airborne risk factors, researchers found that the percentage of COPD that was attributable to workplace risk factors was 10.7 per cent, but this increased to 52.6 per cent among occupationally exposed workers who had never smoked (Bergdahl et al., 2004). Importantly, Murgia and Gambelunghe (2021) argue that COPD is a significantly underdiagnosed disease and, even when it is diagnosed, occupational factors are often overlooked, meaning that many cases go uncompensated.

In many instances it is hard to disentangle workplace and lifestyle risk factors in illness causation. For example, work-related stress is linked to impaired sleep (Åkerstedt, 2006) which is, in turn, associated with high body mass index and obesity (Gangwisch et al., 2005; Bjorvatn et al., 2007). Poor sleep is also an identified risk factor for cardiovascular disease and diabetes (Spiegel et al., 2005; Gangwisch et al., 2006; Gottlieb et al., 2006). Thus, work-related stress (an occupational risk factor) can contribute in complex ways to illnesses typically considered to be associated with living an unhealthy lifestyle. Similarly, it is widely reported that workplace exposures can "potentiate" the effect of smoking (a lifestyle health risk). A great deal of research has focused on the combined risks of asbestos exposure and smoking, with research finding that non-smokers' exposure to asbestos, or smoking without being exposed to asbestos are both linked to increased lung cancer mortality. However, when taken together, exposure to asbestos and smoking have an interactive effect resulting in a substantially increased incidence of lung cancer mortality (Markowitz et al., 2013; Frost et al., 2011). Similar patterns in the occurrence of lung disease have been found when tobacco smoking is combined with exposure to wood dust in the workplace (Barcenas et al., 2005).

O'Neill et al. (2007) highlight the complex challenges in managing workers' exposures to hazardous substances when workers can be exposed to multiple (and interacting) health hazards at the same time, as well as changing exposures over their working lives. Simultaneous exposure to different occupational hazards or environmental conditions can substantially increase the likelihood of harm. For example, exposure to airborne pollutants (including working in a dusty environment) can negatively affect workers' innate lung defence mechanisms (known as the mucociliary clearance system) enabling other harmful airborne substances to enter the body more easily (O'Neill et al., 2007). O'Neill et al. (2007) argue that current exposure standards and risk control regimes do not adequately reflect these interactive effects or the complexity of exposures to occupational health hazards.

2.4 Deciding on appropriate risk controls for occupational health hazards

Notwithstanding these complexities, occupational health and safety legislation establishes the same responsibilities for managing risks to workers' health as those that apply to managing safety risks. In countries that have adopted the UK model of Robens-style occupational health and safety legislation, employers and others have general duties to eliminate hazards or, where this is not possible, to reduce risk so far as is reasonably practicable.

Within this regulatory framework, the concept of the hierarchy of control (HoC) is used to inform decision-making about how to control health (and safety) risks in a given situation. The HoC arranges occupational health risk controls in a descending order of effectiveness based on the understanding that making the work environment safer and healthier is more effective than trying to change the behaviour of workers. The levels of the HoC are:

- elimination: this is the most effective form of control because the elimination of a hazard poses no risk to workers or the public;
- substitution: this involves replacing the hazard with a less harmful alternative;
- engineering controls: these isolate or separate people from hazards;
- administrative controls: these include measures designed to change the way workers undertake a task;
- personal protective equipment (PPE): this is generally regarded as the least effective control measure as it relies on the individual to use it.

Although much emphasised and visible on a worksite, it is widely understood that PPE should always be seen as a "last resort" and always supplemented with higher level controls in the hierarchy.

Example controls for the risk of exposure to diesel exhaust emissions are shown in Table 2.1 below. Diesel exhaust is classified by the International Agency for Research on Cancer (IARC) as definitely carcinogenic to humans. Diesel exhaust emissions are made up of gaseous components and particulate matter, each of which can have health effects on their own but which, in combination, are known to produce complicated effects on the cardiovascular, respiratory and neurological systems, as well as causing cancer (Landwehr et al., 2021). Diesel exhaust is a problem in construction and has been linked to lung function decline in tunnel workers (Bakke et al., 2004) and lung cancer mortality in truck drivers (Järvholm & Silverman, 2003). It is therefore widely recommended that diesel exhaust emissions be eliminated or, at least, reduced as far as possible.

Occupational exposure limits have been established for diesel exhaust. For example, the Australian Institute of Occupational Hygienists recommends an

TABLE 2.1 Example hierarchy of control for diesel exhaust emission

Risk control classification	Example control measure
Elimination	• Replace diesel-powered plants with electrically driven, propane, compressed natural gas or petrol-fuelled vehicles
Substitution	• Use lower diesel emission engines/cleaner fuels (e.g., low sulphur diesel) or more fuel-efficient engines
Engineering controls	• Install engine exhaust filters • Install a local tailpipe exhaust ventilation • Install other ventilation techniques such as dilution ventilations or local extraction ventilation • Use other ventilation, such as exhaust gas recirculation, catalytic converters or selective non-catalytic reduction • Use diesel emissions "after treatment" systems • Fit exhaust gas recirculation systems • Use enclosed cabins in vehicles with filtered air • Provide fresh air by using controls like a canopy air curtain • Separate areas in which diesel engines are operating
Administrative controls	• Reduce the number of employees directly exposed and their period of exposure (e.g., through rotation or work schedules) • Prohibit/restrict unnecessary idling of engines • Restrict the total engine horsepower and number of diesel-powered equipment in defined areas • Allocate areas without any diesel engine operation and personnel travel • Set up speed limits and put one-way traffic routes into place to reduce the level of traffic • Perform regular maintenance of all diesel-powered machines and equipment • Perform annual training for workers • Perform routine cleaning or replacement of air filters, regular tuning of the engine • Monitor emissions and record backpressure on exhaust treatment devices at each routine service
PPE	• Use respiratory protective equipment

Source: RMIT University, 2018.

exposure limit of 100 micrograms (μg) per cubic metre (measured as elemental carbon) as a time-weighted average over 8 hours (AIOH, 2017). However, Landwehr et al. (2021) argue that this level is still too high for an occupational exposure standard because it does not take into account workers with asthma or allergies and is well above diesel exhaust concentrations in studies that found an elevated risk of lung cancer.

2.5 Occupational cancer

Construction workers are at significant risk of occupational cancer. A UK study of the burden of occupational cancer found that approximately 8,000 cancer deaths (in 2005) and 13,500 cancer registrations (in 2004) in Great Britain could be attributed to occupational exposure (HSE, 2020c). The study estimated the proportion of cancer cases associated with exposure to substances identified by the International Agency for Research on Cancer as either known (Group 1) or probable (Group 2A) carcinogens.

Figure 2.1 shows occupational cancer deaths arising from exposure to the top ten carcinogens in 2005 compared to 2014–18 (based on annual average estimates). The majority of occupational cancer deaths were attributed to exposure to asbestos and these deaths increased between 2005 and 2014–18. Other major contributors to occupational cancer death were exposures to silica and diesel engine exhaust.

The HSE (2020c) reports that construction workers were proportionally more likely to experience occupational cancer than workers from any other industry. Construction workers accounted for more than 40 per cent of occupational cancer deaths in 2005. Due to the long latency period of occupational cancers, past exposures to asbestos and silica were the predominant causes of death from

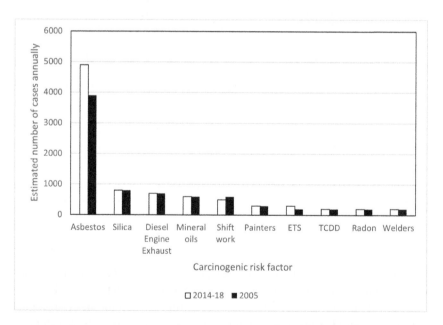

FIGURE 2.1 Carcinogens associated with occupational cancer deaths in the UK

Note: ETS – Environmental Tobacco Smoke, TCDD – 2,3,7,8-Tetrachlorodibenzodioxin.

Source: HSE, 2020c.

lung cancer and mesothelioma. Mesothelioma is most commonly experienced by carpenters, plumbers and electricians. The HSE (2020a) reports that 17 per cent of mesothelioma cases are related to past asbestos exposure in carpentry and, in particular, the use of insulation board containing brown asbestos in building construction. In a study of lung cancer mortality in the USA, Dement et al. (2020) found that the risk of lung cancer death associated with spending five years in construction was comparable to known risk factors of having a personal cancer history, a family history of cancer or a diagnosis of COPD. Dement et al. (2020) analysed a large sample longitudinal data set to show that, by including occupational exposures in modelling construction workers' lung cancer mortality, they were able to identify 86 per cent of participants who would eventually die from lung cancer, compared with only 51 per cent when considering only workers' age and smoking history.

Exposure to solar radiation was also commonly identified as a risk factor for painters and decorators and exposure to coal tar and pitches was identified as a risk factor for roofers, road surfacers, roadmen and paviors in new cancer registrations recorded in 2004 (HSE, 2020c). The HSE study also reported that, although deaths attributed to asbestos exposure would begin to decline after 2020 in the UK, the construction industry would continue to experience the largest number of occupational cancer cases in the future. Projected estimates suggest silica, diesel engine exhaust, solar radiation, shiftwork and working as painters and welders will be linked to the majority of occupational cancer cases among UK construction workers in the future. The link between shiftwork and occupational cancer is noteworthy and related to working time arrangements discussed in Chapter 4 of this book.

Case example 2.1 highlights the importance of taking a global approach to the management of occupational cancer risks.

CASE EXAMPLE 2.1 GLOBAL INTERVENTIONS TO IMPROVE OCCUPATIONAL HEALTH: THE CASE OF ASBESTOS

The importance of a global response to the management of occupational cancer risks is highlighted by the case of asbestos. Asbestos accounts for approximately half of the world's occupational cancer deaths and cancer risk is reported even when workers are exposed to very low levels of asbestos (WHO, 2014).

The World Health Organization (2014) reports that 90 per cent of chrysotile asbestos is used in cement building materials, which is a particular problem because the size of the global construction workforce means that large numbers of people are exposed. It can also be hard to control exposure to airborne contaminants in construction workplaces and exposures can also increase as building materials are damaged or deteriorate over time (WHO, 2014).

According to the World Health Organization (2014), approximately 125 million people in the world remain exposed to asbestos at the workplace and at least 107,000 people die each year from occupational lung cancer, mesothelioma and asbestosis caused by exposure to asbestos at work.

International efforts have been made to eliminate asbestos-related diseases. For example, the International Labour Organization (ILO) Convention no 162 concerning Safety in the Use of Asbestos focused on prevention of occupational exposure to asbestos and established the principle of ensuring workers' exposure to asbestos remains below a specific limit (Lin et al., 2019). Subsequently, in 2003, the Thirteenth Session of the Joint International Labour Organization (ILO)/World Health Organization (WHO) Committee on Occupational Health recommended special attention be paid to the elimination of asbestos-related diseases and, in 2007, the World Health Assembly called for global campaigns to eliminate asbestos-related diseases. Lin et al. (2019) studied the effectiveness and impact of international initiatives and found that individual countries' adoption of international Conventions relating to the reduction of asbestos-related harm play an important role in facilitating the implementation of total asbestos bans in countries around the world, highlighting the importance and effectiveness of international programmes and agreements.

The World Health Organization report on chrysotile asbestos (the most widespread form of asbestos in use globally) states that "the most efficient way to eliminate asbestos-related diseases is to stop the use of all types of asbestos." The WHO is also committed to working with individual countries to reduce the burden of asbestos-related illness and death by: "providing information about solutions for replacing asbestos with safer substitutes and developing economic and technological mechanisms to stimulate its replacement, taking measures to prevent exposure to asbestos in place and during asbestos removal (abatement), improving early diagnosis, treatment and rehabilitation services for asbestos-related diseases and establishing registries of people with past and/or current exposure to asbestos" (WHO, 2014, p.4).

The manufacture and use of all types of asbestos have been banned in some 68 countries. However, workers in countries in which asbestos has been banned from use can still be exposed as a result of historical use of asbestos products in existing buildings (for example, during renovation, maintenance or demolition). In the context of global supply networks for building products it is also difficult to ensure that imported products do not contain asbestos. Australian trade union organisations recently called for a global ban on the use of asbestos when it was found in a number of imported materials and products in use in the Australian construction industry (Australian Broadcasting Corporation, 2021).

Asbestos is still widely used in many countries in the world. The World Health Organization observes the use of asbestos is still common in many developing countries and in the Asia Pacific region. However, the OECD countries of Mexico and the United States have also not yet banned the use of asbestos.

Importantly, because of the long latency period between exposure and illness, even if asbestos production and use completely stopped everywhere in the world now, the global burden of asbestos-related illness and death would still not decline for several decades (WHO, 2014).

The case of asbestos illustrates how difficult it is to prevent exposure to harmful substances, even when they are irrefutably linked to fatal illnesses such as occupational cancers.

2.6   Exposure to respirable silica

In 1930, a landmark International Labour Organization (ILO) conference held in Johannesburg highlighted the health risks associated with being exposed to and inhaling particles of respirable crystalline silica (Sauvé, 2015). However, a broad awareness of the extent and impacts associated with exposure to respirable silica in the construction industry did not develop until as late as the 1990s (Sauvé, 2015). It is now widely recognised that construction workers are a high-risk group for health problems associated with exposure to respirable silica. For example, a World Health Organization project investigating the Global Burden of Disease found that after mining (23%), construction has the second highest percentage of workers exposed to silica (19%) (Driscoll et al., 2004).

Exposure to respirable crystalline silica can cause silicosis, which is an irreversible, fibrotic lung disease caused by the inhalation of respirable crystalline silica. Silicosis is a progressive and potentially lethal disease that constitutes a major public health issue around the world (Hoy et al., 2021). Exposure to respirable crystalline silica is also associated with increased risk for lung infection (e.g., tuberculosis), lung cancer, emphysema, autoimmune diseases, and kidney disease (Nij & Heederik, 2005).

In 1997, crystalline silica was classified as a carcinogen for humans by the International Agency for Research on Cancer (Nij & Heederik, 2005). Hoy et al. (2021) observe that, although occupational exposure limits (OELs) for crystalline silica have been established in many regions of the world, the extent to which they protect workers is limited due to inconsistency – in some low and middle-income countries there is no legislated exposure limit, and OELs established in other areas are often in excess of the recommendation of the American Conference of Governmental Industrial Hygienists of an OEL for respirable crystalline silica of 0.025 mg/m³. Moreover, even when OELs are established by legislation, compliance with these levels is hindered by low levels of surveillance and enforcement (Hoy et al., 2021). Indeed, research shows that exposure to respirable crystalline silica in the construction industry frequently exceeds established OELs (Flanagan et al., 2003; Akbar-Khanzadeh & Brillhart, 2002; Nij et al., 2003; van Deurssen et al., 2014). One US study suggests that overexposure of construction workers to respirable crystalline silica ranges between 65 and 100 per cent (Rappaport et al., 2003)

The International Labour Organization (ILO)/World Health Organization (WHO) Global Program for the Elimination of Silicosis was established in 1995 and focuses on both primary and secondary control of respirable crystalline silica exposure. While secondary prevention focuses on surveillance of the work environment and of workers, primary prevention seeks to eliminate or reduce silica dust at the source (Beaucham et al., 2012). Although primary prevention controls are available, it is widely reported that respiratory protective equipment is the most widely used form of risk control adopted to prevent harm associated with respirable crystalline silica exposure, which may not be sufficient in the absence of other forms of control (Nij et al., 2003). This is in spite of evidence that dust emissions can be substantially reduced through the use of control measures such as the use of local exhaust ventilation systems (Akbar-Khanzadeh & Brillhart, 2002) or wet dust suppression when undertaking high-risk work tasks such as cutting concrete (Summers & Parmigiani, 2015). Importantly, though, the efficacy of control measures in workplace settings can also be impacted by organisational and psychosocial factors, and measures designed to reduce exposures to respirable crystalline silica should take account of barriers to adoption in the work environment (van Deurseen et al., 2014).

One of the challenges associated with managing the risk of exposure to respirable crystalline silica in construction workplaces is that the construction workforce is not homogeneous and exposures vary depending on tasks performed, environmental conditions and tools and materials used (Nij et al., 2004). For this reason, task-based hazard and potential exposure analysis needs to be used to determine appropriate controls.

Importantly, although exposure to respirable crystalline silica is an "ancient" occupational health problem in the construction industry, workers are also affected by emergent risks (Hoy et al., 2018). One such case is the use of engineered stone which has, in recent years, become increasingly fashionable in the construction of stone benchtops in kitchens and bathrooms.

Case example 2.2 considers the use of engineered stone, the harm associated with the use of this product, and how this harm can be managed.

CASE EXAMPLE 2.2 TO BAN OR NOT TO BAN? THE CASE OF ENGINEERED STONE

Safe Work Australia (2021) defines engineered stone as material that "is (a) created by combining and heat curing natural stone materials that contain crystalline silica (such as quartz or stone aggregate) with chemical constituents (such as water, resins or pigments), and (b) can be manipulated through mechanical processes to manufacture other products (such as kitchen benchtops)" (p.6).

Compared to natural stone, engineered stone contains more silica – potentially up to 97 per cent compared to up to 45 per cent for granite (Safe Work Australia, 2021). Higher levels of crystalline silica in engineered stone substantially increase health risks to workers (for example, cutting, grinding, trimming, drilling, sanding and polishing engineered stone). These processes generate respirable dust containing crystalline silica which, when breathed in over time, can cause fatal lung disease (Safe Work Australia, 2021).

Recent analyses of silicosis risk among stone fabrication workers have revealed "outbreaks" of silicosis among workers who work with engineered stone (ABC, 2019). For example, following screening of 659 stonemasons who work with engineered stone in Queensland Australia, 21.4 per cent (141 of 659) were diagnosed with silicosis (Newbigin et al., 2019). In the first year of a health screening programme in Victoria, 86 (36 per cent) of 239 screened stonemasons were diagnosed with silicosis (Hoy et al., 2021). The average age of these workers was 41.8 years and 72 of the 86 were employed in the stone benchtop industry at the time of diagnosis. The others indicated they were no longer working in the industry at the time of diagnosis (Hoy et al., 2021). Hoy et al. (2021) compare the 86 cases identified over a 12-month period to the average of 8 silicosis compensation claims per year in Victoria for the 10 years prior to the health-screening study.

Studies of silicosis attributable to exposure to engineered stone report a short latency period, accelerated occurrence of extensive lung damage and experience of illness in relatively young workers (Leso et al., 2019; Hoy et al., 2021). These characteristics are explained by the high levels of respirable dust generated in some activities and the intensity of exposure (Hoy et al., 2018). Leso et al. (2019) also identify the possibility that dusts produced when working with engineered stone may have specific properties due to the combination of crushed rock and polymeric resins, which potentially increase toxicity and occupational health risk.

León-Jiménez et al. (2020) report an accelerated decline in lung function and a rapid progression to progressive massive fibrosis (PMF) in a sample of Spanish construction workers exposed to silica from engineered stone. Initially (at diagnosis) 6.6 per cent of cases were classified as having PMF but, after cessation of exposure, this rose to 37.7 per cent over a four-year follow-up period (León-Jiménez et al., 2020). A more rapid deterioration in lung function was also observed in silicosis cases associated with engineered stone (León-Jiménez et al., 2020). Thus, silicosis associated with engineered stone appears aggressive compared to silicosis arising as a result of exposure to natural stone.

A retrospective Australian study was conducted of 78 stonemasons diagnosed by their treating respiratory physicians as suffering from either accelerated ($n = 36$) or chronic ($n = 42$) silicosis focused on the presence of occupational risk factors, i.e., whether a person (i) worked with artificial stone products for >50% of their total tenure; (ii) used personal protective equipment (PPE) for <50% of their total tenure; and/or (iii) performed >50% of their work using dry-cutting techniques (Newbigin et al., 2019). The average age of the stonemasons was 34.1 years (range: 23–63) and their average tenure in stonemasonry was 12.9 years (range: 2–45). Most of the stonemasons (68%) reported all three occupational risk factors. All participants indicated the presence of at least one risk factor and 87% indicated they performed more than half of their work using a dry-cutting method (Newbigin et al., 2019). This is consistent with the review of international research undertaken by Leso et al. (2019) which showed that basic preventive measures for controlling occupational exposure (e.g., general or mounted-tool local exhaust ventilation systems or wet-cut methods to suppress dust) were not in place or not implemented properly and full/suitable protective equipment was either not available or not used correctly.

Rose et al. (2019) also report the majority of stone fabrication workers diagnosed with silicosis in the USA were migrant (Hispanic) workers, many of whom worked in small businesses in which low levels of safety awareness, a lack of expertise and low levels of investment in exposure-control technologies substantially increase health risks.

Engineered stone has been compared to asbestos (Fritschi & Reid, 2019). Several Australian organisations (including unions, the Cancer Council, the Thoracic Society of Australia & New Zealand, Lung Foundation Australia, the Australian Institute of Health and Safety, the Public Health Association of Australia and the Australian and New Zealand Society of Occupational Medicine) have supported a ban on the manufacture and use of high silica engineered stone (Fellner, 2021). Fritschi and Reid (2019) point out that alternative (silica-free) products are available for use (e.g., Betta Stone, an environmentally sustainable countertop material made from recycled glass).

However, industry and government stakeholders argue that the danger associated with engineered stone products can be managed through the implementation of effective risk controls within workplaces. This is reflected in recent legislative changes in New South Wales, Queensland and Victoria. As of 2019, in Victoria, employers, self-employed people or people who manage or control a workplace must ensure a power tool is not used to cut, grind or abrasively polish engineered stone, unless the tool: (i) has an integrated water delivery system that supplies a continuous feed of water (on-tool water suppression), or (ii) is fitted with on-tool extraction attached to a HEPA filtered dust class H vacuum cleaner (or similar system that captures the dust generated). If these controls are not reasonably practicable, the use of power tools must be controlled through local exhaust ventilation (LEV). In Victoria, people cutting, grinding or polishing engineered stone with a power tool must also be provided with respiratory protective equipment that: (i) is designed to protect the wearer from the inhalation of airborne contaminants entering the nose, mouth and lungs; and (ii) complies with AS/NZS 1716 – Respiratory protective devices.

However, the efficacy of these control measures has been questioned, with the Australian Cancer Council suggesting they are unlikely to be rigorously implemented in small workplaces. Further, wet cutting alone may not reduce respirable crystalline silica (RCS) levels to safe levels. For example, an international study found dry cutting of engineered stone to generate an RCS concentration of 44.6 milligrams per cubic metre (mg/m³) over 30 minutes of sampling. This decreased to 4.85 mg/m³ when wet blade cutting was used and to 0.69 mg/m³ when wet blade cutting was combined with local exhaust ventilation (Cooper et al., 2015).

To put these concentration levels into perspective, in its recent Code of Practice on managing the risks of RCS in the use of engineered stone, Safe Work Australia established an eight-hour time-weighted average (TWA) exposure standard for RCS of 0.05 mg/m³ (Safe Work Australia, 2021).[1] It is also reported that short-term exposure to concentrations of RCS above 2 mg/m³ is proportionally more risky than longer-term cumulative exposures at lower concentrations (Buchanan et al., 2003). This means that wet blade cutting, without local exhaust ventilation, may still put workers at considerable risk. Hoy et al. (2018) therefore argue that eight-hour standards do not provide adequate guidance concerning the risk posed by short-duration but high-intensity exposure to RCS.

As with all occupational health hazards, it is critical that the most effective controls available are selected based upon the previously described hierarchy of control. Table 2.2 classifies example controls for the risk of airborne contaminants according to their position in the hierarchy.

2.7 Occupational hearing loss

Unlike many dust-related diseases, hearing loss does not result in early mortality. The loss of hearing, however, is a serious disability which can contribute to social isolation, reduced confidence, poor mental health and declining cognitive

TABLE 2.2 Example control measures for airborne health hazards in construction

Risk control classification	Risk control
Elimination	• eliminate airborne hazards (however, this is often not possible especially when working with sand/concrete, when undertaking tunnelling activities or when removing asbestos)
Substitution	• use garnet as a substitute for sand • use aluminium oxide polishing powders instead of silica powders • use pilled solids instead of powders • use wet processes instead of dry processes • vacuum instead of sweep
Engineering controls	• implement barrier protections at the entrance to the working area • use ventilation systems (local exhaust ventilation systems are available such as enclosing hoods, high-velocity low-volume hoods and exterior hoods) • use industrial vacuum cleaners • use water or fine mist suppression to control dust cloud (additional water dust suppression should be applied for tasks which are outside during dry weather or to control dust in mines) • install a conveyor belt wash box where conveyor belts are in use • implement dampeners to increase the air flow • provide fresh air by using controls like a canopy air curtain to cover roof bolters operators and enclosed cabin filtration systems • use sticky floor mats to reduce the amount of dust or debris transferred to other working areas • use thickened substances such as pastes and gels to cover the surfaces being worked on
Administrative controls	• maintain good housekeeping and signage • restrict time of exposure • do not perform dust-generating tasks, such as dry brush sweeping, and the use of compressed air or reuse of vacuum filters • do not carry out dust-generating work on high wind days • reduce the time spent in the dusty areas by job rotation • train the workers how to use PPE correctly and which PPE is appropriate for the task • inform workers about risk of exposures and instruct them how to protect themselves • conduct health monitoring regularly • forbid drinking, eating and smoking while working in areas where asbestos may occur • remove disposable shoe covers or overalls before leaving the working area (if covers aren't used, contaminated shoes and clothing should be cleaned before leaving)

TABLE 2.2 Cont.

Risk control classification	Risk control
	• provide washing facilities as close as possible to the working area, including mild skin cleansers and clean soft paper or towels for drying
	• encourage workers to wash areas of their skin which might have been exposed and to use pre-work creams, if necessary, before starting work or after a break
	• avoid dust-generating activities on high wind days when working outdoors
	• remove construction debris through an approved route, if possible during off-peak times (the debris should be covered and netted when removed)
	• conduct health monitoring including a physical examination of the worker with a focus on the respiratory system
	• conduct additional training or awareness programmes to increase workers' understanding of the risk with a specific task, environment or material-related activity
PPE	• provide appropriate filters for workers (P1 filters are for mechanically generated particulates like silica or asbestos, P2 filters are for thermally and mechanically generated particulates like metal fumes, P3 requires a full-face mask and can be used for all particulates including highly toxic materials like beryllium)
	• provide coveralls, respiratory protective equipment, footwear and gloves in addition to other control measures, when working with asbestos
	• provide hand protection creams
	• use closed eye goggles for any kind of overhead or demolition work

Source: RMIT University, 2018.

function (Chen et al., 2020; Lewkowski et al., 2019). Nelson et al. (2005) report that 16 per cent of disabling hearing loss experienced by adults worldwide is attributed to exposure to noise at work (Nelson et al., 2005).

Noise-induced hearing loss (NIHL) is one of the most frequently experienced occupational diseases among construction workers (van der Molen et al., 2016). NIHL is reported to have a high prevalence among construction workers. For example, NIHL is experienced by 15% of construction workers in the Netherlands (Leensen et al., 2011), 37% in Australia (Kurmis & Apps, 2007) and between 23% and 58% in the USA (Masterson et al., 2013; Dement et al., 2018). However, the definition of NIHL varies from country to country, making direct comparisons difficult (Lie et al., 2016). Research in the USA shows that, although the general all-industry incidence of NIHL is reported to be reducing, the percentage of workers affected by NIHL remains high in construction (Masterson et al., 2015).

Also, Chen (2020) observe that NIHL is more prevalent in developing countries, suggesting that the global problem may be more significant than is reflected by studies conducted in Europe, the USA and Australia.

In many countries, standard exposure levels for noise have been established. For example, in the USA the Occupational Safety and Health Administration establishes a permissible exposure limit of 90 dBA for an eight-hour time-weighted average (TWA) with a 5 decibel (dB) exchange rate and an action level of 85 dBA for an eight-hour TWA. A hearing conservation programme must be implemented for workers whose exposure to noise is equal to or exceeds this action level. The National Institute for Occupational Health and Safety's (NIOSH) recommended exposure limit (REL) is 85 dBA with a 3 dB exchange rate. The exchange rate refers to the number of dB increases at which the allow-able exposure time is halved (Chen et al., 2020).

However, heavy machinery and equipment, transport vehicles, power and hand tools used in construction often produce noise levels that exceed recommended or maximum permissible exposure limits (Hong, 2005). Evidence suggests that, in many cases, construction workers continue to be exposed to noise levels in excess of exposure standards. For example, a large study of construction work practices in the USA found that construction workers were exposed to noise levels that exceeded the NIOSH REL in three-quarters of the work shifts for which full-shift measurements of noise exposure were available (Neitzel et al., 2011). Ironworkers had the highest exposure and insulation workers had the lowest exposure to occupational noise but, importantly, seven of the eight trades included in the study recorded average exposures that exceeded the REL for noise (Nietzel et al., 2011).

In Australia, Lewkowski et al. (2018) developed a questionnaire–algorithm to identify construction workers who are exposed to noise levels that exceed the Australian National Standard for Occupational Noise (an $L_{Aeq,8h}$ of 85 dBA or above). The questionnaire captured information about an individual's work activities, use of noise reduction methods, background environment and shift length. This data is then cross-referenced with a database containing task-based measures of noise taken from previous studies. Questionnaire-derived noise exposure estimates for 100 construction workers were compared to exposure data captured by a personal noise dosimeter over a whole work shift. The ques-tionnaire method demonstrated an excellent ability to estimate whether a worker had exceeded the national standard exposure level over their shift, suggesting it is a useful way to understand exposure to noise in complex environments, such as construction sites (Lewkoswski et al., 2018).

There is strong and consistent evidence that, compared to other workers who are not exposed to high levels of occupational noise, construction workers are a high-risk group for NIHL. In the Netherlands, construction workers exposed to site-based noise were found to have significantly greater hearing loss than a com-parison group of workers who were not noise exposed, i.e. those that had office-based jobs (Leensen et al., 2011). Leensen et al. (2011) found noise exposure to

be a stronger predictor of NIHL than noise intensity and, in a follow-up longitudinal analysis of construction workers' hearing threshold levels, an average
annual deterioration in hearing of 0.54 dB per year was observed (Leensen et al.,
2015). This deterioration was larger with increasing noise exposure. Similarly,
in the USA, Dement et al. (2005) examined health surveillance data and found
that construction trade workers engaged at Department of Energy nuclear sites
were at substantially higher risk of material hearing impairment than workers
in an external population with jobs in which noise exposure is <80 dBA, when
controlling for age-related effects. For the purpose of this analysis, material
hearing impairment was defined in accordance with NIOSH guidelines, i.e.,
a "biaural average threshold greater than 25 dB calculated as the articulation
index weighted average across frequencies of 1, 2, 3, and 4 kHz" (Dement et al.,
2005, p.350). The odds of construction workers experiencing material hearing
impairment increased more than two-fold with exposure to loud or very loud
noise between 50% and 69% of the time, in comparison to workers exposed
to loud or very loud noise less than 50% of the time. Construction workers
exposed to loud or very loud noise for more than 70% of the time were 2.7 times
more likely to experience material hearing impairment. A longitudinal study of
noise exposure and hearing damage in construction apprentices in the USA also
revealed changes in hearing thresholds associated with noise exposure over a
ten-year period (Seixas et al., 2012). These changes were greater than expected.
Seixas et al. (2012) suggest this may be explained by the fact that the apprentices
already had a degree of hearing loss at the outset of the study and were, therefore, potentially more susceptible to further noise-related hearing decline. The
implication of this finding is that programmes to prevent NIHL need to be
implemented early in the working lives of construction workers as exposure to
work and recreational noise levels can affect hearing thresholds at an early age.

The important point to note is that NIHL is irreversible but preventable. For
example, Dement et al. (2005) point to programmes implemented in Sweden and
Canada that have effectively implemented hearing protection programmes that
reduced the percentage of construction workers with NIHL. Key activities in the
prevention of NIHL include monitoring noise exposure levels in the workplace
and implementing appropriate risk controls.

Daniell et al. (2006) considered the scope and effectiveness of hearing protection programmes across a number of high-risk industries in the USA, including
road construction. Hearing loss prevention programmes were found to be
incomplete across all industries included in the study. While most companies
conducted noise measurements, records were not typically kept and there was
little management consideration of ways to control noise (Daniell et al., 2006).

Many hearing protection programmes implemented in construction still focus
heavily on the use of hearing protection devices (HPDs) (Daniell et al., 2006).
Though important in noisy settings, HPD provision and use should be seen as a
secondary protection measure because HPDs are only effective to the extent that
they are used correctly in all appropriate situations (Chen et al., 2020). In fact,

self-reported use of HPDs among construction workers is low and the extent to which they provide the advertised level of protection when used in the workplace has also been questioned. For example, Leensen et al. (2011) report that only 77% of Dutch construction workers exposed to daily noise levels exceeding 80 dB(A) report that they wear hearing protection devices (HPDs) at work, indicating that 23% of the exposed workers do not use protective equipment. Similarly, Hong (2005) found that a high-risk group of machinery operators report using HPDs for only 48% of the time they are exposed to high noise levels. Neitzel & Seixas (2005) found considerable variation between trades in terms of usage of HPDs: e.g., operating engineers spent 49% of minutes in each shift exposed to noise levels greater than 85 dBA but used HPDs for 59% of this time; ironworkers spent 38% of minutes in each shift exposed to noise levels greater than 85 dBA but used HPDs for only 9% of this time (Neitzel & Seixas, 2005). Neitzel and Seixas (2005) also undertook field tests to evaluate the attenuation achieved by ear plugs when used by construction workers. On average, more than 50% of the stated noise reduction rating was achieved for three types of ear plug. However, variability in attenuation was high, being lowest at a frequency of 500 Hz. When considering attenuation performance and use together, Neitzel and Seixas (2005) conclude that HPDs provide negligible effective protection for construction workers, reinforcing the importance of reducing the risk of NIHL through other forms of control.

As with all workplace health and safety issues, the hierarchy of control (HoC) should be applied when deciding how to control the risk of occupational noise. Thus, wherever possible, noise should be eliminated or reduced at source through substitution or engineering controls. Administrative controls, including undertaking routine audiometric examination of workers and providing education on the prevention of NIHL and the use of personal protective equipment, are also recommended (Chen et al., 2020). Most importantly, though, the risk of NIHL is reduced if noise levels are reduced to below 80 dBA.

The best way to control the risks associated with occupational noise is to eliminate noise at source or replace noisy work processes, tools or machinery with methods and equipment that produce less noise. In the USA, NIOSH implemented a programme called "Buy Quiet." The objective of this programme was to encourage businesses to purchase or hire equipment that is quieter to reduce workplace noise levels. This could either be at point of business start-up or when equipment is being replaced. To support the programme, NIOSH developed a database containing noise performance data for power tools in common use, by make and model. It was anticipated that by raising customer awareness and creating an increased demand for quiet equipment, manufacturers would be encouraged to invest effort and resources into designing equipment that produces substantially less noise.

Engineering controls can also substantially reduce noise levels associated with equipment use. For example, Saleh et al. (2017) described an experiment in which commercially available sound-dampening mats were installed between the engine compartment and cabins in three types of plant used in construction (an asphalt roller, a grader and a mobile crawler crane). Sound levels were measured before and after the installation and the results indicated that sound pressure levels could be significantly reduced by the installation of the sound-dampening mats. However, when the machinery was operating at full throttle, sound pressure levels still exceeded 80 dBA when the mats were installed.

2.8 Other factors contributing to occupational hearing loss

Although occupational hearing loss is usually understood to be related to exposure to noisy workplaces, there is also evidence that occupational hearing loss can be caused by exposure to occupational hazards other than noise, such as ototoxic chemicals and lead (Lie et al., 2016). Ototoxic chemicals include organic solvents which, when absorbed into the bloodstream, can damage the inner ear and/or the auditory nerve pathways to the brain, resulting in hearing loss and tinnitus.

Lewkowski et al. (2019) report on an Australian Workplace Exposure Survey (AWES) that focused on hearing. This survey explored Australian workers' exposure to both occupational noise and ototoxic chemicals. In order to assess exposure to ototoxic chemicals, a priority list of all substances identified as being ototoxic or possibly ototoxic was collated from multiple international databases. Next, rules were developed to classify specific work tasks as involving exposure to ototoxic chemicals. These rules were then applied to data collected during interviews with more than 5,000 Australian workers. Over half of the workers in the sample (51%) were exposed to one or more ototoxic chemicals, with 85% of those exposed at a medium or probable high level.

Co-exposure to both ototoxic chemicals and noise were examined with 80% of workers exposed to a full-shift noise level that exceeds the $L_{Aeq,8h}$ limit of 85 dBA, also being exposed to an ototoxic chemical at a medium or probable high level (Lewkowski et al., 2019). This co-exposure is concerning because there is emerging evidence to indicate that the odds of hearing loss is more than doubled for workers exposed to ototoxic chemicals and noise, compared to those just exposed to occupational noise (Choi & Kim, 2014). Among construction workers in the AWES study, 86% were exposed to ototoxic chemicals and 42% were co-exposed to ototoxic chemicals and noise exposure in excess of the $L_{Aeq,8h}$ limit of 85 dBA (Lewkowski et al., 2019). In the USA, a longitudinal study of construction workers' hearing has also linked hearing loss to exposure to both noise and organic solvents (Dement et al., 2018).

2.9 Products causing occupational skin disease

Construction workers are susceptible to occupational skin disease that can be caused by exposure to a wide variety of substances, including wet cement, epoxy resins and hardeners, acrylic sealants, bitumen or asphalt, solvents used in paints, glues or other surface coatings, petrol, diesel, oils and greases, degreasers, descalers and detergents. In Sweden, Meding et al. (2016) report occupational skin disease can prevent people from working, with painters, cement workers and plumbers at particularly high risk. Despite moves to regulate the supply of certain construction materials (see case example 2.3) to reduce the risks of occupational skin disease, skin disease is still a serious occupational health issue for many construction workers (Kaukiainen et al., 2005).

CASE EXAMPLE 2.3 REGULATING PRODUCT SUPPLY TO REDUCE OCCUPATIONAL ILL HEALTH

Cement contains water-soluble hexavalent chromium (chromate), which can penetrate the skin and cause a severe allergic reaction referred to as occupational allergic contact dermatitis (OACD). OACD is a debilitating skin condition that is common among construction workers in many countries around the world (Kridin et al., 2016). OACD significantly reduces workers' quality of life and can lead to economic hardship and early retirement (Roto et al., 1996; Wong et al., 2015). Winder and Carmody (2002) argue the toxicity of cement and concrete is underestimated by many builders and these products should, in fact, be treated as hazardous materials. OACD occurs when the skin is sensitised to contact with a chemical. Sensitisation to a chemical can occur the first time a worker is exposed or after a long period of repeated contact. However, once sensitised, contact with even a small amount of the chemical will produce an allergic reaction.

Steps to reduce the harmful effects of exposure to chromate in cement were introduced in Scandinavian countries 30-plus years ago. In 1983 Denmark passed legislation to require addition of ferrous sulphate to cement to reduce the hexavalent form of chromium to a trivalent form (chromium III), which is less soluble and does not readily permeate the skin (Wong et al., 2015). Finland and Germany introduced similar legislation in 1987 and 2000 respectively. Research evidence suggests that these steps were effective in reducing chromate sensitisation and OACD associated with cement exposure (Roto et al., 1996; Geier et al., 2011).

In 2003, European Union (EU) Directive 2003/53/EC required all member countries of the EU to reduce the chromate content in cement (European Union, 2003). The directive required laws to be passed in member countries that specifically targeted the production and supply of cement products to prohibit the sale of products containing more than 0.0002% (2 parts per million) of soluble chromium by dry weight of cement when hydrated. Importantly, all suppliers selling products in EU countries irrespective of where these products are manufactured need to comply with these laws.

Analysis of the incidence of OACD in the UK and France before and after the introduction of the legislation has revealed significantly lower incidence of

OACD following the changes among groups of workers engaged in construction and/or exposed to cement compared to non-exposed control groups (Stocks et al., 2012; Bensefa-Colas et al., 2017). However, in the absence of European style regulation, many construction workers (including those in Australia) may be exposed to harmful chromates which could be avoided through modification to manufacture and supply (Dear, 2020; Wong et al., 2015).

2.10   Musculoskeletal disorders

Musculoskeletal disorders (MSDs) are injuries or disorders of the muscles, nerves, tendons, joints, cartilage, and spinal discs. MSDs are described as work-related when "the work environment and performance of work contribute significantly to the condition; and/or the condition is made worse or persists longer due to work conditions" (Centers for Disease Control and Prevention, 2022). Commonly experienced types of work-related MSDs include back injury, carpal tunnel syndrome and arthritis. Construction workers are a high-risk group for work-related musculoskeletal disorders (WMSDs). For example, Boschman et al. (2012) report 67% of bricklayers and 57% of supervisors in a random sample of construction workers experience MSDs, the majority of which are attributed to work. Severe WMSDs can lead to functional impairment, permanent disability and early retirement among construction workers (Inyang et al., 2012). Risk factors commonly associated with WMSDs in construction include repetition, force, awkward posture, vibration, and contact stress (Wang et al., 2015).

Work-related MSDs are understood to occur when physical workload required by a job exceeds the physical capacity of a worker's body. Physical workload is influenced by the work tasks being performed, technologies being used, characteristics of the work environment, and the way that work is organised (Figure 2.2). Consequently, when considering ways to reduce the risk of WMSDs, consideration should be given to the way construction work is designed, organised and performed in the context of the worksite environment.

The risk of WMSD was investigated in the Australian construction industry using a whole-body system of wearable sensors to take biomechanical measurements when workers were performing everyday work tasks, such as jack-hammering, shotcreting, steel-fixing, cable-pulling and shovelling. The results of this assessment revealed that workers are frequently exposed to static postures and repetitive movements that are potentially damaging, such as working with a bent back for a prolonged amount of time and flexing and extending the wrist. However, the study also revealed that these risks could be substantially reduced through the use of ergonomically designed equipment and/or alternative technologies (Lingard et al., 2017). The opportunity to reduce significant MSD risk in steel-fixing is described in case example 2.4.

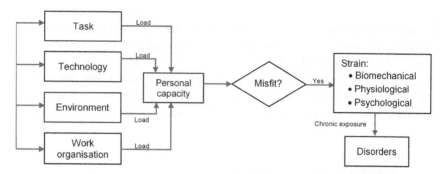

FIGURE 2.2 Factors that contribute to the development of work–related MSDs
Source: Karsh et al., 2001.

CASE EXAMPLE 2.4 TYING STEEL REINFORCEMENT BARS

Tying steel reinforcement bars is a high-risk activity for musculoskeletal injury to the back and upper extremities (Vi, 2003). Back injuries in workers engaged in tying steel reinforcement bars are attributed to frequently working in stooped postures, manually lifting heavy materials, often from toe to hip level, and working on poor walking surfaces (Niskanen, 1985; Tak et al., 2011; Umer et al., 2017). Importantly, WMSD risk exposure in steel tying varies significantly depending upon the specific work context, i.e., the nature of the structure being constructed and the site environment (Buchholz et al., 2003). This is because trunk posture (and the need for bending) varies according to the height at which work is performed. Steel tying is also a high-risk activity for WMSDs affecting the hand, wrist or fingers (Forde et al., 2005).

Australian data captured using a whole-body system of wearable sensors showed that the movements required to fix steel in place using a traditional pincer-cutter tool produce a high risk for WMSD of the wrist. When using a pincer-cutter, wrist flexion values ranged from 29.5 to 33.7 degrees. WorkSafe Victoria's *Manual Handling Code of Practice* recommends that, where the fingers are bent or applying higher forces (for example, gripping), flexion in excess of 15 degrees presents an elevated risk of injury when undertaking a task for more than 2 hours over a whole shift, or continually for more than 30 minutes at a time (WorkSafe Victoria, 2000). Wrist rotation was also a risk for WMSD when using the traditional pincer-cutter tool. However, both wrist rotation and flexion were significantly reduced by the use of a power-typing tool that eliminated the need to manually twist and tie the wire into place.

The analysis also revealed that trunk inclination data (forward flexion and extension in the sagittal plane) exceeded 50 degrees when fixing steel with a traditional pincer-cutter tool between ground level and hip height. WorkSafe

Victoria's *Manual Handling Code of Practice* identifies working with a trunk inclination greater than 20 degrees combined with undertaking a task for more than 2 hours over a whole shift, or continually for more than 30 minutes at a time, as a risk factor for work-related MSDs (WorkSafe Victoria, 2000). Trunk flexion was significantly reduced through the use of a long-handled steel tying tool (but still averaged more than 20 degrees when steel was being tied between ground level and hip height).

Source: *Lingard et al. (2019)*

The opportunity to select tools and equipment that reduce the risk of WMSD in the construction industry is significant. However, the industry has a low uptake of ergonomically designed equipment (Kramer et al., 2009; Glimskär & Lundberg, 2013). Van der Molen et al. (2005a) attribute this to the way that construction work is organised, in particular the reliance on temporary employment and multilevel contracting. The adoption of new ways of working that reduce the risk of WMSDs in construction is dependent on industry norms, organisation-level purchasing policies and appropriate consideration of risk inherent in work tasks at a project level (Kramer et al., 2010). Barriers to adoption can be reduced where it can be shown that solutions improve quality and production efficiency, while also reducing the risk of WMSDs (van der Molen, 2005b; Boatman et al., 2015).

2.11 Conclusion

It is sometimes said that the construction industry shouts safety but whispers health. Construction workers are exposed to a wide array of occupational health hazards and experience a disproportionately high incidence of many debilitating (and some fatal) occupational diseases. This chapter has highlighted the magnitude of the problem and laid out some of the challenges that need to be overcome in order to achieve better outcomes in the management of occupational health in the construction industry. Governments have a part to play in ensuring that appropriate standards are established and that product and materials supply networks are appropriately regulated to reduce worker exposure to harmful substances. Design professionals should be cognisant of the properties of products they specify and should consider the potential health implications of design decision-making. The potential occupational health impacts associated with specific construction methods and technologies should also be considered when designing how construction work will be performed. While there may be merit in organisational wellness strategies designed to assist workers to adopt health-promoting behaviours, such strategies do not satisfy or negate the principal duty of care borne by all construction organisations, which is to protect workers from harm arising from contributing to business operations. The evidence suggests that the construction industry has considerable room for improvement in relation to ensuring that workers' health is not harmed as a result of their work.

2.12 Discussion and review questions

1 In what circumstances does workers' health become an organisational (rather than an individual) responsibility?
2 What should be the balance between individual and organisational responsibility for workers' health?
3 What is the hierarchy of control (HoC), and why is it helpful in selecting control measures for occupational health risk?
4 What are the barriers or challenges associated with reducing the risk of work-related illness in the construction industry?
5 How can governments, employers, managers, designers, manufacturers and suppliers of tools, plant and materials contribute to the reduction of occupational health risks in the construction industry?

2.13 Acknowledgements

The work presented in case example 2.4 was jointly funded by WorkSafe Victoria and the Major Transport Infrastructure Program, Department of Economic Development, Jobs, Transport and Resources, Victorian Government.

Note

1 Members of Safe Work Australia (the body that sets Australia's national policy on Workplace Exposure Standards) have recently determined that the exposure standard for RCS measured as a time weighted average over eight hours should be halved to 0.025 mg/m3. If enacted, this would become effective over a three-year transition period (Bence, 2023).

References

Akbar-Khanzadeh, F., & Brillhart, R. L. (2002). Respirable crystalline silica dust exposure during concrete finishing (grinding) using hand-held grinders in the construction industry. *Annals of Occupational Hygiene*, 46(3), 341–346.
Åkerstedt, T. (2006) Psychosocial stress and impaired sleep. *Scandinavian Journal of Work, Environment & Health*, 32 (6), 493–501.
Australian Broadcasting Corporation (2019). *Silicosis Surge Prompts More Calls for a Ban on Engineered Stone Products.* Accessed 14 November 2021: www.abc.net.au/news/2019-09-16/silicosis-surge-prompts-call-for-ban-on-engineered-stone-product/11516138
Australian Broadcasting Corporation (2021). *Calls for More Testing after Asbestos Found in Imported Toys and Building Materials.* Accessed 12 November 2021 from: www.abc.net.au/news/2021-11-09/asbestos-found-in-imported-toys-and-building-materials/100604278,

Australian Institute of Occupational Hygienists (AIOH) (2017). *Diesel Particulate Matter and Occupational Health Issues – Position Paper*. Australian Institute of Occupational Hygienists.

Bakke, B., Ulvestad, B., Stewart, P., & Eduard, W. (2004). Cumulative exposure to dust and gases as determinants of lung function decline in tunnel construction workers. *Occupational and Environmental Medicine*, 61(3), 262–269.

Barcenas, C. H., Delclos, G. L., El-Zein, R., Tortolero-Luna, G., Whitehead, L. W., & Spitz, M. R. (2005). Wood dust exposure and the association with lung cancer risk. *American Journal of Industrial Medicine*, 47(4), 349–357.

Bence, T. (2023), Australian Institute of Occupational Hygienists: Statement on Silicosis Prevention, https://www.aioh.org.au/news/a-message-to-members-from-aioh-president-tracey-bence/, accessed 1 April 2023.

Bensefa-Colas, L., Stocks, S. J., McNamee, R., Faye, S., Pontin, F., Agius, R. M.,... & Momas, I. (2017). Effectiveness of the European chromium (vi) directive for cement implementation on occupational allergic contact dermatitis occurrence: assessment in France and the UK. *British Journal of Dermatology*, 177(3), 873–876.

Bergdahl, I. A., Toren, K., Eriksson, K., Hedlund, U., Nilsson, T., Flodin, R., & Järvholm, B. (2004). Increased mortality in COPD among construction workers exposed to inorganic dust. *European Respiratory Journal*, 23(3), 402–406.

Bjorvatn, B., Sagen, I. M., Oyane, N., Waage, S., Fetveit, A., Pallesen, S., & Ursin, R. (2007) The association between sleep duration, body mass index and metabolic measures in the Hordaland Health Study. *Journal of Sleep Research*, 16(1), 66–76.

Boatman, L., Chaplan, D., Teran, S., & Welch, L. S. (2015). Creating a climate for ergonomic changes in the construction industry. *American Journal of Industrial Medicine*, 58(8), 858–869.

Boschman, J. S., Van der Molen, H. F., Sluiter, J. K., & Frings-Dresen, M. H. W. (2012). Musculoskeletal disorders among construction workers: a one-year follow-up study. *BMC Musculoskeletal Disorders,* 13(1), 1.

Buchanan, D., Miller, B. G., & Soutar, C. A. (2003). Quantitative relations between exposure to respirable quartz and risk of silicosis. *Occupational and Environmental Medicine*, 60(3), 159–164.

Buchholz, B., Paquet, V., Wellman, H., & Forde, M. (2003). Quantification of ergonomic hazards for ironworkers performing concrete reinforcement tasks during heavy highway construction. *AIHA Journal*, 64(2), 243–250

Centers for Disease Control and Prevention (2022). *Work-Related Musculoskeletal Disorders and Ergonomics*. Accessed 25 July 2022 from: www.cdc.gov/workplacehealthpromotion/health-strategies/musculoskeletal-disorders/index.html#:~:text=Musculoskeletal%20disorders%20(MSD)%20are%20injuries,to%20the%20condition%3B%20and%2For,

Chen, K. H., Su, S. B., & Chen, K. T. (2020). An overview of occupational noise-induced hearing loss among workers: epidemiology, pathogenesis, and preventive measures. *Environmental Health and Preventive Medicine*, 25(1), 1–10.

Choi, Y. H., & Kim, K. (2014). Noise-induced hearing loss in Korean workers: co-exposure to organic solvents and heavy metals in nationwide industries. *PloS one*, 9(5), e97538.

Cooper, J. H., Johnson, D. L., & Phillips, M. L. (2015). Respirable silica dust suppression during artificial stone countertop cutting. *Annals of Occupational Hygiene*, 59(1), 122–126.

Daniell, W. E., Swan, S. S., McDaniel, M. M., Camp, J. E., Cohen, M. A., & Stebbins, J. G. (2006). Noise exposure and hearing loss prevention programmes after 20 years of regulations in the United States. *Occupational and environmental medicine*, 63(5), 343–351.

Dear, K., Palmer, A., & Nixon, R. (2020). Allergic chromate dermatitis to cement in Australia: an ongoing problem. *Occupational and Environmental Medicine, 77*(9), 658–658.

Decopaint (2000). *Study on the Potential for Reducing Emissions of Volatile Organic Compounds (Voc) Due to the Use of Decorative Paints and Varnishes for Professional and Non-Professional Use.* Accessed 25 July 2022: https://ec.europa.eu/environment/archives/air/pdf/paint_solvents/decopaint.pdf

Dement, J. M., Ringen, K., Hines, S., Cranford, K., & Quinn, P. (2020). Lung cancer mortality among construction workers: implications for early detection. *Occupational and Environmental Medicine, 77*(4), 207–213.

Dement, J., Ringen, K., Welch, L., Bingham, E., & Quinn, P. (2005). Surveillance of hearing loss among older construction and trade workers at Department of Energy nuclear sites. *American Journal of Industrial Medicine, 48*(5), 348–358.

Dement, J., Welch, L. S., Ringen, K., Cranford, K., & Quinn, P. (2018). Hearing loss among older construction workers: Updated analyses. *American Journal of Industrial Medicine, 61*(4), 326–335.

Driscoll, T., Steenland, K., Prüss-Üstün, A., Nelson, D. I., & Leigh, J. (2004). *Occupational Carcinogens: Assessing the Environmental Burden of Disease at National and Local Levels.* World Health Organization.

European Union (2003). Directive 2003/53/EC of the European Parliament and of the Council of 18 June 2003 amending for the 26th time Council Directive 76/769/EEC relating to restrictions on the marketing and use of certain dangerous substances and preparations (nonylphenol, nonylphenol ethoxylate and cement), *Official Journal.* L 178, 24–27. Accessed 19 July 2022 from: https://op.europa.eu/en/publication-detail/-/publication/c2ee507b-0b20-48a2-8917-4f853b6a8804/language-en,

Fellner, C. (2021) *Ban on Popular Benchtops Being Considered as Wave of Deadly Illness Sparks Alarm,* Sydney Morning Herald. Accessed 14 November 2021: www.smh.com.au/national/ban-on-popular-benchtops-being-considered-as-wave-of-deadly-illness-sparks-alarm-20210416-p57jxy.html,

Flanagan, M. E., Seixas, N., Majar, M., Camp, J., & Morgan, M. (2003). Silica dust exposures during selected construction activities. *AIHA Journal, 64*(3), 319–328.

Forde, M. S., Punnett, L., & Wegman, D. H. (2005). Prevalence of musculoskeletal disorders in union ironworkers. *Journal of Occupational and Environmental Hygiene, 2*(4), 203–212.

Fritschi, L., & Reid, A. (2019), Engineered stone benchtops are killing our tradies. Here's why a ban's the only answer, The Conversation. Accessed 14 November 2021 from: https://theconversation.com/engineered-stone-benchtops-are-killing-our-tradies-heres-why-a-bans-the-only-answer-126489,

Frost, G., Darnton, A., & Harding, A. H. (2011). The effect of smoking on the risk of lung cancer mortality for asbestos workers in Great Britain (1971–2005). *Annals of Occupational Hygiene, 55*(3), 239–247.

Gangwisch, J. E., Heymsfield, S. B., Boden-Albala, B., Buijs, R. M., Kreier, F., Pickering, T. G., Rundle, A. G., Zammit, G. K., & Malaspina, D. (2006). Short sleep duration as a risk factor for hypertension: analyses of the first National Health and Nutrition Examination Survey. *Hypertension, 47*(5), 833–839.

Gangwisch, J. E., Malaspina, D., Boden-Albala, B., & Heymsfield, S. B. (2005). Inadequate sleep as a risk factor for obesity: Analyses of the NHANES I. *Sleep, 28*(10), 1289–96.

Geier, J., Krautheim, A., Uter, W., Lessmann, H., & Schnuch, A. (2011). Occupational contact allergy in the building trade in Germany: Influence of preventive measures and changing exposure. *International Archives of Occupational and Environmental Health, 84*(4), 403–411.

Glimskär, B., & Lundberg, S. (2013). Barriers to adoption of ergonomic innovations in the construction industry. *Ergonomics in Design*, 21(4), 26–30.

Gottlieb, D. J., Redline, S., Nieto, F. J., Baldwin, C. M., Newman, A. B., Resnick, H. E., & Punjabi, M. D. (2006). Association of usual sleep duration with hypertension: The Sleep Heart Health Study. *Sleep*, 29(8), 1009–1014.

Health and Safety Executive (HSE) (2020a). *Costs to Britain of Workplace Fatalities and Self-Reported Injuries and Ill Health, 2018/19*. Accessed 22 November 2021 from: www.hse.gov.uk/statistics/pdf/cost-to-britain.pdf.

Health and Safety Executive (HSE) (2020b). *Construction Statistics in Great Britain, 2020*. Accessed 9 November 2021 from: www.hse.gov.uk/statistics/industry/construction.pdf.

Health and Safety Executive (HSE) (2020c). *Work-related Chronic Obstructive Pulmonary Disease (COPD) Statistics in Great Britain, 2020*. Accessed 11 November 2021 from: www.hse.gov.uk/statistics/causdis/copd.pdf.

Health and Safety Executive (HSE). (2021). *Occupational Cancer Statistics in Great Britain, 2021*. www.hse.gov.uk/statistics/causdis/cancer.pdf, accessed 27 September 2022.

Hong, O. (2005). Hearing loss among operating engineers in American construction industry. *International Archives of Occupational and Environmental Health*, 78(7), 565–574.

Hoy, R. F., Baird, T., Hammerschlag, G., Hart, D., Johnson, A. R., King, P.,... & Yates, D. H. (2018). Artificial stone-associated silicosis: A rapidly emerging occupational lung disease. *Occupational and Environmental Medicine*, 75(1), 3–5.

Hoy, R. F., Glass, D. C., Dimitriadis, C., Hansen, J., Hore-Lacy, F., & Sim, M. R. (2021). Identification of early-stage silicosis through health screening of stone benchtop industry workers in Victoria, Australia. *Occupational and Environmental Medicine*, 78(4), 296–302.

Inyang, N., Al-Hussein, M., El-Rich, M., & Al-Jibouri, S. (2012). Ergonomic Analysis and the Need for Its Integration for Planning and Assessing Construction Tasks. *Journal of Construction Engineering and Management*, 138(12), 1370–1376.

Järvholm, B., & Burdorf, A. (2017). Effect of reduced use of organic solvents on disability pension in painters. *Occupational and Environmental Medicine*, 74(11), 827–829.

Järvholm, B., & Silverman, D. (2003). Lung cancer in heavy equipment operators and truck drivers with diesel exhaust exposure in the construction industry. *Occupational and Environmental Medicine*, 60(7), 516–520.

Jones, W., Gibb, A., Haslam, R., & Dainty, A. (2019). Work-related ill-health in construction: The importance of scope, ownership and understanding. *Safety Science*, 120, 538–550.

Karsh, B.-T., Moro, F. B. P., & Smith, M. J. (2001). The efficacy of workplace ergonomic interventions to control musculoskeletal disorders: A critical analysis of the peer-reviewed literature. *Theoretical Issues in Ergonomics Science*, 2(1), 23–96.

Kaukiainen, A., Riala, R., Martikainen, R., Akila, R., Reijula, K., & Sainio, M. (2004). Solvent-related health effects among construction painters with decreasing exposure. *American Journal of Industrial Medicine*, 46(6), 627–636.

Kaukiainen, A., Riala, R., Martikainen, R., Estlander, T., Susitaival, P., & Aalto-Korte, K. (2005). Chemical exposure and symptoms of hand dermatitis in construction painters. *Contact Dermatitis*, 53(1), 14–21.

Kramer, D. M., Bigelow, P. L., Carlan, N., Wells, R. P., Garritano, E., Vi, P., and Plawinski, M. (2010). Searching for needles in a haystack: Identifying innovations to prevent MSDs in the construction sector. *Applied Ergonomics*, 41(4), 577–584.

Kramer, D., Bigelow, P., Vi, P., Garritano, E., Carlan, N., & Wells, R. (2009). Spreading good ideas: A case study of the adoption of an innovation in the construction sector. *Applied Ergonomics*, 40(5), 826–832.

Kridin, K., Bergman, R., Khamaisi, M., & Weltfriend, S. (2016). Chromate allergy in northern Israel in relation to exposure to cement and detergents. *Dermatitis*, 27(3), 131–136.

Kurmis, A. P., & Apps, S. A. (2007). Occupationally-acquired noise-induced hearing loss: a senseless workplace hazard. *International Journal of Occupational Medicine and Environmental Health*, 20(2), 127–136.

Landwehr, K. R., Larcombe, A. N., Reid, A., & Mullins, B. J. (2021). Critical review of diesel exhaust exposure health impact research relevant to occupational settings: Are we controlling the wrong pollutants? *Exposure and Health*, 13(2), 141–171.

Leensen, M. C. J., Van Duivenbooden, J. C., & Dreschler, W. A. (2011). A retrospective analysis of noise-induced hearing loss in the Dutch construction industry. *International Archives of Occupational and Environmental Health*, 84(5), 577–590.

Leensen, M. C., & Dreschler, W. A. (2015). Longitudinal changes in hearing threshold levels of noise-exposed construction workers. *International Archives of Occupational and Environmental Health*, 88(1), 45–60.

León-Jiménez, A., Hidalgo-Molina, A., Conde-Sánchez, M. Á., Pérez-Alonso, A., Morales-Morales, J. M., García-Gámez, E. M., & Córdoba-Doña, J. A. (2020). Artificial stone silicosis: Rapid progression following exposure cessation. *Chest*, 158(3), 1060–1068.

Leso, V., Fontana, L., Romano, R., Gervetti, P., & Iavicoli, I. (2019). Artificial stone associated silicosis: A systematic review. *International Journal of Environmental Research and Public Health*, 16(4), 568.

Lewkowski, K., Heyworth, J. S., Li, I. W., Williams, W., McCausland, K., Gray, C.,... & Fritschi, L. (2019). Exposure to noise and ototoxic chemicals in the Australian workforce. *Occupational And Environmental Medicine*, 76(5), 341–348.

Lewkowski, K., McCausland, K., Heyworth, J. S., Li, I. W., Williams, W., & Fritschi, L. (2018). Questionnaire-based algorithm for assessing occupational noise exposure of construction workers. *Occupational and Environmental Medicine*, 75(3), 237–242.

Lie, A., Skogstad, M., Johannessen, H. A., Tynes, T., Mehlum, I. S., Nordby, K. C.,... & Tambs, K. (2016). Occupational noise exposure and hearing: a systematic review. *International Archives of Occupational and Environmental Health*, 89(3), 351–372.

Lin, R. T., Chien, L. C., Jimba, M., Furuya, S., & Takahashi, K. (2019). Implementation of national policies for a total asbestos ban: A global comparison. *The Lancet Planetary Health*, 3(8), e341–e348.

Lingard, H., Bird, S., Lythgo, N., Selva-Raj, I., & Troynikov, O. (2017). *Musculoskeletal Risk in the Rail Construction Sector*. RMIT University: Melbourne.

Lingard, H., Raj, I. S., Lythgo, N., Troynikov, O., & Fitzgerald, C. (2019). The impact of tool selection on back and wrist injury risk in tying steel reinforcement bars: A single case experiment. *Construction Economics and Building*, 19(1), 1–19.

Markowitz, S. B., Levin, S. M., Miller, A., & Morabia, A. (2013). Asbestos, asbestosis, smoking, and lung cancer. New findings from the North American insulator cohort. *American Journal of Respiratory and Critical Care Medicine*, 188(1), 90–96.

Masterson, E. A., Deddens, J. A., Themann, C. L., Bertke, S., & Calvert, G. M. (2015). Trends in worker hearing loss by industry sector, 1981–2010. *American Journal of Industrial Medicine*, 58(4), 392–401.

Masterson, E. A., Tak, S., Themann, C. L., Wall, D. K., Groenewold, M. R., Deddens, J. A., & Calvert, G. M. (2013). Prevalence of hearing loss in the United States by industry. *American Journal of Industrial Medicine*, 56(6), 670–681.

Meding, B., Wrangsjö, K., Burdorf, A., & Järvholm, B. (2016). Disability pensions due to skin diseases: a cohort study in Swedish construction workers. *Acta Dermato-Venereologica*, 96(2), 232–236.

Murgia, N., & Gambelunghe, A. (2021). Occupational COPD – The most under-recognized occupational lung disease? *Respirology*, 27, 399–410.

Neitzel, R. L., Stover, B., & Seixas, N. S. (2011). Longitudinal assessment of noise exposure in a cohort of construction workers. *Annals of Occupational Hygiene*, 55(8), 906–916.

Neitzel, R., & Seixas, N. (2005). The effectiveness of hearing protection among construction workers. *Journal of Occupational and Environmental Hygiene*, 2(4), 227–238.

Nelson, D. I., Nelson, R. Y., Concha-Barrientos, M., & Fingerhut, M. (2005). The global burden of occupational noise-induced hearing loss. *American Journal of Industrial Medicine*, 48(6), 446–458.

Newbigin, K., Parsons, R., Deller, D., Edwards, R., & McBean, R. (2019). Stonemasons with silicosis: Preliminary findings and a warning message from Australia. *Respirology*, 24(12), 1220–1221.

Nij, T. E., & Heederik, D. (2005). Risk assessment of silicosis and lung cancer among construction workers exposed to respirable quartz. *Scandinavian Journal of Work, Environment & Health*, 31(2), 49–56.

Nij, T. E., Hilhorst, S., Spee, T. O. N., Spierings, J., Steffens, F., Lumens, M., & Heederik, D. (2003). Dust control measures in the construction industry. *Annals of Occupational Hygiene*, 47(3), 211–218.

Nij, T. E., Höhr, D., Borm, P., Burstyn, I., Spierings, J., Steffens, F.,... & Heederik, D. (2004). Variability in quartz exposure in the construction industry: implications for assessing exposure-response relations. *Journal of Occupational and Environmental Hygiene*, 1(3), 191–198.

Niskanen, T. (1985), Accidents and minor accidents of the musculoskeletal system in heavy (concrete reinforcement work) and light (painting) construction work. *Journal of Occupational Accidents*, 7, 17–32.

O'Neill, R., Pickvance, S., & Watterson, A. (2007). Burying the evidence: How Great Britain is prolonging the occupational cancer epidemic. *International Journal of Occupational and Environmental Health*, 13(4), 428–436.

Rappaport, S. M., Goldberg, M., Susi, P. A. M., & Herrick, R. F. (2003). Excessive exposure to silica in the US construction industry. *Annals of Occupational Hygiene*, 47(2), 111–122.

Ringen, K., Dement, J., Welch, L., Dong, X. S., Bingham, E., & Quinn, P. S. (2014). Risks of a lifetime in construction. Part II: Chronic occupational diseases. *American Journal of Industrial Medicine*, 57(11), 1235–1245.

RMIT University, Control Measures for Occupational Health Risks Relevant to Civil Construction Work. file:///C:/Users/Helen/Downloads/control-measures-occupational-health-risks-relevant-civil-construction-work%20(5).pdf, accessed 27 September 2022.

Rose, C., Heinzerling, A., Patel, K., Sack, C., Wolff, J., Zell-Baran, L.,... & Harrison, R. (2019). Severe silicosis in engineered stone fabrication workers – California, Colorado, Texas, and Washington, 2017–2019. *Morbidity and Mortality Weekly Report*, 68(38), 813.

Roto, P., Sainio, H., Reunala, T., & Laippala, P. (1996). Addition of ferrous sulfate to cement and risk of chromium dermatitis among construction workers. *Contact Dermatitis*, 34(1), 43–50.

Safe Work Australia (2021). *Managing the Risks of Respirable Crystalline Silica from Engineered Stone in the Workplace: Code of Practice.* Safe Work Australia.

Saleh, S., Woskie, S., & Bello, A. (2017). The use of noise dampening mats to reduce heavy-equipment noise exposures in construction. *Safety and Health at Work*, 8(2), 226–230.

Sauvé, J. F. (2015). Historical and emerging workplaces affected by silica exposure since the 1930 Johannesburg conference on Silicosis, with special reference to construction. *American Journal of Industrial Medicine*, 58(S1), 67–71.

Seixas, N. S., Neitzel, R., Stover, B., Sheppard, L., Feeney, P., Mills, D., & Kujawa, S. (2012). 10-Year prospective study of noise exposure and hearing damage among construction workers. *Occupational and Environmental Medicine*, 69(9), 643–650.

Sherratt, F. (2016). Shiny happy people? UK construction industry health: Priorities, practice and public relations. In *Proceedings of the 32nd annual ARCOM conference* (Vol. 1, pp.447–456).

Snashall, D. (2005). Occupational health in the construction industry. *Scandinavian Journal of Work, Environment & Health*, 31, 5–10.

Snashall, D. (2007). Preventing occupational ill health in the construction industry. *Occupational and Environmental Medicine*, 64(12), 789–790.

Spiegel, K., Knutson, K., Leproult, R., Tasali, E., & Van Cauter, E. (2005). Sleep loss: A novel risk factor for insulin resistance and type 2 diabetes. *Journal of Applied Physiology*, 99(5), 2008–2019.

Stocks, S. J., McNamee, R., Turner, S., Carder, M., & Agius, R. M. (2012). Has European Union legislation to reduce exposure to chromate in cement been effective in reducing the incidence of allergic contact dermatitis attributed to chromate in the UK? *Occupational and Environmental Medicine*, 69(2), 150–152.

Summers, M. P., & Parmigiani, J. P. (2015). A water soluble additive to suppress respirable dust from concrete-cutting chainsaws: a case study. *Journal of Occupational and Environmental Hygiene*, 12(4), D29–D34.

Tak, S., Buchholz, B., Punnett, L., Moir, S., Paquet, V., Fulmer, S.,... & Wegman, D. (2011). Physical ergonomic hazards in highway tunnel construction: overview from the Construction Occupational Health Program. *Applied Ergonomics*, 42(5), 665–671.

Ulvestad, B., Lund, M. B., Bakke, B., Thomassen, Y., & Ellingsen, D. G. (2015). Short-term lung function decline in tunnel construction workers. *Occupational and Environmental Medicine*, 72(2), 108–113.

Umer, W., Li, H., Szeto, G. P. Y., & Wong, A. Y. L., 2017. Identification of biomechanical risk factors for the development of lower-back disorders during manual rebar tying. *Journal of Construction Engineering and Management*, 143(1), 04016080.

van der Molen, H. F., de Vries, S. C., Stocks, S. J., Warning, J., & Frings-Dresen, M. H. (2016). Incidence rates of occupational diseases in the Dutch construction sector, 2010–2014. *Occupational and Environmental Medicine*, 73(5), 350–352.

van der Molen, H. F., Koningsveld, E., Haslam, R., and Gibb, A. (2005a). Editorial. Ergonomics in building and construction: time for implementation. *Applied Ergonomics*, 36(4), 387–389.

van der Molen, H. F., Sluiter, J. K., & Frings-Dresen, M. H. W. (2005b). Behavioral change phases of different stakeholders involved in the implementation process of ergonomics measures in bricklaying. *Applied Ergonomics*, 36(4), 449–459.

Van Deurssen, E., Pronk, A., Spaan, S., Goede, H., Tielemans, E., Heederik, D., & Meijster, T. (2014). Quartz and respirable dust in the Dutch construction industry: A baseline exposure assessment as part of a multidimensional intervention approach. *Annals of Occupational Hygiene*, 58(6), 724–738.

Vi, P. (2003). Reducing risk of musculoskeletal disorders through the use of rebar-tying machines. *Applied Occupational and Environmental Hygiene*, 18(9), 649–654.

Wang, D., Dai, F., & Ning, X. (2015). Risk Assessment of Work-Related Musculoskeletal Disorders in Construction: State-of-the-Art Review. *Journal of Construction Engineering and Management,* 141(6), 04015008.

Winder, C., & Carmody, M. (2002). The dermal toxicity of cement. *Toxicology and Industrial Health*, 18(7), 321–331.

Wong, C. C., Gamboni, S. E., Palmer, A. M., & Nixon, R. L. (2015). Occupational allergic contact dermatitis to chromium from cement: Estimating the size of the problem in Australia. *Australasian Journal of Dermatology*, 56(4), 290–293.

WorkSafe Victoria (2000). *Code of Practice for Manual Handling*. Melbourne: Victorian WorkCover Authority.

WorkSafe Victoria (2021). *Changes to Protect Victorians Working with Engineered Stone*. Accessed 14 November 2021 from: www.worksafe.vic.gov.au/changes-protect-vic torians-working-engineered-stone

World Health Organization (2014). *Chrysotile Asbestos*. Accessed 13 November 2021 from: www.who.int/ipcs/assessment/public_health/chrysotile_asbestos_summ ary.pdf.

3

WORK-RELATED FACTORS IMPACTING CONSTRUCTION WORKERS' PSYCHOLOGICAL HEALTH

3.1 Introduction

Some industries and occupations are more stressful than others (Bültmann et al., 2001) and, consequently, mental ill health can "cluster within high-risk industries and occupations" (Roche et al., 2016, p.280). In this chapter we examine evidence for the relationship between work and psychological health and consider features of working in the construction industry that are likely to contribute to the relatively low level of psychological health observed in the construction workforce in many countries.

We describe policy interventions that seek to ensure that workplace risk factors with the potential to affect workers' psychological health are systematically identified, assessed and controlled in appropriate ways. We examine limitations inherent in some types of mental health programmes that focus on providing individual workers with resources to better cope with adverse conditions of work. Consistent with occupational health and safety discourse, we suggest that construction organisations need to focus their efforts and energies on eliminating or reducing work-related factors rather than focusing on "fixing" individual workers. The different approach that is adopted to control safety risks compared to controlling risks with the potential to cause psychological harm is summed up in the following observation made by one of our industry partners: "In safety we stop people from falling into holes by covering these holes or erecting barriers to stop people from falling in, but, in psychological health we let people fall first and then try to pull them out once they are in trouble. We need to stop them falling in the first place."

The need to look more carefully at the quality of work in the construction industry and to think about how to design organisational and project environments that are free of adverse conditions is a recurring theme in this chapter. The

DOI: 10.1201/9780367814236-3

prevention of psychological harm through effective risk management is a legal responsibility of employers and persons in charge of business undertakings. The prevention of psychological harm should therefore be afforded the same attention as the prevention of workplace accidents or elimination/reduction of risks to physical health (see Chapter 2). However, construction organisations have paid far less attention to addressing psychosocial risks that are known to contribute to work stress and psychological harm. Given the stressful nature of work and prevalence of mental ill health in the construction industry, there is an urgent need to address this imbalance.

3.2 The relationship between job quality and psychological health

Work plays an important role in people's lives. It provides people with an income that helps sustain their material standard of living and supports social and psychological wellbeing (Butterworth et al., 2011a). Epidemiological studies indicate a strong, positive association between unemployment and poor psychological health outcomes, including higher rates of overall mortality and suicide among unemployed men and women than among those in employment or the general population (Jin et al., 1995). However, although employment is usually associated with having better psychological health, the quality of work that people do is also very important (Findlay et al., 2013). Extensive research shows that unfavourable working environments, characterised by poor quality work, are harmful for psychological health (Niuwenhuijsen et al., 2010; Stansfeld & Candy, 2006; Netterstrom et al., 2008).

The prevalence of common mental disorders (CMDs) is actually similar for people in poor quality jobs to those who are unemployed (Butterworth et al., 2013). Poor quality work may therefore be as bad for psychological health as unemployment.

Job quality has been defined as "sets of work features which foster the wellbeing of the worker" (Strazdins et al., 2010, p.2052). While there is no universally agreed set of components for job quality, it is often understood to be reflected by the presence or absence of adverse conditions, including job demands and complexity, imbalance between effort and reward, low levels of job control, exposure to health and safety risks and insecurity of employment (Green, 2006; Strazdins et al., 2004).

Job quality is a determinant of sickness absence. In one Australian study the presence of adverse job conditions (i.e., low job security, low job control, high job demands and complexity and a perception of unfair pay) was examined as a determinant of sickness absence. Compared to people with no adverse job conditions, people with one, two or more than two adverse job conditions were found to take 26%, 28% and 58% more sickness absence respectively (Milner et al., 2015).

Analysis of data collected in longitudinal cohort studies in Australia and the UK also reveals that when people who change jobs move into jobs in which they are exposed to more adverse conditions, they experience a subsequent increase in self-reported mental health problems and diagnosed mental disorders (Butterworth et al., 2011a, 2013). These relationships were found for people in unskilled and professional roles. Importantly the same causal relationship was not found for physical health. While adverse job quality appears to contribute to a deterioration in mental health over time, Butterworth et al. (2011a) explain that the association between poor physical health and low job quality reflects the likelihood that poor physical health acts as a barrier to entry into high quality jobs.

Poor job quality is reported to be particularly harmful to the psychological health of older workers and can also have inter-generational effects (Welsh et al., 2016). For example, Strazdins et al. (2010) found that children of mothers and fathers in poor quality jobs showed a significantly higher incidence of emotional and behavioural difficulties than other children, even when controlling for income, parents' education, family structure and work hours.

The relationship between job quality and psychological health was explored in a sample of manual/non-managerial construction workers, drawn from the same longitudinal cohort study of Australian workers (the Household, Income and Labour Dynamics in Australia data set). This is the same data set used by Butterworth et al. (2011a) and Milner et al. (2015) in their analyses. The analysis revealed that mental health declines in manual/non-managerial workers when exposed to adverse job conditions irrespective of their age. However, the decline is more marked and rapid in mid-aged workers who experience two or more adverse conditions. This may be explained by the fact that mid-life is a complex stage of development and mid-age workers are more likely than younger or older workers to be juggling work with family demands and to have more significant financial responsibilities. While the mental health of younger construction workers (up to the age of 25 years) was significantly affected by low job security and unfairness of effort and reward, the mental health of mid-aged (25–45 years of age) and older workers (46 or more years of age) was also negatively affected by high job demands and complexity and high work intensity (Pirzadeh et al., 2022). Differences between younger, older and mid-age workers' experiences highlight the need to understand and address factors that impact psychological health and wellbeing over the life course.

3.3 Theories linking work with psychological health

A number of key theories have been developed to explain the relationship between job characteristics and mental health:

- job demand-control (JD-C) model,
- job demands-resources (JD-R) model, and
- effort-reward imbalance (ERI) model.

A common feature of these theories is that they explain the link between work and psychological health in terms of the combined effects of the demands inherent in the job, and other factors that are believed to be protective or supportive of healthy functioning (i.e., job control, social support or resources).

The job demand–control (JD-C) theory is often cited to explain the relationship between work conditions and psychological health (Karasek, 1979). The JD-C theory describes two key dimensions of the psychosocial work environment, i.e., job demands and job decision latitude (Karasek, 1979). Job demands are psychological stressors present in the work environment, while job decision latitude reflects the extent to which someone has control over their work (Karasek, 1979). According to the JD-C model, jobs can be divided into four types: 1) high-strain jobs, characterised by high demands and low decision latitude, are considered to be the most problematic in relation to mental strain and health outcomes; 2) active jobs, involving simultaneously high demands and decision latitude, are associated with average levels of mental strain and are likely to facilitate employee development; 3) passive jobs, characterised by low demands and low decision latitude, are associated with average levels of mental strain but can be demotivating; and 4) low-strain jobs, combining low demands and high decision latitude, involve lower than average levels of mental strain and lower risk of ill health (Karasek, 1979).

The JD-C theory is supported by empirical evidence (Häusser et al., 2010). Drawing on the JD-C model, job demands and complexity, and job control have previously been linked to workers' experiences of psychological health (Butterworth et al., 2011a, 2013; Leach et al., 2010; Stansfeld & Candy, 2006).

The JD-C model was subsequently extended by Karasek and Theorell (1990) to incorporate social support as a third factor affecting workers' stress, strain and health impacts. Thus, it is argued that the most negative health outcomes will be found in workers whose jobs are high in demands, low in control and low in social support.

The job demands-resources (JD-R) model explains work stress as arising from an imbalance between:

- job demands, defined as physical, psychological, social or organisational aspects of a job that require workers to expend effort and energy and therefore create a physiological or psychological "cost" for workers, and
- job resources, defined as physical, psychological, social or organisational aspects of a job that support goal achievement, reduce demands or stimulate learning, growth and development (Bakker & Demerouti, 2007).

The effort-reward imbalance (ERI) theory posits that an imbalance between (high) effort and (low) reward causes a strain reaction that negatively affects workers' health (Siegrist, 1996). This model assumes that work is underpinned by a norm of reciprocity whereby efforts are rewarded commensurately with rewards, which can be in the form of money, esteem, career opportunities or job security (Siegrist et al., 2004). However, sometimes workers' efforts exceed perceived rewards and this imbalance between high "costs" and low "gains" can lead to a state of sustained strain reactions in the autonomic nervous system and ultimately produce emotional distress (Siegrist, 1996). This is particularly evident when workers have few alternatives in the labour market, for example because they are low in skill or have restricted mobility (Siegrist et al., 2004).

According to Siegrist (2012, p.3), three hypotheses are derived from the ERI model:

1. An imbalance between high effort and low reward (non-reciprocity) increases the risk of reduced health over and above the risk associated with each one of the components.
2. Overcommitted people are at increased risk of reduced health (whether or not this pattern of coping is reinforced by work characteristics).
3. The highest risks of reduced health are expected in people who are characterised by conditions (1) and (2).

The ERI model is supported by empirical research (van Vegchel et al., 2005). Based on the ERI model, fair pay and job security have been previously linked to mental health (Butterworth et al., 2011a, 2011b; Milner et al., 2015).

The combined effects of the JD-C and ERI models on workers' health are reportedly stronger than their separate effects (De Jonge et al., 2000; Rydstedt et al., 2007).

3.4 Work-related stress in construction work

During the UN General Assembly in September 2015, decent work and the four pillars of the Decent Work Agenda – employment creation, social protection, rights at work, and social dialogue – became central dimensions of the 2030 Agenda for Sustainable Development. Goal 8 of the 2030 Agenda seeks to "promote sustained, inclusive and sustainable economic growth, full and productive employment and decent work for all" (ILO, 2015, p.18). Despite the recognition of the importance of decent work for sustainable global development, the negative impact of work stress is far reaching and is now considered as a social phenomenon in urgent need of attention due to its cost at the individual, organisational, and societal levels (Hassard et al., 2018). The human costs of workplace stress include the emotional strain and reduction in quality of life experienced by affected individuals, and a decline in the quality of relationships with spouse, children and other family members. There are also significant financial burdens on individuals, organisations and societies. At the individual level the impacts of work stress may be related to increased medical and insurance costs and reduced income. At the organisational level, the financial implications of work-related stress are associated with a reduction in productivity, increased levels of absenteeism, and employee turnover (Hassard et al., 2014).

Work stress has been defined as "the adverse reaction people have to excessive pressures or other types of demand placed on them at work" (HSE, 2019, p.3). The Health and Safety Executive (2019) also distinguish between pressure and stress. According to this distinction, experiencing some pressure at work can be motivating but the experience of excessive pressure can cause stress.

The JD-C theory has been used to explain the relationship between conditions of work and work-related stress among construction industry workers (Bowen et al., 2014). A recent report undertaken on behalf of the Chartered Institute of Building revealed that construction industry workers are worse off than workers in other industries in terms of experiencing:

- poor work–life balance
- high workload
- excessive travel time
- technology overload, and
- unrealistic deadlines (Cattell et al., 2017).

Work speed and quantity of work have also been linked to symptoms of depression in bricklayers and construction supervisors, while low participation in decision making and low levels of supervisor support were linked with symptoms of depression in supervisors (Boschman et al., 2013). Job autonomy is reported to be especially beneficial for older construction workers as a protective factor against mental ill health (Zaniboni et al., 2016). Low job control and high demands have also been identified as risk factors for suicide among Australian men (Milner et al., 2016).

The construction industry possesses characteristics with the potential to amplify the impact of work on mental ill health. Construction work is project-based, and work hours are long and inflexible. The impact of working time on workers' psychological health is discussed in Chapter 4. However, construction also has other characteristics that make it stressful.

Co-worker/supervisor support and job insecurity have also been linked to stress-related disorders in male workers (Nieuwenhuijsen et al., 2010). The delivery of construction projects is heavily reliant on winning competitive tendering opportunities and projects are delivered through a complicated multitiered subcontracting system. Intense competition for contracts, coupled with low profit margins and incentive payment systems, increases the pressure experienced throughout the supply chain. Flexible employment practices have increased workforce casualisation and concerns about job security have been linked to construction workers' psychological wellbeing (Turner & Lingard, 2016). Mayhew and Quinlan (2006) report long work hours, stressed and chronically fatigued workers in similar multitiered subcontracting arrangements in the Australian trucking industry. The health impacts of subcontracting have also been reported in international studies in which subcontracted workers are reported to be three times more likely to experience anxiety or depression,

TABLE 3.1 Risk factors for mental ill health in construction

Risk factor category	Example
Job demand	Work overload / quantity of work
	Hours worked
Job control	Little opportunity to participate in decision making
Family	Work–home conflict
Welfare and socioeconomic	Job insecurity
Work hazard	Occupational injury/hazard
	Musculoskeletal pain/injuries
Coping mechanism	Substance abuse
	Alcohol abuse
Work support	Minimal social support from co-workers
	Criticism
	Lack of feedback
Workplace injustice	Gender discrimination
	Harassment/bullying

Source: Chan et al., 2020.

and to miss work due to illness, compared to directly employed workers (Min et al., 2013). Milner et al. (2017) analysed coronial findings to identify the stressors precipitating death by suicide in a sample of Australian construction workers. Transient work conditions, concerns about job insecurity and feelings of pressure were all identified as precipitating factors in these deaths (Milner et al., 2017).

The research conducted in the construction industry is consistent with studies linking conditions of work with job strain and mental ill health in other industries (Cohidon et al., 2012). However, the industry's characteristics (discussed above) create conditions in which workers are at a particularly high risk of mental ill health. Research has found that adverse work conditions (high demands, low control and job insecurity) influence mental health independently of one another. This means that jobs that combine two or three adverse conditions present a higher mental health risk, than jobs in which only one risk factor is present (Strazdins et al., 2011).

It is now well established that construction workers can suffer from a wide range of work factors which can contribute to mental ill health (Chan et al., 2020; Sun et al., 2022). Chan et al. (2020) undertook a systematic review of risk factors for mental ill health in construction and the results are summarised in Table 3.1. Risk factors comprised job demand as the highest ranked risk factor, followed by low job control, family, welfare and socioeconomic conditions, work hazards, use of coping mechanisms, the availability of work support, and workplace injustice.

In a meta-analysis review examining the relationship between psychosocial hazards and mental health in the construction industry, Sun et al. (2022) found that construction professionals (e.g., project managers, architects, engineers) and construction trade workers experienced similar adverse effects caused by psychosocial hazards on mental health. Some differences were found between construction professionals and trade workers for psychosocial hazards and their impact on mental health. For example, high job demands (e.g., role overload, interpersonal conflict, job insecurity) generally affected the mental health of construction trade workers more strongly than that of construction professionals. Low job control was found to affect the mental health of construction professionals more strongly than that of construction trade workers. Lack of job support had a similar impact on the mental health of both construction trade workers and professionals.

The findings of Sun et al. (2022) raise an important point regarding the exposure to psychosocial hazards and the impact on mental health. The construction workforce is not a homogeneous group. Instead, experience of risk factors is nuanced and can be driven by occupation, gender, age, and worksite and we explore these in more detail throughout the book. For example, in Chapter 5 we examine the risk factors to which women are exposed and how this can affect their health, and in Chapter 8 we explore young workers' health and wellbeing and specific risk factors that construction workers experience during the early stage of their career.

3.5   Psychosocial hazards and the management of risk

The International Labour Office (ILO) first defined psychosocial factors at work as "interactions between and among work environment, job content, organisational conditions and workers' capacities, needs, culture, personal extra-job considerations that may, through perceptions and experience, influence health, work performance and job satisfaction" (ILO, 1986, p.3).

Since this initial conceptualisation, the language of occupational health and safety risk management has been adopted to describe psychosocial factors and their potential to cause harm. Specifically, the term "psychosocial hazard" is used to refer to aspects of the design and management of work and its social and organisational context that have the potential to cause harm (Leka & Jain, 2010) and "psychosocial risk" describes the potential of psychosocial hazards to cause harm (Leka et al., 2015).

Work stress (discussed above in relation to the construction industry) has been identified as an outcome of exposure to psychosocial hazards in the work environment. Importantly, stress can be experienced when the risk of harm occurring is present, even if that harm has not yet occurred. For example, workers who have been exposed to workplace violence can experience stress if they believe the risk has not been effectively controlled, even if the violence has not re-occurred (Safe Work Australia, 2022a).

Psychological harm that can occur as a result of exposure to psychosocial hazards in the workplace includes conditions such as anxiety, depression, posttraumatic stress disorder (PTSD) and sleep disorders (Safe Work Australia,

2022a). Exposure to psychosocial hazards is also linked to physical health conditions, including musculoskeletal disorders (Answer et al., 2021), cardiovascular conditions (Santosa et al., 2021) and diabetes (Hackett & Steptoe, 2016), and can be a factor in fatigue-related workplace incidents causing physical injury (Safe Work Australia, 2022a).

Some commonly identified psychosocial hazards are:

- *Job content* – a lack of variety or short work cycles, fragmented or meaningless work, under use of skills, high uncertainty, continuous exposure to people through work
- *Workload and work pace* – work overload or under load, machine pacing, high levels of time pressure, continually subject to deadlines
- *Work schedule* – shift working, night shifts, inflexible work schedules, unpredictable hours, long or unsociable hours
- *Control* – low participation in decision making, lack of control over workload, pacing, etc.
- *Environment & equipment* – inadequate equipment availability, suitability or maintenance; poor environmental conditions such as lack of space, poor lighting, excessive noise
- *Organisational culture & function* – poor communication, low levels of support for problem solving and personal development, lack of definition of, or agreement on, organisational objectives
- *Interpersonal relationships at work* – social or physical isolation, poor relationships with superiors, interpersonal conflict, lack of social support, bullying, harassment
- *Role in organisation* – role ambiguity, role conflict, and responsibility for people
- *Career development* – career stagnation and uncertainty, under-promotion or over-promotion, poor pay, job insecurity, low social value to work, and
- *Home-work interface* – conflicting demands of work and home, low support at home, dual career problems (Leka and Jain, 2010, p.5).

Poorly managed organisational change, inadequate reward and recognition, poor organisational justice, witnessing, investigating or being exposed to traumatic events or materials and exposure to workplace violence or aggression have also been identified as psychosocial hazards in the workplace (Safe Work Australia, 2022b).

Leka et al. (2015) identified challenges to the practical management of psychosocial risk in workplaces, as follows:

- psychosocial risk is poorly understood by industry stakeholders who do not appreciate that existing legislative frameworks include requirements for the management of psychosocial risk;
- industry stakeholders do not appreciate that effective management of psychosocial risk can (in addition to reducing harm) also improve positive

outcomes for organisations (e.g., work engagement, improved quality and performance); and

- methods and tools for assessing and managing psychosocial risk are perceived to be difficult to use, particularly by small-to-medium sized enterprises.

The management of psychosocial risk has been required by mainstream occupational health and safety legislation for many years, in the European Union under the European Union Framework Directive 339/89/EEC (Leka et al., 2011) and countries in which the UK Robens-style model of health and safety regulation has been implemented (Johnstone et al., 2011). General obligations in these regimes require employers to manage all types of risks to workers' health and safety, including psychosocial risks. However, although they are clearly covered by general duties requirements, Johnstone et al. (2011) describe challenges associated with the enforcement of Australian occupational health and safety legislation in relation to psychosocial risk. In a qualitative study of government-employed health and safety inspectors, legal requirements for psychosocial risks were perceived to be insufficiently clear to enable effective enforcement and agency managers lacked confidence that enforcement action in relation to psychosocial issues would be successful in the courts.

Arguments have been made in favour of establishing regulations with clear and specific requirements for the management of psychosocial risk. In August 2022, Safe Work Australia released a set of model regulations and a model Code of Practice (CoP) on managing psychosocial hazards at work. The CoP provides guidance on how to comply with the laws, including how to manage the risks to psychological health in the workplace. Safe Work Australia is a national body that develops policy to improve occupational health and safety and workers' compensation arrangements across Australia.

To have effect, these model regulations and CoP need to be implemented by States/Territories as, in Australia, occupational health and safety is regulated (for the most part) by States and Territories.

The Safe Work Australia model CoP establishes a risk management process for psychosocial risk that comprises the following steps:

- Identify hazards – find out what could cause harm
- Assess risks – consider how serious the harm could be
- Control risks – implement the most effective controls that are reasonably practicable in the workplace context, and
- Review control measures – monitor risk to ensure controls are working as expected.

Consultation between employers and workers is important throughout all steps in the risk management process. The importance of consulting workers in identifying and assessing the risk posed by psychosocial hazards is arguably even greater than for physical occupational health and safety hazards. Research shows that managers and workers perceive psychosocial risks differently (Houtman et al., 2020). This may be because psychosocial risks are less "visible" and, consequently, they may be under-estimated by managers, who might also regard psychosocial risks as being sensitive and more relevant to individuals rather than the organisation. Effective consultation is therefore important to understand hazards present in a work environment and the risks posed by these hazards to workers.

When consulting workers in relation to psychosocial hazards and risks, it is important to recognise that workers may describe hazards using different terminology. There is anecdotal evidence to suggest that psychosocial risk mitigation programmes implemented in the construction industry have been hampered by the use of language that workers do not easily understand. Managers implementing these programmes describe how they have had to "translate" psychosocial risk concepts into language that workers relate to. The Safe Work Australia CoP also suggests workers may talk about a range of different feelings in relation to their work (e.g., feeling burnt out, exhausted, anxious, scared, humiliated, degraded, undermined, angry, confused, distressed or traumatised) that may be caused by exposure to psychosocial risks (Safe Work Australia, 2022a). It is therefore important to listen to workers and identify underlying work-related factors that contribute to these feelings. For example, a feeling of anger may be caused by organisational policies being applied unfairly or a feeling of fear might be caused by interacting with an aggressive co-worker. It is also important to consider whether the workplace culture supports harmful behaviour or whether different psychosocial hazards in a work environment interact with one another to increase the potential for harm.

Understanding the nature and extent of psychosocial risks in a workplace can be difficult and multiple sources of information can be used. Incident reports and data relating to complaints, absenteeism, turnover and issues raised and discussed in health and safety committee meetings and toolbox talks, etc. can provide indicators of the presence of psychosocial hazards. Observing the work environment to see how people work (e.g., are they rushed?) and interact (e.g., is communication sufficient and respectful?) can also provide useful insights into the quality of the psychosocial work environment. The extent to which psychosocial hazards are present in a workplace can also be measured using anonymous employee perception surveys. The advantage of anonymous surveys is that they can overcome workers' concerns that they may be identified and victimised as consequence of reporting the presence of psychosocial risk in a workplace. For example, the UK's Health and Safety Executive has developed a Work-Related Stress Indicator Tool that is used to assess risk associated with six areas of work design that are associated with poor health: demands; control; support; relationships; role; and change (Edwards et al., 2008).

The traditional hierarchy of control (HoC) concept was developed for application to physical health and safety risks. The HoC arranges risk control measures in a descending order of effectiveness (see Chapter 2 for examples of the application of the HoC to physical health risks). In relation to the selection of control measures for psychosocial risks the same principles as embodied in the HoC apply. That is, wherever possible hazards should be eliminated. If it is not possible to eliminate a hazard, then psychosocial risks should be minimised by changing the environment in which work takes place, considering making changes to job/work design, the systems of work and/or the physical work environment. These controls correspond in some ways to the technological controls of substitution, isolation and engineering in the traditional HoC because they seek to make the workplace intrinsically safer. Further down the hierarchy are controls that focus on human behaviour within the work environment, such as implementing safe work systems and procedures and encouraging desirable worker behaviours. Safe Work Australia (2022a) provide examples of possible controls for different psychological risks, noting that the selection of controls should always be based upon an assessment of the risks present in a specific workplace.

3.6 ISO 45003

Published in 2021, ISO 45003, *Occupational health and safety management – Psychological health and safety at work – Guidelines for managing psychosocial risks* provides guidance on the management of psychosocial risks and promotion of wellbeing at work, as part of an organisation's occupational health and safety management system. ISO 45003 groups psychosocial hazards into three categories as follows: (i) aspects of work organisation, (ii) social factors at work, and (iii) work environment, equipment and hazardous tasks. Examples of these are provided in Table 3.2.

ISO 45003 requires that organisations first understand their internal and external contexts to fully understand their operating environment, including the needs and expectations of their workers and other relevant stakeholders, and the factors that could affect the effectiveness of management processes implemented for psychosocial risk. For example, in the construction industry organisational factors, such as hierarchical systems of subcontracting and unfavourable contractual conditions governing the client-contractor relationship, may influence the experience and management of psychosocial risk. Construction workers may also be exposed to psychosocial risks arising from the work environment, equipment and tasks they perform – for example, working in conditions of extreme heat or cold and in unfavourable work environments characterised by exposure to high levels of noise and other physical health or safety hazards. The social environment in construction work is also shaped by the highly male-dominated work environment and prevailing masculine culture.

Once the organisational context for managing psychosocial risk is understood, ISO 45003 requires organisations to establish strong leadership commitment to the management of psychosocial risk (as part of the organisation's occupational health and safety management activities) and ensure that the management of psychosocial risk is addressed in organisational policy documents. ISO 45003 requires that organisational roles, responsibilities and authorities relating to the

TABLE 3.2 Psychosocial hazard types and examples

Aspects of work organisation	*Social factors at work*	*Work environment, equipment and hazardous tasks*
Roles and expectations, e.g., ambiguous roles, conflicting roles or roles that involve a duty of care for other persons	Interpersonal relationships, e.g., poor communication, interpersonal conflict, harassment, bullying and victimisation.	Inadequate equipment availability, suitability, reliability, maintenance or repair.
Job autonomy and control, e.g., little opportunity to participate in decision making, little control over workload, etc.	Leadership, e.g., lack of clear vision and objectives, abuse of power, etc.	Poor workplace conditions such as lack of space, poor lighting and excessive noise.
Job demands, e.g., having too much to do within a certain time or with a set number of workers, conflicting demands and deadlines, lack of task variety or performing highly repetitive tasks, etc.	Organisational/workgroup culture, e.g., poor communication, low levels of support for problem solving and personal development, etc.	Lack of the necessary tools, equipment or other resources to complete work tasks.
Organizational change management, e.g., lack of practical support provided to assist workers during transition periods, etc.	Recognition and reward, e.g. imbalance between workers' effort and formal and informal recognition and reward.	Working in extreme conditions or situations, such as very high or low temperatures, or at height.
Remote and isolated work, e.g., working in locations that are far from home, family, friends and usual support networks, working alone without social/human interaction at work (working at home), etc.	Career development, e.g., career stagnation and uncertainty, under-promotion or over-promotion, lack of opportunity for skill development.	Working in unstable environments such as conflict zones.
	Support, e.g., lack of support from supervisors and co-workers, lack of access to support services.	
	Supervision, e.g., lack of constructive performance feedback and evaluation processes, lack of support and/or resources to facilitate performance improvement, misuse of digital surveillance.	

Workload and work pace, e.g., work overload or underload, high levels of time pressure, continually subject to deadlines, etc.

Working hours and schedule, e.g., shift work, inflexible work schedules, unpredictable hours, long or unsociable hours, etc.

Job security and precarious work, e.g., uncertainty regarding work availability, possibility of redundancy or temporary loss of work with reduced pay, non-standard employment, etc.

Civility and respect, e.g., lack of trust, honesty, respect, civility and fairness in interactions (internal and external to the organisation).

Work–life imbalance, e.g., work tasks, roles, schedules or expectations that cause conflicting demands of work and home, impact the ability to recover, etc.

Violence at work, i.e., incidents involving an explicit or implicit challenge to health, safety or well-being, such as abuse, threats, assault (physical, verbal or sexual) including gender-based violence.

Harassment, i.e., unwanted, offensive, intimidating behaviours (sexual or non-sexual in nature) which relate to characteristic(s) of the targeted individual, such as race, gender identity, religion, etc.

Bullying and victimisation, i.e., repeated unreasonable behaviours which can present a risk to health, safety and well-being at work, such as social or physical isolation, name-calling, insults and intimidation, etc.

Source: Adapted from ISO 45003: Occupational health and safety management – Psychological health and safety at work – Guidelines for managing psychosocial risks.

management of psychosocial risk are clearly established and robust processes for consulting workers about psychosocial risks and how best to manage them are also implemented.

Reflecting on the definition of the organisational context, ISO 45003 requires that specific plans be developed in regard to how psychosocial hazards are to be dealt with to prevent psychological injury and ill health, as well as strategies for workers returning to work following an injury/illness. Planning processes should also identify opportunities for improvement, including promotion of wellbeing at work. Wellbeing at work is defined in ISO45003 as "fulfilment of the physical, mental, social and cognitive needs and expectations of a worker related to their work."

Thus, ISO 45003 references both prevention of negative outcomes and promotion of positive outcomes for workers' psychological health. Organisations are also required to develop, review and maintain systems, processes and reporting structures focused on the management of psychosocial risks. Based on understanding what could create or affect the management of psychosocial risk within a particular operating context, ISO 45003 requires that organisations set appropriate objectives, determine how these objectives will be met and demonstrate a commitment to continual improvement that, where possible, goes beyond fulfilling minimum legal requirements.

ISO 45003 requires that hazards (sources of harm) be identified before appropriate risk control measures are selected. Moreover, processes for hazard identification need to be proactive and ongoing to ensure that changes to operational context or conditions that change hazard exposures are understood and dealt with. When assessing the risk (i.e., potential for harm) posed by psychosocial hazards, ISO 45003 specifically requires that organisations compare groups of workers that differ in exposure to hazards. For example, in the construction context, professional/managerial and manual/non-managerial workers are likely to be at risk of harm from different psychosocial risk factors. Subcontracted workers and direct employees may also be exposed to different hazards, particularly those relating to job security and employment conditions.

ISO 45003 also requires risks to be assessed with due consideration to the interaction of psychosocial risks with risks from other identified hazards and to consider the diversity of the workforce and the needs of particular groups in determining the risk of harm. Some worker groups may be particularly vulnerable to some psychosocial risk factors, such as young and inexperienced workers being frequently exposed to bullying behaviours. Women workers are also a minority group in the construction industry and are likely to experience psychosocial risk differently to male workers (see also Chapter 5).

ISO 45003 requires organisations to establish, provide and maintain resourcing (considering human, financial, technological and other resource requirements) to ensure plans relating to the management of psychosocial risk are properly implemented and objectives are met. In particular, organisations are required to actively develop workforce competence in relation to the identification and management of psychosocial risks and ensure workers are familiar with processes for reporting hazards or raising concerns. Importantly, workers' needs, experience, language skills and literacy should be considered in the design and delivery of any training or development activity undertaken.

Traditional training approaches are not always effective in the construction industry and alternative methods may be more effectively used to develop competency in certain "soft skills" relevant to the management of psychosocial risk, as illustrated in case example 3.1.

CASE EXAMPLE 3.1 DIGITAL ROLE PLAY GAME TO DEVELOP SUPERVISORS' AND APPRENTICES' COMMUNICATION SKILLS

Role play is a well-established approach to developing soft skills, such as how to best communicate in particular situations and displaying empathy (Lane et al., 2007; Ma et al., 2021). Role play involves playing a role in a specific situation or scenario. The role played can reflect a participant's own role or the role of another person, and learning is enhanced because roles are played in a safe environment, permitting participants to experiment and learn with no risk of irreversible consequences (Ladousse, 1987). Digital role play games are increasingly used to help users to improve interpersonal skills (e.g., communication, negotiation, leadership).

A recent Australian study used a participatory approach to develop a digital role play game to help apprentices and their supervisors to develop better ways to communicate with one another in the workplace. Specific communication characteristics included as learning objectives in the digital role play game included: demonstrating empathy, using emotional intelligence, respecting personal boundaries, communicating with respect, the difference between being assertive and being aggressive, and being supportive and approachable.

The digital role play game was developed in consultation with young men and women engaged in construction industry apprenticeship training and was based on their real life stories (lived experiences).

Scenarios were developed and trainees (players) are asked to navigate through these scenarios by making turn-based decisions, which lead to different outcomes. Every outcome demonstrates the importance of effective communication in improving the safety, health and wellbeing of young workers. Figure 3.1 shows a screenshot from the digital role play game.

Trainees have commented that this type of approach to developing interpersonal communication skills is more engaging and effective than classroom-based training methods and that they are more likely to feel confident dealing with difficult workplace situations having played the game.

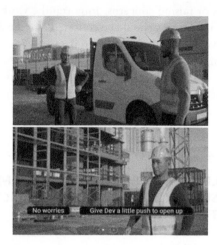

FIGURE 3.1 A screenshot from the digital role play game

With regard to the operational planning and control of psychosocial risk, organisations are required by ISO 45003 to eliminate hazards and reduce risks by considering the best fit between tasks, structures and work processes and the needs of workers, as well as to design and manage work in ways that prevent psychosocial risk and promote wellbeing at work. Risk assessments should take into account existing controls in place for psychosocial risk and the adequacy and effectiveness of these controls. Where new controls are needed the hierarchy of control should be used to guide the selection of these. ISO 45003 also suggests that a combination of primary, secondary and tertiary controls be implemented (see also Table 3.2). ISO 45003 specifically states that organisations should implement controls for psychosocial risk related to work organisation, which often involves a redesign of work processes (not just the adjustment of tasks). Control measures that address psychosocial risks related to social factors and to work environment, equipment and hazardous tasks should also be implemented.

ISO 45003 acknowledges that organisational and work-related change (to objectives, activities, work processes, leadership, work tasks and working conditions) can affect existing psychosocial risks or create new ones. Organisational change processes need to be carefully managed so that risks to psychological health and safety are identified and controlled. Risks posed by the procurement of products and services and the outsourcing of work (for example, engaging subcontractors) can also have an effect on psychosocial risks experienced by workers. ISO 45003 requires organisations to consider the effects of procurement and outsourcing on psychosocial risk exposure and ensure risks are managed effectively. ISO 45003 also requires organisations to manage the psychosocial risk associated with exposure to or experience of emergency situations in workplaces

TABLE 3.3 Example metrics/indicators for the management of psychosocial risk

Category	Example indicators
Work hours	Contract enforcing work hours restrictions
	Percentage of overtime
	Average hours worked per worker per month
Understanding the prevalence of mental health issues	Employee engagement surveys, health and safety culture surveys or regular pulse surveys focused on mental health
	Facilitated focus groups to gather feedback on psychological health and safety and organisational climate around mental health reporting
Raising awareness about psychological health	Extent of information sharing on psychosocial risk management processes (e.g., feedback, experiences, outcomes, improvement opportunities)
Return-to-work monitoring	Number of workers returned to pre-work hours and duties after being off with a mental illness, recovery duration, and identifying trends and any relationship to initiatives and processes in place
Psychological risk exposure	Percentage of workers reporting being exposed to psychosocial hazards at their workplace in the last 12 months (including: bullying, undesired sexual attention, feeling that work drains so much energy that it has a negative effect on private life; employees unable to express their views and feelings; feeling of lacking any influence on what they do at work)
Psychological risk control	Percentage of worksites that provide free or subsidised clinical assessments for depression by a provider, followed by directed feedback and clinical referral when appropriate
	Percentage of worksites that provide educational materials on stress management
	Percentage of identified psychosocial risks that have been eliminated or reduced through work design

(for example witnessing safety incidents) and to design and implement appropriate rehabilitation and return-to-work programmes to support workers who have been absent from work due to exposure to psychosocial hazards.

A systematic approach to performance monitoring and review is required by ISO 45003 to determine whether the organisation's objectives with regard to the management of psychosocial risk are being met and organisational policy is being followed. Effective performance monitoring, using qualitative and quantitative and leading and lagging metrics, helps organisations to determine if risk controls are having the desired effect in reducing psychosocial risk. Table 3.3 shows some example metrics that could be used.

ISO 45003 requires organisations to perform internal audits to evaluate their performance in managing psychological risk on a regular basis. These audits should evaluate compliance with policy (and legislation) and identify opportunities to improve the management of psychosocial risk. Opportunities with the greatest potential to reduce psychosocial risk and/or improve worker wellbeing should be prioritised.

3.7 Workplace mental health programmes

There is an increasing emphasis on the workplace as a point of intervention for targeting the prevention of mental illness and the promotion of psychological wellbeing (Harvey et al., 2014). The workplace is seen to be an effective point of intervention for mental health promotion programmes, particularly among men who are reported to have lower levels of mental health literacy and be less likely than women to seek help for personal difficulties (Roche et al., 2016).

Roche et al. (2016) argue that:

- large numbers of people can be accessed through workplace interventions,
- workplaces already contain existing infrastructure and frameworks to support the implementation of mental health and wellbeing programmes, and
- addressing mental health as part of workplace occupational health and safety management activities reduces stigma and encourages help-seeking behaviour in relation to mental health.

Some initiatives have already been implemented and are having a positive impact in the construction industry. For example, the Mates in Construction programme provides a training/peer support programme that is widely accepted in the construction industry and is effectively changing attitudes towards mental health and help-seeking behaviour (Ross et al., 2019).

While changing attitudes and behaviour in relation to mental ill health is important, long-term prevention measures also need to target the construction industry's culture and entrenched practices that contribute to the emergence of mental ill health. Dextras-Gauthier et al. (2012) argue that the behaviours, structures and processes that produce adverse conditions of work are shaped by the values, assumptions and beliefs inherent in an industry or organisational culture. They argue that "when dealing with mental health issues, including burnout, depression, and psychological distress, managers need to tread further upstream to identify those elements of organizational culture that are ultimately causing ill health" (Dextras-Gauthier et al., 2012, p.97).

Safe Work Australia (2019) also clarifies the role played by health promotion programmes that focus on promoting a healthy lifestyle, personal development and learning, and non-work-related health behaviours. These initiatives do not protect workers from harmful exposure to workplace psychosocial (or physical) hazards and are therefore not a substitute for a systematic management process for psychosocial risks.

With the growing recognition that job stress can have adverse outcomes for individuals and organisations, literature on interventions seeking to address job stress has rapidly expanded (LaMontagne et al., 2007; Karanika-Murray & Biron, 2015). Organisational stress and wellbeing interventions are diverse and said to operate at three levels (Hurrell, 2005; LaMontagne et al., 2007):

- primary interventions eliminate or reduce job stressors,
- secondary interventions alter the way that workers perceive or respond to job stressors, and
- tertiary interventions treat and rehabilitate workers with job stress-related illness.

While primary prevention is generally more effective than secondary prevention, and secondary is generally more effective than tertiary prevention, it is acknowledged these prevention approaches are not mutually exclusive and should be used in combination (LaMontagne et al., 2007).

Primary-level interventions are proactive and aim to prevent exposure to job stressors. Interventions at this level address sources of stress in the workplace through modifications to the physical or psychosocial work environment or through organisational changes (LaMontagne et al., 2007). Examples of primary preventive interventions include job redesign, changes in work pacing, enhancement of social support, and the formation of joint labour/management health and safety committees. Most primary preventive interventions are directed at the organisation or the work environment, but some can also be directed at individuals when addressing stressors rather than stress responses.

Secondary-level interventions aim to modify an individual's response to or perception of stressors. Secondary interventions target the individual with "the justifiable underlying assumption that addressing individuals' responses to stressors should be done in addition to removing or reducing stressors" (LaMontagne et al., 2007, p.225). Examples of secondary prevention interventions include stress management training to assist workers to either modify or control their perception of stressful situations, such as the development of meditation skills.

Tertiary interventions focus on treating stress-related illness, and aim to minimise the effects of stress-related problems once they have occurred through management or treatment of symptoms or disease and to reintegrate the affected worker back into the workforce. These include counselling (such as in the form of employee assistance programmes), rehabilitation, return-to-work, and other programmes (LaMontagne et al., 2007).

There is alignment between the three intervention levels and the HoC framework (LaMontagne et al., 2007), as interventions and controls are in descending order of likely effectiveness and protectiveness. In Table 3.4, we outline the intervention and hierarchy of control levels and corresponding control measures for time pressures or fast-paced work which is a common job demand experienced by construction workers. Control measures at the primary and secondary levels

TABLE 3.4 Control measures for time pressures or fast-paced work

	Intervention level	Hierarchy of control	Control measure
Most effective	Primary: eliminate or reduce job stressors	Control at the source through removal or designing out the hazard through: • Elimination • Substitution • Isolation • Engineering controls	Schedule tasks to avoid intense or sustained high job demands (e.g., schedule non-urgent work for quieter periods) Plan the workforce so there is an adequate number of appropriately skilled staff to do the work and so that tasks utilise workers' skills
	Secondary: alter the way that workers perceive or respond to job stressors	Control at the worker level through: • Administrative controls • Training and education • PPE	Have regular conversations about work expectations, workloads, deadlines and instructions to ensure job demands are understood and can be managed Time management training Stress management training
Least effective	Tertiary: treat and rehabilitate workers with job stress-related illness	Control at the level of illness through: • Treatment • Rehabilitation	Employee Assistance Programme Therapy

Source: Adapted from LaMontagne et al., 2007.

are drawn from *Managing Psychosocial Hazards at Work: Code of Practice* (Safe Work Australia, 2022a). We have added time management training as it is a commonly utilised control used to assist workers with planning and managing their work time, and stress management training which is also a commonly utilised control to manage workers' response to stress. Table 3.4 highlights that, importantly, control measures/interventions are most effective when they are directly aligned with addressing the specific hazard.

Training and education are positioned at the individual level in the HoC framework and are not usually associated with elimination of the hazard. However, in some instances training and education may lead to hazard elimination. For example, we refer to the elimination of harmful behaviour that women in construction can experience. Harmful behaviour is identified as a psychosocial hazard and incorporates:

- violence and aggression
- bullying
- harassment including sexual harassment or gender-based harassment, and
- conflict or poor workplace relationships and interactions (Safe Work Australia, 2022a).

In 2022, the Victorian Government released a Respect Code for the construction industry. The Respect Code aims to create safe and respectful workplaces for women where safety, inclusiveness and wellbeing are paramount (Victorian Government, 2022). Implementation of the Respect Code seeks to change individuals' behaviour towards women. In this instance, training and educating workers on respectful workplace behaviour and acceptable standards functions as a primary intervention and is aligned with controlling the hazard through elimination. Together with training and education, implementing practices in which disrespectful behaviour by an individual has consequences contributes to a control system with the potential to eliminate harmful behaviour.

Case example 3.2 describes the development of Mental Health Action Plans in civil construction organisations which aimed to drive reductions in work-related stress factors, prevent burnout and improve mental health.

CASE EXAMPLE 3.2 POSITIVE PLANS – POSITIVE FUTURES PROGRAM

The Civil Contractors Federation (CCF) of Victoria (Australia) received funding from WorkSafe Victoria under the WorkWell Mental Health Improvement Fund. The project aimed to make mental health a priority in construction workplaces. The CCF Chief Executive at the time commented: "We have cultural heritage plans, energy efficiency plans and COVID-safe plans but we think it is time for construction businesses to have a mental health action plan" (Plumbing Connection, 2021). The Positive Plans – Positive Futures Program engages civil construction organisations to develop Mental Health Action Plans to drive reductions in work-related stress factors, prevent burnout and improve mental health (Construction Advisor, 2021). The work commenced with a third-party survey undertaken in each participating organisation that provided insights into factors in the working environment and business that could impact mental health, including job demands, access to management, and communication (Roads & Infrastructure, 2022). This data was used to develop Mental Health Action Plans targeting specific areas of need within each organisation. Construction companies participating in the programme were supported with resources developed by WorkSafe Victoria, regular engagement in capacity building activities and knowledge-sharing opportunities, facilitated by CCF personnel. The Safety Health Environment and Quality (SHEQ) Systems Manager at one participating organisation commented: "In my experience, if you were to search mental health online, it tends to go directly to a diagnosed mental health condition. We really want to focus on the wellness side, and what are the practical things that you can do to stay well, to be able to manage the normal stresses in your life" (Roads & Infrastructure, 2022). This organisation focused their initial efforts on integrating mental health terminology and concepts into their health and safety and human relations management systems, providing information in accessible format and language that workers could understand and building up trust to encourage people to seek help if they needed help. Toolbox style information sessions were also held on topics identified as being relevant to workers' stress, including financial counselling and budgeting. The SHEQ Systems Manager commented: "We're more understanding and considerate of each other. Our behaviour has changed and there's now an extra level of sincerity and compassion that people are starting to show. Our employees are able to say 'look, I'm just not in the right headspace today, I can't concentrate on this particular task'. That is critical in a high-risk industry such as our own" (Roads & Infrastructure, 2022). The CCF suggests that participating organisations can use their Mental Health Action Plans to demonstrate (when tendering for work) that opportunities to reduce stress have been adequately considered in project planning and resourcing decision-making. Companies also report regularly against their Mental Health Action Plans to determine the extent to which psychosocial risk factors are being effectively managed. To support organisations in the implementation of the Positive Plans – Positive Futures Program, the CCF ran Regional Roadshows and convened annual Mental Health Summits that were attended by 300-plus business owners and senior managers. This information sharing was considered to be a critical success factor because, as the Positive Plans – Positive Futures Project Manager explained: "We know that managing mental health in the workplace can be a complex issue. Not knowing where to start can put businesses off doing anything about it" (Roads & Infrastructure, 2022).

3.8 Conclusion

Construction workers are a high-risk group for work-related stress due to the nature and organisation of work tasks. The impacts of work-related stress are felt by the worker and their family members, the company, and the wider construction industry. There is now growing awareness that companies can and should proactively protect both the physical and psychological health of workers. ISO 45003 (*Occupational health and safety management – Psychological health and safety at work – Guidelines for managing psychosocial risks*) provides companies with guidance on the management of psychosocial risks and promotion of psychological wellbeing at work, as part of an organisation's occupational health and safety management system. Integrating psychosocial risk management more effectively into strategic policy and business decision-making will help to create construction work environments, that are supportive, sustainable and inclusive.

3.9 Discussion and review questions

1. What are the key theories linking psychological health with work? What are the key differences between these theories?
2. What work-related factors do construction workers experience that have the potential to affect their psychological health?
3. What actions can construction organisations take to protect workers' psychological health?

3.10 Acknowledgements

The work presented in case example 3.1 was funded by icare New South Wales and supported by the Master Builders Association of New South Wales and the NSW Centre for Work Health and Safety. The work presented in case example 3.2 was funded by the Civil Contractors Federation (Victoria) as part of their WorkSafe Victoria WorkWell Mental Health Improvement Fund grant.

References

Anwer, S., Li, H., Antwi-Afari, M. F., & Wong, A. Y. L. (2021). Associations between physical or psychosocial risk factors and work-related musculoskeletal disorders in construction workers based on literature in the last 20 years: A systematic review. *International Journal of Industrial Ergonomics*, 83, 103113.

Bakker, A. B., & Demerouti, E. (2007). The Job Demands-Resources model: State of the art. *Journal of Managerial Psychology*, 22(3), 309–328.

Boschman, J. S., Van der Molen, H. F., Sluiter, J. K., & Frings-Dresen, M. H. W. (2013). Psychosocial work environment and mental health among construction workers. *Applied Ergonomics*, 44(5), 748–755.

Bowen, P., Edwards, P., Lingard, H., & Cattell, K. (2014). Occupational stress and job demand, control and support factors among construction project consultants. *International Journal of Project Management*, 32(7), 1273–1284.

Bültmann, U., Kant, I., van Amelsvoort, L. G., van den Brandt, P. A., & Kasl, S. V. (2001). Differences in fatigue and psychological distress across occupations: results from the Maastricht Cohort Study of Fatigue at Work. *Journal of Occupational and Environmental Medicine*, 43, 976–983.

Butterworth, P., Leach, L. S., McManus, S., & Stansfeld, S. A. (2013). Common mental disorders, unemployment and psychosocial job quality: Is a poor job better than no job at all? *Psychological Medicine*, 43(8), 1763.

Butterworth, P., Leach, L. S., Rodgers, B., Broom, D. H., Olesen, S. C., & Strazdins, L. (2011a). Psychosocial job adversity and health in Australia: analysis of data from the HILDA Survey. *Australian and New Zealand Journal of Public Health*, 35(6), 564–571.

Butterworth, P., Leach, L. S., Strazdins, L., Olesen, S. C., Rodgers, B., & Broom, D. H. (2011b). The psychosocial quality of work determines whether employment has benefits for mental health: Results from a longitudinal national household panel survey. *Occupational and Environmental Medicine*, 68(11), 806–812.

Cattell, K. S., Bowen, P. A., Cooper, C. L., & Edwards, P. J. (2017). *The State of Well-Being in the Construction Industry*. Chartered Institute of Building.

Chan, A. P. C., Nwaogu, J. M., & Naslund, J. A. (2020). Mental ill-health risk factors in the construction industry: Systematic review. *Journal of Construction Engineering and Management*, 146(3), 04020004.

Cohidon, C., Santin, G., Chastang, J. F., Imbernon, E., & Niedhammer, I. (2012). Psychosocial exposures at work and mental health: potential utility of a job-exposure matrix. *Journal of Occupational and Environmental Medicine*, 54(2), 184–191.

Construction Advisor (2021). Positive Plans, Positive Futures Project – Working To Improve Mental Health In Construction. Accessed 2 September 2022 from: www.constructionadvisor.com.au/positive-plans-positive-futures/

De Jonge, J., Bosma, H., Peter, R., & Siegrist, J. (2000). Job strain, effort-reward imbalance and employee well-being: A large-scale cross-sectional study. *Social Science & Medicine*, 50(9), 1317–1327.

Dextras-Gauthier, J., Marchand, A., & Haines III, V. (2012). Organizational culture, work organization conditions, and mental health: A proposed integration. *International Journal of Stress Management*, 19(2), 81–104.

Edwards, J. A., Webster, S., Van Laar, D., & Easton, S. (2008). Psychometric Analysis of the UK Health and Safety Executive's Management Standards Work-related Stress Indicator Tool. *Work & Stress*, 22(2), 96–107.

Findlay, P., Kalleberg, A. L., & Warhurst, C. (2013). The challenge of job quality. *Human Relations*, 66(4), 441–451.

Green, F. (2006). *Demanding Work: The Paradox of Job Quality in the Affluent Economy*. Princeton University Press.

Hackett, R. A., & Steptoe, A. (2016). Psychosocial factors in diabetes and cardiovascular risk. *Current Cardiology Reports*, 18(10), 1–12.

Harvey, S. B., Joyce, S., Tan, L., Johnson, A., Nguyen, H., Modini, M., & Growth, M., (2014), *Developing a Mentally Healthy Workplace: A Review of the Literature,* A report for the National Mental Health Commission and Mentally Healthy Workplace Alliance, University of New South Wales, Sydney.

Hassard, J., Teoh, K. R. H., Visockaite, G., Dewe, P., & Cox, T. (2018). The cost of work-related stress to society: A systematic review. *Journal of Occupational Health Psychology*, 23(1), 1–17.

Hassard, J., Teoh, K., Cox, T., Dewe, P., Cosmar, M., Gründler, R. A. , Flemming, D., Cosemans, B., & Van den Broek, K. (2014). Calculating the Cost of Work-Related Stress and Psychosocial Risks. Technical Report. Publications Office of the European Union, Luxembourg. Downloaded from: https://eprints.bbk.ac.uk/id/eprint/20923/

Häusser, J. A., Mojzisch, A., Niesel, M., & Schulz-Hardt, S. (2010). Ten years on: A review of recent research on the Job Demand–Control (-Support) model and psychological well-being. *Work & Stress*, 24(1), 1–35.

Health and Safety Executive (2019). *Tackling Work-Related Stress Using the Management Standards Approach,* The Stationery Office, Norwich. Accessed 6 September 2022 from: www.hse.gov.uk/pubns/wbk01.pdf,

Houtman, I., van Zwieten, M., Leka, S., Jain, A., & de Vroome, E. (2020). Social dialogue and psychosocial risk management: Added value of manager and employee representative agreement in risk perception and awareness. *International Journal of Environmental Research and Public Health,* 17(10), 3672.

Hurrell, J. (2005). Organizational stress intervention. In J. Barling, E. K. Kelloway and M. R. Frone (Eds.), *Handbook of Work Stress.* SAGE Publications (pp.623–646).

International Labour Organization (ILO) (1986). *Psychosocial Factors at Work: Recognition and Control. Report of the Joint ILO/WHO Committee on Occupational Health,* ninth session, Geneva, 18–24 September 1984.

International Labour Organization (ILO) (2015). *Transforming Our World: The 2030 Agenda for Sustainable Development.* International Labour Organization.

International Organization for Standardization (ISO) (2021). *Occupational health and safety management – Psychological health and safety at work – Guidelines for managing psychosocial risks* (ISO Standard No. 45003:2021). Accessed 20 June 2022 from: www.iso.org/obp/ui/#iso:std:iso:45003:ed-1:v1:en

Jin, R. L., Shah, C. P., & Svoboda, T. J. (1995). The impact of unemployment on health: A review of the evidence. *Canadian Medical Association Journal,* 153(5), 529.

Johnstone, R., Quinlan, M., & McNamara, M. (2011). OHS inspectors and psychosocial risk factors: Evidence from Australia. *Safety Science,* 49(4), 547–557.

Karanika-Murray, M., & Biron, C. (2015). Introduction – Why do some interventions derail? Deconstructing the elements of organizational interventions for stress and well-being. In M. Karanika-Murray & C. Biron (Eds.), *Derailed Organizational Interventions for Stress and Well-Being: Confessions of Failure and Solutions for Success.* Springer Netherlands (pp. 1–15).

Karasek, R. A. (1979). Job Demands, Job Decision Latitude, and Mental Strain: Implications for Job Redesign. *Administrative Science Quarterly,* 24(2), 285–308.

Karasek, R., & Theorell, T. (1990). *Healthy Work. Stress, productivity and the reconstruction of work life.* Basic Books: New York.

Ladousse, G. P. (1987). *Role-play.* Oxford University Press.

LaMontagne, A.D., Keegel, T., & Vallance, D. (2007). Protecting and promoting mental health in the workplace: Developing a systems approach to job stress. *Health Promotion Journal of Australia,* 18 (3), 221–228.

Lane, C., & Rollnick, S. (2007). The use of simulated patients and role-play in communication skills training: a review of the literature to August 2005. *Patient Education and Counseling,* 67(1–2), 13–20.

Leach, L. S., Butterworth, P., Strazdins, L., Rodgers, B., Broom, D. H., & Olesen, S. C. (2010). The limitations of employment as a tool for social inclusion. *BMC Public Health,* 10(1), 1–13.

Leka, S., & Jain, A. (2010). *Health impact of psychosocial hazards at work: An overview.* World Health Organization. https://apps.who.int/iris/handle/10665/44428

Leka, S., Jain, A., Widerszal-Bazyl, M., Żołnierczyk-Zreda, D., & Zwetsloot, G. (2011). Developing a standard for psychosocial risk management: PAS 1010. *Safety Science,* 49(7), 1047–1057.

Leka, S., Van Wassenhove, W., & Jain, A. (2015). Is psychosocial risk prevention possible? Deconstructing common presumptions. *Safety Science,* 71, 61–67.

Ma, Z., Huang, K. T., & Yao, L. (2021). Feasibility of a Computer Role-Playing Game to Promote Empathy in Nursing Students: The Role of Immersiveness and Perspective. *Cyberpsychology, Behavior, and Social Networking*, 24(11), 750–755.

Mayhew, C., & Quinlan, M. (2006). Economic pressure, multi-tiered subcontracting and occupational health and safety in Australian long-haul trucking. *Employee Relations*, 28(3), 212–229.

Milner, A., Butterworth, P., Bentley, R., Kavanagh, A. M., & LaMontagne, A. D. (2015). Sickness absence and psychosocial job quality: an analysis from a longitudinal survey of working Australians, 2005–2012. *American Journal of Epidemiology*, 181(10), 781–788.

Milner, A., Maheen, H., Currier, D., & LaMontagne, A. D. (2017). Male suicide among construction workers in Australia: A qualitative analysis of the major stressors precipitating death. *BMC Public Health*, 17(1), 584.

Milner, A., Page, K., Witt, K., & LaMontagne, A. (2016). Psychosocial working conditions and suicide ideation. *Journal of Occupational and Environmental Medicine*, 58(6), 584–587.

Min, K. B., Park, S. G., Song, J. S., Yi, K. H., Jang, T. W., & Min, J. Y. (2013). Subcontractors and increased risk for work-related diseases and absenteeism. *American Journal of Industrial Medicine*, 56(11), 1296–1306.

Netterstrøm, B., Conrad, N., Bech, P., Fink, P., Olsen, O., Rugulies, R., & Stansfeld, S. (2008). The relation between work-related psychosocial factors and the development of depression. *Epidemiologic Reviews*, 30(1), 118–132.

Nieuwenhuijsen, K., Bruinvels, D., & Frings-Dresen, M. (2010). Psychosocial work environment and stress-related disorders, a systematic review. *Occupational Medicine*, 60(4), 277–286.

Pirzadeh, P., Lingard, H., & Zhang, R. P. (2022), Job Quality and Construction Workers' Mental Health: A Life Course Perspective, *Journal of Construction Engineering and Management*. In press.

Plumbing Connection (2021). https://plumbingconnection.com.au/ccf-vic-building-cap ability-in-construction/, accessed 2 September 2022

Roads & Infrastructure, (2022). https://roadsonline.com.au/a-journey-for-positive-men tal-health-with-nvc-precast/, accessed 2 September 2022.

Roche, A. M., Pidd, K., Fischer, J. A., Lee, N., Scarfe, A., & Kostadinov, V. (2016). Men, work, and mental health: A systematic review of depression in male-dominated industries and occupations. *Safety and Health at Work*, 7(4), 268–283.

Ross, V., Caton, N., Gullestrup, J., & Kõlves, K. (2019). Understanding the barriers and pathways to male help-seeking and help-offering: A mixed methods study of the impact of the Mates in Construction Program. *International Journal of Environmental Research and Public Health*, 16(16), 2979.

Rydstedt, L. W., Devereux, J., & Sverke, M. (2007). Comparing and combining the demand-control-support model and the effort reward imbalance model to predict long-term mental strain. *European Journal of Work and Organizational Psychology*, 16(3), 261–278.

Safe Work Australia (2019). Work-related Psychological Health and Safety: A systematic approach to meeting your duties. National guidance material. Safe Work Australia.

Safe Work Australia (2022a). Managing Psychosocial Hazards at Work: Code of Practice. Safe Work Australia.

Safe Work Australia (2022b). www.safeworkaustralia.gov.au/safety-topic/managing-hea lth-and-safety/mental-health/psychosocial-hazards, accessed 5 September 2022.

Santosa, A., Rosengren, A., Ramasundarahettige, C., Rangarajan, S., Chifamba, J., Lear, S. A.,... & Yusuf, S. (2021). Psychosocial risk factors and cardiovascular disease and death in a population-based cohort from 21 low-, middle-, and high-income countries. *JAMA network open*, 4(12), e2138920–e2138920.

Siegrist, J. (1996). Adverse health effects of high-effort/low-reward conditions. *Journal of Occupational Health Psychology*, 1(1), 27–41.

Siegrist, J. (2012). *Effort-Reward Imbalance at Work: Theory, Measurement and Evidence.* Department of Medical Sociology, University of Düsseldorf.

Siegrist, J., Starke, D., Chandola, T., Godin, I., Marmot, M., Niedhammer, I., & Peter, R. (2004). The measurement of effort–reward imbalance at work: European comparisons. *Social Science & Medicine*, 58(8), 1483–1499.

Stansfeld, S., & Candy, B., (2006). Psychosocial work environment and mental health – a meta-analytic review. *Scandinavian Journal of Work, Environment & Health*, 32(6), 443–462.

Strazdins, L., D'Souza, R. M., Clements, M., Broom, D. H., Rodgers, B., & Berry, H. L. (2011). Could better jobs improve mental health? A prospective study of change in work conditions and mental health in mid-aged adults. *Journal of Epidemiology & Community Health*, 65(6), 529–534.

Strazdins, L., D'Souza, R. M., Lim, L. L. Y., Broom, D. H., & Rodgers, B. (2004). Job strain, job insecurity, and health: rethinking the relationship. *Journal of Occupational Health Psychology*, 9(4), 296.

Strazdins, L., Shipley, M., Clements, M., Obrien, L. V., & Broom, D. H. (2010). Job quality and inequality: Parents' jobs and children's emotional and behavioural difficulties. *Social Science & Medicine*, 70(12), 2052–2060.

Sun, C., Hon, C. K. H., Way, K. A., Jimmieson, N. L., & Xia, B. (2022). The relationship between psychosocial hazards and mental health in the construction industry: A meta-analysis. *Safety Science,* 145, 105485.

Turner, M., & Lingard, H. (2016). Improving workers' health in project-based work: job security considerations. *International Journal of Managing Projects in Business*, 9(3), 606–623.

Van Vegchel, N., De Jonge, J., Bosma, H., & Schaufeli, W. (2005). Reviewing the effort–reward imbalance model: Drawing up the balance of 45 empirical studies. *Social Science & Medicine*, 60(5), 1117–1131.

Victorian Government (2022). *Respect Code Building and Construction Industry.* Accessed 9 September 2022 from: www.vic.gov.au/respect-code-building-and-construction-industry

Welsh, J., Strazdins, L., Charlesworth, S., Kulik, C. T., & Butterworth, P. (2016). Health or harm? A cohort study of the importance of job quality in extended workforce participation by older adults. *BMC Public Health*, 16(1), 1–14.

Zaniboni, S., Truxillo, D. M., Rineer, J. R., Bodner, T. E., Hammer, L. B., & Krainer, M. (2016). Relating age, decision authority, job satisfaction, and mental health: a study of construction workers. *Work, Aging and Retirement*, 2(4), 428–435.

4

WORKING TIME, HEALTH AND WELLBEING

4.1 Introduction

This chapter will discuss different approaches to working time and their associated effects on the health and wellbeing of workers in the Australian construction industry. It will review how time is understood in project-based construction work, and look at the connection between long work hours and health and wellbeing and consider the effects of long hours in the construction context. It will also outline the factors related to balancing time spent at work (or on work-related activities) and non–work activities and consider the role played by gender in shaping workers' experiences of balancing work and non-work life. The chapter considers the way that work hours are distributed over the working week and explores alternative ways of scheduling work that may help construction workers to achieve a better life balance. These alternatives include a compressed working week operating between Monday and Friday, or reduced working hours during Monday to Friday and offset with working on Saturday. The right to disconnect from the pressures and activity of work after leaving the worksite is discussed, as are the new-found flexible working regimes that have become normalised during the COVID-19 pandemic. The chapter ends with a consideration of the factors that shape working time within the construction industry.

4.2 Time in project-based construction work

Time performance (i.e., completion of work to a pre-determined timeline) is considered an essential determinant of success in construction projects (Serrador & Turner, 2015). Soderlund (2005) argues that project deadlines are a "fundamental organisational rationale for project organising" (p.381) and project

DOI: 10.1201/9780367814236-4

management teams play a role in setting the pace of work, changing the time orientations of workers to respond to project milestones, and monitoring the "rhythms" of the project to identify and resolve activities that may be out of step with requirements. Soderlund (2005) acknowledges that the work of project managers involves putting pressure on project participants to ensure timelines are met, which can create the feeling that project-based work is "constantly under time pressure" (p.384). Furthermore, when unexpected project events threaten time-related goal attainment, workers experience this as stressful (Gällstedt, 2003). Limited time resources affect project workers' wellbeing (Nordqvist et al., 2004) and create psychological distress (Zika-Viktorsson et al., 2006). Unexpected delays can also contribute to an intensification of work, increase required work pace, and have a damaging impact on workers' health (Tuchsen et al., 2005).

4.3   Long work hours, health and wellbeing

Long hours of work have important implications for work–life balance, mental and physical health (Charlesworth et al., 2011; Fagan & Walthery, 2011). For example, long hours are associated with heightened stress, burnout, anxiety and depression (Artazcoz et al., 2009; Bannai & Tamakoshi, 2014; Dinh et al., 2017). Australian research by Milner et al. (2017) reports that long, inflexible and unsocial hours contribute to the high suicide rates experienced in the construction industry. Multiple studies have also found a direct link between long work hours and chronic diseases, such as cardiovascular disease and diabetes (Van der Hulst, 2003; Artazcoz et al., 2009). Importantly, in 2021 the World Health Organization and International Labour Organization published research indicating that, in 2016, 398,000 people died from stroke and 347,000 from heart disease as a result of having worked at least 55 hours a week. Moreover, the number of deaths from heart disease and stroke due to working long hours increased by 42 and 19 per cent respectively between 2000 and 2016 (World Health Organization, 2021).

Furthermore, the risk of workplace injury increases as work hours rise due to fatigue and burnout (Dembe et al., 2005; Kecklund, 2005; Dong, 2005). Lombardi et al. (2010) found that rates of workplace injury increased from 2.03 per 100 workers for those working less than 20 hours per week to 3.71 for 50–60 hours, and 4.34 for those working more than 100 hours per week (Lombardi et al., 2010). In the USA, research shows that construction workers working more than eight hours per day were 1.57 times more likely to be injured than those working between seven and eight hours per day (Dong, 2005).

Health-related impacts of long hours are attributed to:

(i) less time to recover from work,
(ii) longer exposure to work-related hazards, and
(iii) interference with time spent in non-work activities (Caruso, 2006).

However, the relationship between work hours and health is not simple and linear. Up to a certain point, paid work hours contribute to good health. Employment provides income required to support health and wellbeing and provides the opportunity for regular social interactions and the creation of shared experiences with people outside the family (Australian Government Productivity Commission, 2019). However, once work hours become long or excessive both physical and mental health can be negatively affected. There are only 24 hours each day, so working long hours shifts time away from care, sleep, exercise and healthy eating, which, in turn, can have adverse social, psychological and physical impacts. Long work hours therefore reduce time allocated to health and reduce participation in beneficial health behaviours. It is noteworthy that long work hours are one of the biggest barriers to healthy eating and physical activity and contribute to time scarcity (Venn & Strazdins, 2017). Devine et al. (2007) report that the time-demands of work interfere with family meals and healthy food choices in a sample of construction labourers. In particular, the experience of negative spillover between work and family life was associated with lower consumption of fruit and vegetables. In the Australian construction context, Lingard and Turner (2015) report that time scarcity impeded healthy eating and physical exercise among project-based workers, even in the context of an organisational health promotion programme focused on improving diet and exercise.

4.4 Long hours of work in construction

Work hours in project-based construction work are notoriously long (Lingard et al., 2010a), particularly in large public infrastructure construction projects which often work "around the clock" to optimise the use of machinery (Personn et al., 2006; Tuschen et al., 2005). Long work hours and overtime work have also been linked to stress at work and at home, fatigue, disrupted sleep, insufficient recovery opportunity and productivity losses in project-based construction work (Beswick et al., 2007; Goldenhar et al., 2003; Alvanchi et al., 2012).

Importantly, long hours of work in construction projects are experienced in conjunction with work overload and poor work–life balance. For example, a report undertaken on behalf of the Chartered Institute of Building (UK) revealed that construction industry workers are worse off than workers in other industries in terms of experiencing higher:

- poor work–life balance
- high workload
- excessive travel time
- technology overload
- unrealistic deadlines (Cattell et al., 2017).

4.5   The balance between work and non-work life

Work–life imbalance is a risk factor for poor health. Kossek et al. (2014) argue that work–life balance is a key component of wellbeing that is important for a sustainable workforce. However, achieving a balance between work and participation in other life domains is difficult in the context of long work hours, inflexible work schedules, demanding, intensive work and a lack of autonomy experienced by workers (Cooklin et al., 2016).

Work–family conflict (WFC), defined as "a form of interrole conflict in which role pressures from the work and family domains are mutually incompatible in some respect" (Greenhaus & Beutell, 1985, p.77) has been consistently linked to indicators of poor health and wellbeing, including job dissatisfaction, life dissatisfaction, turnover intention, general wellbeing, psychological strain, psychiatric disorders, substance abuse and problem drinking (Netemeyer et al., 1996; Boyar et al., 2003; O'Driscoll et al., 2003; Grant-Vallone & Donaldson, 2001; Hammer et al., 2004; Frone, 2000; Grzywacz & Marks, 2000; Allen et al., 2000; Wang et al., 2007).

Cooklin et al. (2016) studied the relationship between mental health and WFC, using a large longitudinal data set collected in Australia. They analysed changes in the experience of WFC over time in relation to mental health experiences. Cooklin et al. (2016) report that Australian working men and women who get "trapped" in a situation of chronic WFC have the lowest levels of mental health, while those who report they "never" experience WFC had the best mental health scores. Men and women who move into a situation of WFC experienced deteriorating mental health, while those who move out of a situation of WFC experience significant improvements in mental health.

In the construction industry, levels of WFC are high (Lingard et al., 2010b). As in other sectors, construction workers who experience high levels of WFC are more likely to experience psychological distress, depression, anxiety, sleep problems, and negative attitudes towards mental health (Bowen et al., 2018; Kotera et al., 2020). Construction workers experiencing WFC also report higher levels of substance misuse and marital dissatisfaction (Tijani et al., 2021).

4.6   The gendered nature of work hours and health

Research suggests that long work hours affect men and women workers differently and reinforce gender and health inequality in industries like construction (Galea et al., 2018). Drawing on data from a large representative sample of Australians in paid work, Dinh et al. (2017) considered the interaction between work hours, gender and health. They found that across all workforce groups, working some time was good for mental health. These benefits arise because jobs provide income, as well as a sense of identity, security, status and inclusion. However, the positive relationship between work hours and mental health only applied up to a threshold limit of 39 hours of paid work per week. When workers worked more than 39 hours a week, their mental health declined. The relationship between work hours and mental health was therefore shaped like an inverted letter "U."

Importantly, the tipping point for women was 34 hours per week, considerably less than it was for men who could work up to 47 hours a week before they experienced any negative impacts to their mental health. This 13-hour difference in weekly work hours means that the average Australian man can work 13 hours more each week than the average Australian woman before mental health is negatively affected. Dinh et al. (2017) explain this in terms of the fact that women are more likely to combine paid work with unpaid care and domestic work. Long hours therefore serve to reinforce traditional gender roles and the division of labour between paid work and care.

The research undertaken by Dinh et al. (2017) also shows that "unencumbered" workers, who do not have responsibility for the care of others and perform minimal domestic work, are able to work more hours before this affects their mental health, irrespective of their gender. Therefore, it is not being a man or a woman that determines the number of hours one can work before mental health deteriorates. Rather, the key determinant is the amount of domestic or care work that someone performs.

Case example 4.1 highlights how women working in construction can be affected by the expectation of long work hours, and how flexible work arrangements have been implemented in construction workplaces to help workers with caring responsibilities.

CASE EXAMPLE 4.1 LENGTH AND FLEXIBILITY OF WORK HOURS IN CONSTRUCTION

Interviews with leaders in the Australian construction industry (undertaken during an investigation of factors influencing mental health in the construction industry) suggest that women in project-based construction roles experience difficulty in juggling long work hours with family responsibility. One industry leader explained: "*I think it stops women entering the industry because they look at it and go, 'Why do I want to work in that industry when I can work somewhere else? And I can't see that I can have a family and be on site and do the hours and still be a mum', which is really sad.*" Another commented: "*So our women report that they love working on site but they cannot see how they can continue to do site-based roles and be a parent.*" However, the industry leaders also noted that some construction companies have implemented flexible work arrangements to support workers with family/caring responsibilities. While the industry leaders stressed that flexible working arrangements are important for men as well as women workers, some cultural barriers prevent men from requesting flexibility to fulfil family obligations: *"We're making sure that the men feel that they can adopt the flexibility programmes as much as the females because ... if you're a female and you say 'I have to leave work to pick up the kids or be with the kids' it's a somewhat more socially acceptable thing to do than, rather than the male that says 'I'm leaving work so I can have dinner with my family' ... So we're trying to break down those barriers."*

The International Labour Organization's (ILO) definition of 48 hours as the safe limit up to which people should work was set in 1919, when the labour market was almost entirely men and families operated on a "man breadwinner–woman homemaker model." Consequently, this work-time threshold did not consider the impacts of domestic or care work. Given emerging evidence that the ILO threshold is not appropriate for a gender-balanced workforce, it should be reconsidered in the interests of protecting the health and wellbeing of all workers with domestic or caring responsibilities. Curbing long work hours and providing greater flexibility can help to improve gender equality and mental health and wellbeing in "long hours" industries like construction.

4.7 Other facets of working time with relevance to health

Working long hours is not the only facet of working time that can affect workers' health and wellbeing (Burke et al., 2010; Strazdins et al., 2011). For example, Adam (1995) identifies the *tempo* and *timing* of work as facets of working time with the potential to affect health and wellbeing. The tempo of work refers to the number of activities to be conducted within a specific timeframe and is sometimes referred to as work pace or intensity. The timing of work reflects when work is scheduled and, in particular, the extent to which the timing of work is compatible with the timing of other life activities, e.g., family routines (Tammelin, 2018).

Hallberg's concept of "synchronous leisure" references the need for work-place strategies to synchronise working time with the different schedules of family carers, especially in the context of dual earner couples with dependent care responsibilities (Hallberg, 2003). When one or both carers are engaged in atypical work schedules that cause involuntary desynchronisations, juggling caring responsibilities is particularly challenging (Brown et al., 2011). In most cases, women workers bear the brunt of these challenges, often being forced to choose between (paid) work and (unpaid) caring. For example, in a study of dual earner couples in which at least one partner worked in the construction industry, Lingard and Francis (2008) describe how adaptive strategies used by couples to cope with long, inflexible work hours are highly gendered. In the majority of cases, women construction workers, or women partners of construction workers choose to reduce their involvement in paid work, thereby perpetuating gender pay gaps and inequality in economic security.

Both tempo and timing of work have been linked to workers' health experiences. For example, increases in work pace associated with lean production management processes have been linked to psychosocial risk factors at work (Koukoulaki, 2014). In addition, workers' wellbeing is reported to be negatively affected if work is scheduled at times that do not fit well with workers' family commitments and personal preferences (Golden et al., 2011). Kristensen et al. (2004) also observe interdependencies between work time, tempo and timing, such that a heavy workload and/or tight deadlines create pressures to work faster, as well as a need to work longer or non-standard hours.

A final facet of work time that has the potential to impact health and wellbeing is the degree to which workers have control over their working time. Härmä (2006) argues that control over work quantity, schedule, pace of work and when rest breaks can be taken are important determinants of wellbeing. This position is also empirically supported by research that shows that negative impacts of overtime on wellbeing, sleep and depressive symptoms depend on whether workers have control over their working hours or schedule (Beckers et al., 2008; Takahashi et al., 2011).

Case example 4.2 reflects data collected from project-based workers in the Australian construction industry. It reflects the extent to which project pressures necessitate long hours of work and the extent to which weekend work is disruptive to family life. It also suggests that low levels of work-schedule control and feelings of being constantly under pressure affect individuals' satisfaction and their long-term commitment to remaining in the construction industry.

CASE EXAMPLE 4.2 LONG WORK HOURS, WORK–LIFE IMBALANCE AND WORK ABILITY AT A ROAD CONSTRUCTION PROJECT

Working time, health and wellbeing experiences of workers working on an upgrade of a major arterial road in a major city in Australia were examined. Survey data was collected on work demands, including working time, work–family conflict and work ability. Work ability is often used to understand wellbeing in the workplace. The concept of work ability was developed by Professor Juhani Ilmarinen in the early 1980s at the Finnish Institute of Occupational Health. It reflects the extent to which a worker's physical and psychological health, as well as social and environmental factors (including working conditions, work and spare time activities), affect the ability to work (Ilmarinen et al., 2015). The majority of survey respondents were professional or managerial workers, rather than manual construction workers.

The average weekly working hours reported by survey participants was 57.6 and average weekly commuting time was 6.9 hours per week. Weekly work hours were significantly and negatively correlated with aspects of work ability, i.e., working conditions, organisation of work, work community and management, and work and non-work activities. This suggests that working long hours significantly affects the environmental and social components of work ability, reducing participants' self-reported ability to work. The survey also revealed that longer weekly work hours were associated with higher reported time- and strain-based work interference with family life. Comments provided by 13 participants on the handwritten survey forms further indicate that long weekly work hours contribute to poor work–life balance, work stress and diminished wellbeing. One participant explained: "*I leave my house at 4.40am and get home 6.45pm onwards.*" Long hours reduced time available for family life: "*Given the long hours/ early starts required on site, I spend limited time with my family during the week.*" Weekend work was identified as being particularly problematic and participants explained that their families were negatively affected: "*One of the biggest issues is weekend work, this really impacts on work/family balance. Long days during the week are manageable, but the weekends really impact both myself and my family.*"

Participants described how unexpected project events create a high-pressure work environment: "*Constantly reacting to changes with time implications means always putting out fires and constantly running on adrenaline*" and time pressure was unrelenting: "*[T]he construction machine keeps turning regardless of whether I have time. Any setbacks/things take longer, etc., increase my workload but we have no additional resources to get us back on track. This leads to rushing/corner cutting and mistakes, thus chewing up additional time.*" The comments also revealed that opportunities for rest and recovery are limited due to resource constraints: "*The workload is not manageable by the small team we have for a 24/7 job.* [The] *culture for taking days in lieu is not there after working 80-hour weeks. Lack of resources therefore no coverage to take a day off.*" Limited resources also created a culture of presenteeism (i.e., remaining at work when unwell or needing a break to recover from work) because: "*No one picks up work when* [someone is] *away sick. Work just builds up – more work when returning.* [I] *put off taking needed sick or annual leave.*" Although the company involved in delivering this project had instigated wellbeing days (a quarterly day off for recovery), survey participants commented that the effectiveness of these recovery days was reduced by project-related time pressures: "*Wellbeing days can seem a little useless when all it does is put you under more pressure for the rest of the week.*"

Eight participants participated in follow-up interviews that explored in more depth the demands that they experience at work, home and in general life. The demands identified as posing the greatest problems for participants occurred in the work domain and many were time-related, such as time spent in paid work and overtime hours, or else related to workload and/or normative expectations of long work hours. Only one home-based demand was identified as being particularly challenging for the interview participants (i.e., time spent in household chores), although this was generally not considered to be as challenging as the work-related time demands. It is important to note that six of the eight interview participants were men and home-related demands may be experienced differently among professional/managerial women working in the construction industry.

The interview participants observed that long work hours are an entrenched component of the construction industry's culture and practice: "*I work 58–60 hours per week. There is an industry expectation of long hours. I have worked in the industry for 35 years and nothing has changed.*" Participants described how working long hours reduces their ability to participate in healthy activities outside work, including sport and social activities: "*I lose opportunities for things outside of work, sports and travel. I can't do what a normal guy in his mid-twenties would do due to work hours. I'm too tired to see friends after work.*" Engaging in health-promoting recovery activities is important and, when long work hours prevent people from psychologically detaching from work and relaxing, stress levels increase: "*Time at work means less time doing what I like – exercising and socialising. I used to play tennis weekly but* [that has] *dropped off, as has my running. However, exercise helps to manage my stress. And stress keeps me awake at night.*"

The interview participants suggested that long work hours required of project-based construction work are complicated and can be attributed to more systemic characteristics of the construction industry's supply arrangements, including clients' demands and expectations: "*I am running on adrenaline with high pressure, high workload, and expectations from the client.*" This was often driven by the client's focus on maintaining traffic flows as the contract with the client stipulated that the major arterial road being upgraded must remain open during the construction project. Interview participants' comments suggested that the lack of control they experience in relation to the work schedule (which is driven by traffic conditions) exacerbated the stress associated with long hours of work at the project. One participant commented: "*Travel volume and client demands drive work schedule. Work hours are often up in the air until the last minute.*" Another participant observed: "*There are constantly programme changes. If we are ahead of schedule, they draw in the schedule. So, if you think you have some breathing space, they bring the time forward.*"

The links to work ability were also reflected in interview participants' comments, with long working hours identified as the reason people leave the construction industry: "*Long hours are not sustainable for me in the long term. I will opt out and have planned my exit plan. A lot of the guys I know in the industry will also opt out and have their exit plan. It's a common thing.*"

4.8 Taxonomy of work schedules: Long hours, overtime and work schedule control

In a 2019 study, Brauner et al. outlined a taxonomy for the design of sustainable work schedules by considering working-time demands (the amount of physical and mental exertion required) in relation to working-time control (an individual's autonomy over the duration/timing of their work). By analysing data from the 2015 BAuA-Working Time Survey of the Federal Institute for Occupational Safety and Health in Germany, Brauner et al. identified six different classes of work schedules:

1. **Flexible extended.** This class did not work shifts but had a high probability of occasionally working on weekends and working overtime (high working-time demands/high working-time control).
2. **Extended shift.** This class had the highest probability of shift work and working overtime (high working-time demands/low working-time control).
3. **Rigid standard.** This class had the lowest probabilities of over-long working hours, frequent change in working hours and control over the beginning/end of work days (low working-time demands/low working-time control)
4. **Flexible standard.** This class had the lowest probability of working on weekends and were very likely to have control over the beginning/end of workdays and taking hours off (low working-time demands/high working-time control)
5. **Rigid all-week.** This class had the highest probability of working on weekends and were unlikely to have control over the beginning/end of workdays and taking hours off (high working-time demands/low working-time control)
6. **Rigid extended.** This class did not work shifts, but were likely to work overtime and on weekends (high working-time demands/low working-time control) (Brauner et al., 2019).

Brauner et al. note that workers with schedules that allowed for high working time control perceived increased health benefits. Of these six classes, "extended shift," "rigid all-week" and "rigid extended" are all characterised by high demand and low control, and can thus be considered as high-strain risk groups (Brauner et al., 2019). Workers in these three risk groups reported the worst health results, as well as the lowest satisfaction regarding balance between work and non-work lives (Brauner et al., 2019). As highlighted in case example 4.2, project-based construction work can be characterised by long work hours, weekend work and low levels of work-schedule control. These characteristics in combination are therefore likely to negatively affect workers' health.

4.9 Working time modifications and reductions

At an organisation or project level, a variety of models have been adopted with the aim of reducing or modifying work hours. Broadly, these include the following:

- reducing the work week, e.g., compressing the work week by reducing the number of days worked each week;
- reducing daily work hours, e.g., reducing the length of work shifts;
- reducing the work month, e.g., working three longer weeks followed by a week off;
- reducing the work year, e.g., introducing additional free time such as annual leave.

Compressed work weeks often redistribute rather than reduce hours, such that the length of the workday is increased, but the number of days worked per week is decreased. Thus, the compressed work week departs from a standard eight-hour working day, traditionally favoured by trade unions, although a cap may still be applied to the number of hours worked each week. Compressed work weeks can take different forms.

Bambra et al. (2008) identify three popular forms as follows:

- 12-hour compressed work week, which involves four 12-hour shifts (day, night) over four days with three or four days off;
- 10-hour compressed work week, which involves four 10-hour shifts followed by three days off;
- the Ottawa system, which involves three or four 10-hour morning or after-noon shifts spread over four days, then two days off. This is then followed by a block of seven 8-hour nights, then six days off.

Given the variety of different forms of compressing the work week, it is perhaps unsurprising that the health benefits associated with compressed work weeks are mixed (Bambra et al., 2008).

One of the critical factors associated with the introduction of working-time reductions or modifications is who bears the costs associated with the changes. In some instances, work-hour reductions for people who are paid by the hour have been accompanied by a commensurate reduction in pay. For example, in 1993, Volkswagen introduced a scheme to reduce work hours to avoid mass redun-dancies during an economic downturn. Weekly hours were reduced from 36 to 28.5 with a corresponding loss of income amounting to a 20 per cent decrease in pay. In order to offset the financial impact, the union negotiated a small increase in the hourly wage of workers as well as increased holiday pay and an annual bonus. However, even with these modifications, annual wages were reduced by 16 per cent (De Spiegelaere & Piasna, 2017). Workers' health and wellbeing were reported to be negatively affected by the changes (De Spiegelaere & Piasna,

2017). In particular, high levels of stress were reported by 75 per cent of the workforce and were particularly prevalent in "white collar" workers (Seifert & Trinczek, 2000).

In some instances, work-hour reductions have been implemented without any reduction in remuneration. Under these arrangements total work hours are reduced but wages are maintained, such that the worker does not incur any financial loss. The costs to business of this strategy are higher, although these costs may be offset by productivity increases and, in some instances, government incentives or subsidies.

One example of a reduction in work hours with no loss of pay occurred at a New Zealand firm that manages company trusts, Perpetual Guardian, in early 2018 (Graham-McLay, 2018). The initiative involved the introduction of a four-day work week, reducing work hours from 37.5 to 30 per week. All other employment conditions, including pay levels, remained unchanged during this six-week trial.

In an assessment of the initiative, Haar (2022) notes that significant improvements were observed in key areas of perceptions of organisational and supervisor support, teamwork, work–life balance, job attitudes, engagement, retention and wellbeing, following the implementation of the four-day week. Workers also reported significantly reduced job demands and stress, and 78 per cent of staff reporting that they were able to balance work and home commitments (compared to 54 per cent before the change in work hours).

4.10 Working-time modifications in the Australian construction industry

The sensitivity of workers to the costs associated with reducing or modifying working time was evident in a series of projects undertaken in the construction industry in Queensland. The different effects of working time modifications or reductions were highlighted in the construction industry in which various project working-time regimes were introduced and evaluated as part of a research project examining the work–life balance experiences of project-based workers.

Project 1

Project 1 implemented a compressed work week at a water infrastructure construction project (a dam upgrade). The compressed work week involved eliminating an 8-hour Saturday shift but extending the working hours from Monday to Friday from 10 to 11.5 hours in the summer months. In winter months the daily work hours were reduced from 11.5 to 10.5 (Lingard et al., 2007). Data was only collected following the implementation of the compressed work week, so no before-and-after comparisons could be made. However, data was also collected from a control group of workers engaged at another construction site being delivered by the construction company involved in project delivery. The control site was working a standard six-day week (Lingard et al., 2007).

A total of 42 workers (23 waged and 19 salaried) completed a survey to gauge their preferences for the compressed work week, as well as their wellbeing, satisfaction with balance between work and non-work life, and perceptions of work–life conflict. Self-reported wellbeing and satisfaction with balance between work and non-work life were generally high. On a 7-point scale, with "7" representing the highest level of wellbeing and "1" representing the lowest level of wellbeing, salaried workers' mean wellbeing rating was 5.4 and waged workers' mean wellbeing rating was 5.5. Both waged and salaried workers at Project 1 also reported high levels of satisfaction with their work life, their non-work life, and the balance between their work and non-work lives. Workers indicated a preference for the five-day week with an average preference score of 1.8, scored on a 7-point scale, where "1" reflected a "very strongly prefer five-day week" and "7" reflected a "very strongly prefer six-day week." No salaried workers but a small number of waged workers indicated they preferred a six-day week.

Interview data in Project 1 supported the benefits of the compressed work week on work–family interaction. Interviews with workers at the six-day week comparison site reported lower levels of satisfaction with the balance between their work and non-work life than at Project 1 working a compressed week.

Project 1 was also completed six months ahead of schedule and significantly under budget. The project manager indicated he thought the compressed work week had improved workers' morale, commitment to the project, and health and safety performance, and reduced the incidence of workplace disputes (both with the union and between individuals).

Project 2

Project 2 implemented a five-day week in another water infrastructure construction project. At this project, the leadership team was focused on improving work–life balance and modified the project schedule from a traditional six-day week to a compulsory five-day week (10-hour shifts daily between Monday and Friday).

Anecdotal evidence suggested that waged workers at the project were not happy with the impact of the change on their remuneration as they lost out on penalty rates paid for work on Saturdays ("time and a half" for the first four hours and "double time" thereafter for Saturday work). The project management team observed that many (approximately 30 per cent) of the waged workers left the site to work at other projects where they could continue to earn penalty rates on Saturdays. Anecdotally, this left less skilled and inexperienced workers at Project 2 which affected productivity and performance. In response, the change to the five-day week was not sustained and the leadership team decided to revert to a six-day work week. However, salaried workers were permitted to have alternate Saturdays off.

Townsend et al. (2012) report that, although waged workers recognised that not working on Saturdays provided them with substantial benefits, including mental and physical recovery and time to spend with their family or engage in non-work activities, many of these waged workers were unhappy about the impact on their weekly remuneration. In contrast, salaried workers, for whom working on Saturday did not attract overtime payments or penalty rates, strongly favoured the five-day week. Townsend et al. (2012) conclude that negotiating and implementing modified working-time arrangements in the construction industry is complicated due to the presence of two distinct groups of workers: salaried workers and waged workers. These groups were observed to have conflicting motivations and interests with regard to reducing work hours and eliminating weekend work.

Project 3

Project 3 involved a road construction project. At this project, survey data was collected from workers before and after the implementation of a compressed work week. A baseline survey was completed by 95 workers at Project 3 before the site changed from a six-day to a five-day working week. The revised roster followed a four-week cycle, such that workers enjoyed two "two-day" weekends, one "one-day" weekend, and one "three-day" weekend every four weeks. Site hours were extended to 6.30am to 5pm on weekdays (a 30-minute earlier start time) and from 6.30am to 3pm on the one Saturday worked each month. Follow-up surveys were conducted to determine whether work–life experiences were different under the new roster. A statistically significant reduction in perceived work-to-home conflict between the baseline and follow-up surveys was found (Lingard et al., 2008).

Qualitative data collected at Project 3 before the introduction of the compressed work week revealed concerns that work negatively affected non-work life among waged and salaried workers. Follow-up interviews revealed that waged and salaried workers were generally happy with the revised working time arrangements, although waged workers still indicated concerns about loss of pay associated with giving up regular Saturday work (Townsend et al., 2011).

Project 4

Project 4 involved another road construction project. At the commencement of the study, the site was working a standard six-day week. Workers at Project 4 were surveyed before the introduction of a modified work schedule to identify their baseline perceptions of the balance they experienced between their work and non-work life. The survey data indicated that most workers at Project 4 believed that their home life did not interfere with work to a great extent, but their work life was perceived to interfere with home life to a far greater extent.

The project leadership team decided to introduce a five-day week. However, although Project 4 was ahead of schedule, the managers were concerned that moving to a five-day week would negatively affect production. In response the five-day week was optional and only available to workers who could demonstrate a "personal need" for the change. To utilise the option, workers also had to demonstrate that their work would not be adversely affected by the changed work schedule. Unlike the compressed work week implemented at the other case study projects, work hours between Monday and Friday were not extended. This meant that waged workers who decided to work five days would be considerably impacted financially.

Fewer than 20 out of more than 300 workers engaged at Project 4 opted to change their work schedules. All workers who changed their schedule were salaried workers. Eight of those who made the change were interviewed after they had done so. Their comments suggest that work–life balance was not significantly improved and that the culture of long hours was maintained at Project 4.

These four case study projects highlight challenges inherent in modifying and especially reducing work hours in the Australian construction industry. Although the elimination of weekend work was viewed favourably by workers at the case study projects, the findings also reveal the existence of two distinct groups of workers within the Australian construction industry. These groups operate in distinct labour markets and experience modified work-time arrangements differently. Managerial, professional, administrative and supervisory workers are salaried, meaning that they are paid a fixed annual salary irrespective of the hours they work each week. In contrast, skilled and unskilled trade workers and labourers (manual/non-managerial workers) are paid an hourly wage. This is based upon an hourly rate up to a standard work week, above which penalty rates (usually one and a half times the standard hourly rate) are paid. This penalty rate also applies to weekend work. Capping hours of work between Monday and Friday and/or eliminating Saturday work has a different impact on remuneration for waged and salaried workers. Reducing work hours, particularly overtime and weekend work, will not change the amount of money earned by salaried workers but could substantially reduce the take-home pay of waged workers.

It is no coincidence that the projects at which the modified working time arrangements were most successful (Projects 1 and 3) opted to implement a compressed work week (i.e., lengthening the workday between Monday and Friday and eliminating Saturday work). This limited the extent to which waged workers' pay was reduced. In comparison, when a standard 10-hour day was maintained and Saturday work was eliminated (as was offered as an option in Project 4), the uptake of the offer was low and no waged workers opted to make the change. At Project 2 the compulsory change from a six-day week to a "10 hours x 5 day" schedule resulted in waged workers leaving the project to work at other projects at which a six-day week was still in place.

Similar unintended consequences were observed at the Thames Tideway Tunnel project in the United Kingdom, at which an initiative to reduce the length of shifts worked underground was not favourably received by all workers (see case example 4.3).

CASE EXAMPLE 4.3 MANAGING WORK HOURS AT THAMES TIDEWAY TUNNEL

The Thames Tideway Tunnel project involves constructing a 25 km tunnel for London's sewerage system to increase its capacity. The project comprises 21 sites along the tunnel route and involves an ambitious timeline with an expected completion date in 2023, allowing the asset to become operational in 2024.

At a very early stage of the project, the project team initiated an innovative health and safety management programme with a health and safety vison about "zero harm, zero incidents and zero compromise in delivering a transformational health and safety performance" (Simons, 2014). The programme involves regular reviews and reflections on health and safety on every site, developing health and safety plans (including a 24-week look ahead), immersive inductions for employees, early safety engagement and health and safety communication assessment.

The project team was particularly keen to manage fatigue. However, it was recognised that the health benefits of shorter work shifts would depend on how workers spent time away from work. Factors affecting the outcomes of working shorter shifts included where workers lived and therefore the distance they travelled to and from work and the way they chose to spend time away from work. While the workers who lived near the site were more accepting of shorter shifts, those who travelled a long distance to work preferred to work longer hours. By working 12-hour shifts, tunnelling workers could work shorter weeks, i.e., completing their work hours in fewer days, commute less and return home for a longer rest period. Working shorter shifts meant that workers needed to spend more time in rented accommodation. Being away from their family and friends, the workers spent their free time on social activities, spent more money on leisure and rested less. The consequence was increased worker dissatisfaction with the new working time arrangements. It was also reported that the reduced pay that workers received as a result of working shorter shifts made jobs at the project less attractive (Smale, 2018).

In 2018, Park Health (specialists in occupational hygiene and fatigue risk management) was engaged by the project team to effectively monitor the shift patterns, manage fatigue and explore the possibility of safely extending work shifts to 12 hours. Based on the analysis of the project data, it was decided to enforce a maximum ten-hour shift length instead of eight hours. It was specified that workers must not spend more than ten hours underground. The ten-hour shift included one hour pre-shift to prepare workers for healthy and safe work and a one-hour post-shift recovery period before leaving the worksite. Contractors needed to develop fatigue management plans and provide them to the project team to ensure measures were in place to prevent workers becoming overly tired.

Other factors to consider were shift rotation and the number of consecutive night shifts or day shifts that contractors worked. As shift rotations can increase fatigue, it was necessary to allocate recovery time to workers.

A key aspect of implementing the change was developing a positive culture of supporting wellbeing on the project which was reinforced by working closely with shift leaders and providing training to develop an awareness of their own fatigue management. As a representative from Park Health explained:

> *Reducing the length of a shift is not a silver bullet when it comes to managing fatigue. The social, cultural and financial needs of the workforce have to be considered alongside their personal wellbeing but, equally, it is the duty of every employee to ensure they get enough rest. An employer cannot make an employee sleep but recognising that and each of us taking responsibility for getting enough rest means we all contribute to a safer working environment for everyone.*
>
> Park Health, 2020

4.11 Recovery and the right to disconnect

Recovery has been identified as an important mechanism explaining how acute stress reactions arising from work can contribute to chronic health impairment (Geurts & Sonnentag, 2006). Insufficient recovery from work over an extended period has, for example, been linked to health status and cardiovascular death (Sluiter et al., 2001; Kivimäki et al., 2006). A need for recovery describes the "sense of urgency that people feel to take a break from their demands, when fatigue builds up" (Demerouti et al., 2009, p.107). Need for recovery has been linked to job demands, including certain types of shift systems and working-time arrangements (Demerouti et al., 2009). Workers who are high in need for recovery report significantly poorer health, and higher levels of insomnia, burnout, stress, depression, sickness absence and working while sick (presenteeism) than workers low in need for recovery (Wentz et al., 2020).

The importance of recovery is often explained by two complementary theories. These are: (i) the effort-recovery model; and (ii) the conservation of resources theory (Sonnentag, 2001).

According to the effort-recovery model (Meijman & Mulder, 1998), the effort spent while working creates load reactions (such as accelerated heart rate, elevated blood pressure and fatigue). In a healthy situation, stress-related load reactions return to pre-stressor levels during after-work hours when the body's physiological responses are changed from a state of activation to one of rest (Demerouti et al., 2009). Recovery occurs when stressors are no longer present and has been described as the process during which fatigue is reduced and a person's functioning returns to "a status of physiological and psychological performance readiness" (Demerouti et al., 2009, p. 91). If stress-related load reactions are reduced – through the recovery process – before the next work period (e.g., day or shift), health will not be negatively affected. However, if complete recovery cannot occur between work periods (for example in the case of long working hours, overtime or when demands continue after hours) a chronic load reaction can accumulate over time, and is a significant risk factor for impaired health and wellbeing (Sonnentag, 2001).

The underlying premise of the conservation of resources (COR) theory is that people seek to obtain, retain and protect resources, defined as "objects, personal characteristics and energies that are either themselves valued for survival, directly or indirectly, or that serve as a means of achieving these resources" (Hobfall, 1998, p.45). According to the COR theory, stress occurs when a person is threatened with resource loss, or fails to regain resources after effort expenditure. Unfavourable work situations can threaten or harm resources by depleting energy and vigour, increasing fatigue and tension, thereby negatively affecting health and functioning in other life domains (Grandey & Cropanzano, 1999). Taking a break from work can restore depleted resources or help people to gain new resources (Sanz-Vergel et al., 2010), thereby mitigating harmful impacts of resource loss. Time away from work enables people to invest time in restoring their resources, for example by engaging in restful or relaxing activities, looking after their health and fitness and drawing on sources of social support from friends and family (Sonnentag, 2001).

Research shows the importance of daily recovery between work hours, for health, wellbeing and performance (Derks & Bakker, 2014). Van Hooff et al. (2007) argue that after-work recovery opportunities may be inadequate in both quantity (amount of time available) and/or quality. The amount of time available for recovery can be affected by long hours of work, including overtime and engaging in weekend work. The quality of recovery can depend upon cognitive processes that prolong physiological activation to job stressors (Geurts & Sonnentag, 2006). For example, Geurts and Sonnentag (2006) describe how rumination, i.e., unintentionally thinking about past stressors or anticipating future stressors, impedes recovery (Demerouti et al., 2009). Being able to switch off and psychologically detach from work is reported to be more difficult when workers experience chronic time pressure (Sonnentag & Bayer, 2005).

The quality of recovery can also depend on what people do in their time away from work. For example, engaging in low-effort (e.g., watching television), social (e.g., meeting friends) or active (e.g., playing sport/exercising) leisure activities are reported to have positive effects on workers' overall evaluations of their wellbeing (Sonnentag, 2001). Van Hooff et al. (2007) report that jobs that require a high level of effort expenditure are associated with more overtime work and less engagement in active leisure (thereby affecting both the quantity and quality of recovery). High-effort jobs are also linked to higher levels of fatigue during evenings and weekends and lower sleep quality during the week (van Hooff et al., 2007). The importance of recovery is likely to be enhanced in jobs in which workers have limited opportunity to take sufficient rest breaks during the working day (Geurts & Sonnentag, 2006). Importantly, engaging in work-related activity after hours is reported to have a negative effect on well-being (Sonnentag, 2001).

How time participating in work and non-work activities is experienced by workers (i.e., whether it is experienced as pleasurable or effortful) is also reported to affect recovery. Van Hooff et al. (2011) report workers' feelings of recovery are enhanced when work and non-work activities are experienced as pleasurable. In contrast, when time spent at work is effortful and unpleasant, recovery is impeded, highlighting the importance of providing well-designed work (van Hooff et al., 2011).

Smartphones and other devices have increased the extent to which people can be interrupted during their non-work time. In some contexts, this may be essential (for example, for on-call workers). In other cases, organisational cultures may shape the acceptability of out-of-hours contact and/or the expectation that workers will respond to work-related matters in their personal time. However, the experience of work-to-home interference and burnout is more severe among workers who report high, compared to low, smartphone use after hours (Derks & Bakker, 2014).

To address the impact of technology on work hours and unpaid overtime, the French government legislated a "right to disconnect" in 2017. Under the French labour code, companies with more than 50 workers have to draw up a charter setting out the hours during which staff are not obliged to send or action emails and receive or return work-related calls (De Spiegelaere & Piasna, 2017). The law does not mandate specific procedures that should be enacted but requires that parties enter negotiations with respective unions to produce agreements protecting employees' right to disconnect (Brin, 2019). Other European countries are considering similar legislation. Most recently, the EU Parliament announced that it will increase efforts to protect employees' "fundamental right to disconnect from work and not be reachable outside work hours" (Butt, 2021, p.1). Noting that teleworking, especially during the COVID-19 pandemic, has blurred the distinction between work and private life, the European Commission is proposing regulation that would "establish minimum requirements for remote working and clarify working conditions, hours and rest periods" (Butt, 2021, p.1).

4.12 Conclusion

Long work hours are known to be harmful for workers, yet long and inflexible work hours have continued to be the norm in construction, where workers suffer from high levels of work–family conflict, burnout and fatigue. Construction organisations can implement work schedules that enable workers to spend quality time with family and allow for sufficient rest and recovery. Yet, taking a one-size-fits-all approach to work hours is problematic as different subsets of the construction workforce experience work hours and related impacts differently. Given the serious effects of long hours of work and low levels of control over working time on workers' health, construction organisations, clients, and unions are urged to take a collaborative approach to changing the long work hours culture of the industry so that workers' health is protected.

4.13   Discussion and review questions

1.   Why do construction organisations continue to require workers to work long hours with little control over their working time? Do you think this needs to change? What would need to change to support work hour reductions in project-based construction work?
2.   What are the types of harm created by long and inflexible hours of work? Should long hours be managed in the same way as other occupational health risks?
3.   Why do long and inflexible work hours affect workers in the construction industry differently? Consider the difference between men and women and waged and salaried workers. How can healthy working time regimes be designed and implemented to protect all workers equally?
4.   How can working time practices be modified so that workers do not experience harmful consequences?

4.14   Acknowledgements

Some of the work presented in this chapter was funded by the Construction Industry Leadership Forum. Some of the work in this chapter was also funded by the Australian Research Council (LP0560581) and the Construction Industry Institute of Australia.

References

Adam, B. (1995). *Timewatch: The Social Analysis of Time.* Cambridge.
Allen, T. D., Herst, D. E. L., Bruck, C. S., & Sutton, M. (2000). Consequences associated with work-to-family conflict: a review and agenda for future research. *Journal of Occupational Health Psychology,* 5(2), 278–308.
Alvanchi, A., Lee, S., & AbouRizk, S. (2012). Dynamics of working hours in construction. *Journal of Construction Engineering and Management,* 138(1), 66–77.
Artazcoz, L., Cortès, I., Escribà-Agüir, V., Cascant, L., & Villegas, R. (2009). Understanding the relationship of long working hours with health status and health-related behaviours. *Journal of Epidemiology & Community Health,* 63(7), 521–527.
Australian Government Productivity Commission. (2019). *Mental Health,* Draft Report, October 2019. Canberra.
Bambra, C., Whitehead, M., Sowden, A., Akers, J., & Petticrew, M. (2008). "A hard day's night?" The effects of Compressed Working Week interventions on the health

and work-life balance of shift workers: A systematic review. *Journal of Epidemiology & Community Health*, 62(9), 764–777.

Bannai, A., & Tamakoshi, A. (2014). The association between long working hours and health: a systematic review of epidemiological evidence. *Scandinavian Journal of Work, Environment & Health*, 40(1), 5–18.

Beckers, D. G., van der Linden, D., Smulders, P. G., Kompier, M. A., Taris, T. W., & Geurts, S. A. (2008). Voluntary or involuntary? Control over overtime and rewards for overtime in relation to fatigue and work satisfaction. *Work & Stress*, 22(1), 33–50.

Beswisk, J., Rogers, K., Corbett, E. Binch, S., & Jackson, K. (2007). *An Analysis of the Prevalence and Distribution of Stress in the Construction Industry*. Health and Safety Executive.

Bowen, P., Govender, R., Edwards, P., & Cattell, K. (2018). Work-related contact, work–family conflict, psychological distress and sleep problems experienced by construction professionals: An integrated explanatory model. *Construction Management and Economics*, 36(3), 153–174.

Boyar, S., Maertz, C., Pearson, A., & Keough, S. (2003). Work-family conflict: A model of linkages between work and family domain variables and turnover intentions. *Journal of Managerial Issues,* 15(2), 175–190.

Brauner, C., Wöhrmann, A., Frank, K., & Michel, A. (2019). Health and work-life balance across types of work schedules: A latent class analysis. *Applied Ergonomics*, 81, 1–10.

Brin, D. (2019). *France and Spain: Right to Disconnect Spreads*. Accessed 1 September 2022 from: www.shrm.org/resourcesandtools/legal-and-compliance/employment-law/pages/global-france-spain-right-to-disconnect.aspx

Brown, K., Bradley, L., Lingard, H., Townsend, K., & Ling, S. (2011). Labouring for leisure? Achieving work-life balance through compressed working weeks. *Annals of Leisure Research*, 14(1), 43–59.

Burke, R. J., Singh, P., & Fiksenbaum, L. (2010). Work intensity: Potential antecedents and consequences. *Personnel Review*, 39(3), 347–360.

Butt, J. (2021). *EU to protect the "Right to Disconnect" from Work*. Accessed 1 September 2022 from: https://myosh.com/blog/2021/02/12/europe-to-protect-the-right-to-disconnect-from-work/>.

Caruso, C. C. (2006). Possible broad impacts of long work hours. *Industrial Health*, 44(4), 531–536.

Cattell, K. S., Bowen, P. A., Cooper, C. L. & Edwards, P. J. (2017). The State of Well-Being in *the Construction Industry*. Chartered Institute of Building.

Charlesworth, S., Strazdins, L., O'Brien, L., & Sims, S. (2011). Parents' jobs in Australia: Work hours polarisation and the consequences for job quality and gender equality. *Australian Journal of Labour Economics*, 14(1), 35–57.

Cooklin, A. R., Dinh, H., Strazdins, L., Westrupp, E., Leach, L. S., & Nicholson, J. M. (2016). Change and stability in work–family conflict and mothers' and fathers' mental health: Longitudinal evidence from an Australian cohort. *Social Science & Medicine*, 155, 24–34.

De Spiegelaere, S., & Piasna, A. (2017). *The Why and How of Working Time Reduction*. European Trade Union Institute.

Dembe, A. E., Erickson, J. B., Delbos, R. G., & Banks, S. M. (2005). The impact of overtime and long work hours on occupational injuries and illnesses: New evidence from the United States. *Occupational and Environmental Medicine*, 62(9), 588–597.

Demerouti, E., Bakker, A. B., Geurts, S. A. E., & Taris, T. W. (2009). Daily recovery from work-related effort during non-work time. In S. Sonnentag, P. L. Perrewé, & D.

C. Ganster (Eds.), *Current Perspectives on Job-Stress Recovery*. Emerald Group Publishing (pp. 85–123).

Derks, D., & Bakker, A. B. (2014). Smartphone use, work–home interference, and burnout: A diary study on the role of recovery. *Applied Psychology*, 63(3), 411–440.

Devine, C., Stoddard, A., Barbeau, E., Naishadham, D., & Sorensen, G. (2007). Work-to-family spillover and fruit and vegetable: Consumption among construction laborers. *American Journal of Health Promotion*, 21(3), 175–182.

Dinh, H., Strazdins, L., & Welsh, J. (2017). Hour-glass ceilings: Work-hour thresholds, gendered health inequities. *Social Science & Medicine*, 176, 42–51.

Dong, X. (2005). Long workhours, work scheduling and work-related injuries among construction workers in the United States. *Scandinavian Journal of Work, Environment & Health*, 31(5), 329–335.

Fagan, C., & Walthery, P. (2011). Job quality and the perceived work-life balance fit between work hours and personal commitments: A comparison of parents and older workers in Europe. In S. Drobnič & A. Guillén (Eds.), *Work-Life Balance in Europe*. Palgrave Macmillan (pp. 69–94).

Frone, M. R. (2000). Work-family conflict and employee psychiatric disorders: The national comorbidity survey. *Journal of Applied Psychology*, 85(6), 888–895.

Galea, N., Powell, A., Loosemore, M., & Chappell, L. (2018). *Demolishing Gender Structures*. University of New South Wales.

Gällstedt, M. (2003). Working conditions in projects: Perceptions of stress and motivation among project team members and project managers. *International Journal of Project Management*, 21(6), 449–455.

Geurts, S. A., & Sonnentag, S. (2006). Recovery as an explanatory mechanism in the relation between acute stress reactions and chronic health impairment. *Scandinavian Journal of Work, Environment & Health*, 32(6), 482–492.

Golden, L., Wiens-Tuers, B., Lambert, S. J., & Henly, J. R., 2011. Working time in the employment relationship: Working time, perceived control and work-life balance. In K. Townsend and A. Wilkinson (Eds.), *Research Handbook on the Future of Work and Employment Relations*. Edward Elgar (pp. 188–211).

Goldenhar, L. M., Hecker, S., Moir, S., & Rosecrance, J. (2003). The "Goldilocks model" of overtime in construction: Not too much, not too little, but just right. *Journal of Safety Research*, 34(2), 215–226.

Graham-McLay, C. (2018). *A 4-day Workweek? A Test Run Shows a Surprising Result*. The New York Times. Accessed 2 September 2022 from: www.nytimes.com/2018/07/19/world/asia/four-day-workweek-new-zealand.html

Grandey, A. & Cropanzano, R. (1999). The conservation of resources model and work–family conflict and strain. *Journal of Vocational Behavior*, 54, 350–70.

Grant-Vallone, E. J., & Donaldson, S. I. (2001). Consequences of work-family conflict on employee well-being over time. *Work & Stress*, 15(3), 214–226.

Greenhaus, J. H., & Beutell, N. J. (1985). Sources of Conflict Between Work and Family Roles. *Academy of Management Review*, 10(1), 76–88.

Grzywacz, J. G., & Marks, N. F. (2000). Reconceptualizing the work-family Interface: An ecological perspective on the correlates of positive and negative spillover between work and family. *Journal of Occupational Health Psychology*, 5(1), 111–126.

Haar, J. (2022). Overview of the Perpetual Guardian 4-day (paid 5) Work Trial. www.4dayweek.com/research-prof-jarrod-haar-quantitative-research, accessed 27 September 2022.

Hallberg, D. (2003). Synchronous leisure, jointness and household labor supply. *Labour Economics*, 10(2), 185–203.

Hammer, T. H., Saksvik, P. O., Nytrø, K., H., T., & Bayazit, M. (2004). Expanding the psychosocial work environment: Workplace norms and work–family conflict as correlates of stress and health. *Journal of Occupational Health Psychology*, 9(1), 83–97.

Härmä, M. (2006). Workhours in relation to work stress, recovery and health. *Scandinavian Journal of Work, Environment & Health*, 32(6), 502–514.

Hobfoll, S. E. (1998). *Stress, Culture, and Community: The Psychology and Philosophy of Stress*. Plenum Press.

Ilmarinen, V., Ilmarinen, J., Huuhtanen, P., Louhevaara, V., & Näsman, O. (2015). Examining the factorial structure, measurement invariance and convergent and discriminant validity of a novel self-report measure of work ability: Work ability – personal radar. *Ergonomics*, 58(8), 1445–1460.

Kecklund, G. (2005). Long workhours are a safety risk – causes and practical legislative implications. *Scandinavian Journal of Work, Environment & Health*, 31(5), 325–327.

Kivimäki, M., Leino-Arjas, P., Kaila-Kangas, L., Luukkonen, R., Vahtera, J., Elovainio, M.,... & Kirjonen, J. (2006). Is incomplete recovery from work a risk marker of cardiovascular death? Prospective evidence from industrial employees. *Psychosomatic Medicine*, 68(3), 402–407.

Kossek, E. E., Valcour, M., & Lirio, P. (2014). Organizational strategies for promoting work–life balance and wellbeing. *Work and Wellbeing*, 3, 295–319.

Kotera, Y., Green, P., & Sheffield, D. (2020). Work-life balance of UK construction workers: relationship with mental health. *Construction Management and Economics*, 38(3), 291–303.

Koukoulaki, T. (2014). The impact of lean production on musculoskeletal and psychosocial risks: An examination of sociotechnical trends over 20 years. *Applied Ergonomics*, 45(2), 198–212.

Kristensen, T. S., Bjorner, J. B., Christensen, K. B., & Borg, V. (2004). The distinction between work pace and working hours in the measurement of quantitative demands at work. *Work & Stress*, 18(4), 305–322.

Lingard, H. C., Francis, V., & Turner, M. (2010a). The rhythms of project life: A longitudinal analysis of work hours and work–life experiences in construction. *Construction Management and Economics*, 28(10), 1085–1098.

Lingard, H., & Francis, V. (2008). An exploration of the adaptive strategies of working families in the Australian construction industry, *Engineering, Construction and Architectural Management*, 15(6), 562–579.

Lingard, H., & Turner, M. (2015). Improving the health of male, blue collar construction workers: A social ecological perspective. *Construction Management and Economics*, 33(1), 18–34.

Lingard, H., Brown, K., Bradley, L., Bailey, C., & Townsend, K. (2007). Improving employees' work-life balance in the construction industry: Project alliance case study. *Journal of Construction Engineering and Management*, 133(10), 807–815.

Lingard, H., Francis, V., & Turner, M. (2010b). Work-family conflict in construction: Case for a finer-grained analysis. *Journal of Construction Engineering and Management*, 136(11), 1196–1206.

Lingard, H., Townsend, K., Bradley, L., & Brown, K. (2008). Alternative work schedule interventions in the Australian construction industry: A comparative case study analysis. *Construction Management and Economics*, 26(10), 1101–111.

Lombardi, D. A., Folkard, S., Willetts, J. L., & Smith, G. S. (2010). Daily sleep, weekly working hours, and risk of work-related injury: US National Health Interview Survey (2004–2008). *Chronobiology International*, 27(5), 1013–1030.

Meijman, T. F., & Mulder, G. (1998). Psychological aspects of workload. In P. J. D. Drenth, & H. Thierry (Eds.), *Handbook of Work and Organizational Psychology*. Psychology Press (Vol. 2, pp. 5–33).

Milner, A., Spittal, M. J., Pirkis, J., Chastang, J. F., Niedhammer, I., & LaMontagne, A. D. (2017). Low control and high demands at work as risk factors for suicide: An Australian national population-level case-control study. *Psychosomatic Medicine*, 79(3), 358–364.

Netemeyer, R. G., Boles, J. S., & McMurrian, R. (1996). Development and validation of work-family conflict and family-work conflict scales. *Journal of Applied Psychology*, 81(4), 400–410.

Nordqvist, S., Hovmark, S., & Zika-Viktorsson, A. (2004). Perceived time pressure and social processes in project teams. *International Journal of Project Management*, 22(6), 463–468.

O'Driscoll, M. P., Poelmans, S., Spector, P. E., Kalliath, T., Allen, T. D., Cooper, C. L., & Sanchez, J. I. (2003). Family-responsive interventions, perceived organizational and supervisor support, work-family conflict, and psychological strain. *International Journal of Stress Management*, 10(4), 326.

Park Health. (2020). Shifting working hours to help stop fatigue. https://parkhs.co.uk/shifting-working-hours-to-help-stop-fatigue/, accessed 27 September 2022.

Persson, R., Helene Garde, A., Schibye, B., & Ørbæk, P. (2006). Building-site camps and extended work hours: A two-week monitoring of self-reported physical exertion, fatigue, and daytime sleepiness. *Chronobiology International*, 23(6), 1329–1345.

Sanz-Vergel, A. I., Demerouti, E., Moreno-Jiménez, B., & Mayo, M. (2010). Work-family balance and energy: A day-level study on recovery conditions. *Journal of Vocational Behavior*, 76(1), 118–130.

Seifert, H., & Trinczek, R. (2000). *New Approaches to Working Time Policy in Germany: The 28, 8 hour Working Week at Volkswagen Company*. WSI Working Papers, 80. Accessed 2 September 2022 from: www.econstor.eu/bitstream/10419/50479/1/314656324.pdf

Serrador, P., & Turner, R. (2015). The relationship between project success and project efficiency. *Project Management Journal*, 46(1), 30–39.

Simons, K. (2014). Karl Simons explains the health and safety approach at the Thames Tideway project. *Safety and Health Practitioner*, 12 November, 2014. Accessed 11 February 2023 from: www.shponline.co.uk/feature/tunnel-vision/.

Sluiter, J. K., Frings-Dresen, M. H., van der Beek, A. J., & Meijman, T. F. (2001). The relation between work-induced neuroendocrine reactivity and recovery, subjective need for recovery, and health status. *Journal of Psychosomatic Research*, 50(1), 29–37.

Smale, K. (2018). Changing Tunnellers' Shift Patterns. *New Civil Engineer*. Accessed 2 September 2022 from: www.newcivilengineer.com/archive/changing-tunnellers-shift-patterns-16-01-2018/

Soderlund, J. (2005). What project management really is about: alternative perspectives on the role and practice of project management. *International Journal of Technology Management*, 32(3–4), 371–387.

Sonnentag, S. (2001). Work, recovery activities, and individual well-being: A diary study. *Journal of Occupational Health Psychology*, 6(3), 196–210.

Sonnentag, S., & Bayer, U. V. (2005). Switching off mentally: Predictors and consequences of psychological detachment from work during off-job time. *Journal of Occupational Health Psychology*, 10(4), 393.

Strazdins, L., D'Souza, R. M., Clements, M., Broom, D. H., Rodgers, B., & Berry, H. L. (2011). Could better jobs improve mental health? A prospective study of change in work conditions and mental health in mid-aged adults. *Journal of Epidemiology & Community Health*, 65(6), 529–534.

Takahashi, M., Iwasaki, K., Sasaki, T., Kubo, T., Mori, I., & Otsuka, Y. (2011). Worktime control-dependent reductions in fatigue, sleep problems, and depression. *Applied Ergonomics*, 42(2), 244–250.

Tammelin, M. (2018). Introduction: Working time, family and wellbeing. In M. Tammelin (Ed.), *Family, Work and Well-being: Emergence of New Issues*. Springer (pp. 1–7).

Tijani, B., Xiaohua, J., & Osei-Kyei, R. (2021). Critical analysis of mental health research among construction project professionals. *Journal of Engineering, Design and Technology*, 19(2), 467–496.

Townsend, K., Lingard, H., Bradley, L., & Brown, K. (2011). Working time alterations within the Australian construction industry. *Personnel Review*, 40(1), 70–86.

Townsend, K., Lingard, H., Bradley, L., & Brown, K. (2012). Complicated working time arrangements: Construction industry case study. *Journal of Construction Engineering and Management*, 138(3), 443–448.

Tüchsen, F., Hannerz, H., & Spangenberg, S., 2005. Mortality and morbidity among bridge and tunnel construction workers who worked long hours and long days constructing the Great Belt Fixed Link. *Scandinavian Journal of Work, Environment & Health*, 31 (Supp. 2), 22–26.

Van der Hulst, M. (2003). Long work hours and health. *Scandinavian Journal of Work, Environment and Health*, 29, 171–188.

Van Hooff, M. L., Geurts, S. A., Beckers, D. G., & Kompier, M. A. (2011). Daily recovery from work: The role of activities, effort and pleasure. *Work & Stress*, 25(1), 55–74.

Van Hooff, M. L., Geurts, S. A., Kompier, M. A., & Taris, T. W. (2007). Workdays, in-between workdays and the weekend: A diary study on effort and recovery. *International Archives of Occupational and Environmental Health*, 80(7), 599–613.

Venn, D., & Strazdins, L. (2017). Your money or your time? How both types of scarcity matter to physical activity and healthy eating. *Social Science & Medicine*, 172, 98–106.

Wang, J. L., Afifi, T. O., Cox, B., & Sareen, J. (2007). Work-family conflict and mental disorders in the United States: Cross-sectional findings from the National Comorbidity Survey. *American Journal of Industrial Medicine*, 50(2), 143–149.

Wentz, K., Gyllensten, K., Sluiter, J. K., & Hagberg, M. (2020). Need for recovery in relation to effort from work and health in four occupations. *International Archives of Occupational and Environmental Health*, 93(2), 243–259.

World Health Organization. (2021). Long working hours increasing deaths from heart disease and stroke: WHO, ILO, www.who.int/news/item/17-05-2021-long-working-hours-increasing-deaths-from-heart-disease-and-stroke-who-ilo, Accessed 27 September 2022.

Zika-Viktorsson, A., Sundström, P., & Engwall, M. (2006). Project overload: An exploratory study of work and management in multi-project settings. *International Journal of Project Management*, 24(5), 385–394.

5

WOMEN'S HEALTH IN CONSTRUCTION

5.1 Introduction

We acknowledge that health is important for all workers, irrespective of gender. In this chapter we specifically respond to the call for more attention on the occupational health of women. Throughout the chapter we focus on the characteristics of work and the workplace and how they can be detrimental to health, particularly for women. We start the chapter by reviewing the health inequality of women from a societal perspective and how this is reflected in occupational health research. We consider gender as a social determinant of health, and how the health of women is affected by their status as a minority group in the male-dominated construction industry. We explore the discrimination–health relationship and how this manifests for women in construction. The psychosocial risk factor of bullying is considered, and the way in which gendered work hazards are perpetuated in the construction industry is outlined and their impact on health is identified. Finally, we explore how construction workplaces designed for males can have a detrimental impact on the health of women. Throughout the chapter we present case examples which illustrate how women in construction can experience work and how it impacts on their health.

5.2 Health inequality: A societal issue

The health of women working in construction has received less attention than the health of men, and this is reflective of a broader societal issue. As recently as 2021, an article was published by the Royal Australian College of General Practitioners (RACGP) (Burrowes, 2021, p.1) stating that "mentally, physically and biologically, men and women are simply not built the same way. It sounds

DOI: 10.1201/9780367814236-5

obvious, but we have only really begun to understand why. These differences have not been reflected accurately in the field of medicine." Burrowes (2021) draws attention to the point that women's health has been underresearched and underdiagnosed, and that women are at higher risk of some of the most challenging health conditions. For example, autoimmune diseases affect approximately 8 per cent of the global population but 78 per cent of those affected are women (Fairweather & Rose, 2004). Women are three times more likely than males to develop rheumatoid arthritis and four times more likely to be diagnosed with multiple sclerosis, an autoimmune disease that attacks the central nervous system (van Vollenhoven, 2009). Women make up two-thirds of people with Alzheimer's disease, and are three times more likely to have a heart attack than men. Women are at least twice as likely to suffer chronic pain conditions such as fibromyalgia, chronic fatigue syndrome and chronic Lyme disease (Burrowes, 2021). Conditions such as these are underresearched and often go undiagnosed and untreated (Dusenbery, 2018; Holdcroft, 2007). Another shortcoming is that gender is not considered in the study of many diseases. For example, women are less likely to experience the "classic" symptoms of a heart attack – symptoms that were discovered in research led by men, in which most of the participants were men (Lyons, 2018). Because the diagnosis method of a heart attack still favours male biology, many women experience a delayed diagnosis or a misdiagnosis and on average, women are diagnosed with heart disease 7–10 years later than men (Maas & Appelman, 2010).

Consistent with the gender bias apparent in medical research, gender bias also exists in the work domain. The deficit around women's occupational health is highlighted by the International Labour Office who state that:

> women's safety and health problems are frequently ignored or not accurately reflected in research and data collection. OSH [Occupational Safety and Health] inquiries seem to pay more attention to problems relating to male-dominated work, and the data collected by OSH institutions and research often fail to reflect adequately the illnesses and injuries that women experience.
>
> *2009, p.93*

The contention outlined by the International Labour Office (2009) is echoed by the European Agency for Safety and Health at Work who state that:

> work-related risks to women's safety and health have been underestimated and neglected compared to men's, regarding both research and prevention. This imbalance should be addressed in research, awareness-raising and prevention activities. Taking a gender-neutral approach in policy and legislation has contributed to less attention and fewer resources being directed towards work-related risks to women and their prevention.
>
> *2013, p.15*

Much of the extant research related to the health of the construction work-force is informed largely by male samples (Nwaogu et al., 2020; Johansson et al., 2019; Sinyai & Choi, 2020). The findings of Sinyai and Choi (2020) illustrate this point. A review of American construction occupational safety and health research published in high-impact, peer-reviewed academic journals between 2002 and 2016 found that less than 2 per cent of the 741 articles focused on women (Sinyai & Choi, 2020).

Research seeking to explore the health of women in construction is fur-ther hampered by workforce participation rates. Women in construction are acknowledged as an underrepresented group in construction. The proportion of women working in construction is low internationally, and little has changed in the past few decades (French & Strachan, 2017). The employment of women in the construction industry has fluctuated between 5 and 15 per cent of the total workforce globally over the last two decades, and the representation of women in craft and trade occupations is even lower (Hasan et al., 2021). For example, in 2020 only 1 per cent of trades and technician positions in the Australian con-struction industry were filled by women (Master Builders Association, 2021). This low figure is consistent across countries such as the UK and USA (French & Strachan, 2017; Slowey, 2019). In Canada, less than 4 per cent of women work in male-dominated trades (Weikle, 2019). The low number of women employed in construction presents researchers with challenges in obtaining sufficient sample sizes to enable viable analysis and results (for example: Stocks et al., 2010). It is probable that the low participation rates of women in construction contributes to the lack of occupational health research focused on the experience of women.

It is important to understand the occupational experiences of women as these differ from the experiences of men. For example, in a US-based study, the causes of non-fatal work-related injuries among men and women differed in several respects. Women suffered more from injuries caused by falls, slips and trips while men experienced twice as many transportation incidents as women. While incidents relating to exposure to hazardous substances increased among women between 2011 and 2013, they decreased among men during the same period. The most marked difference was in women's experience of injury arising from violence, which was substantially more prominent as a causal factor for non-fatal injury among women than among men (Rios et al., 2017). Workplace violence has also been a prominent cause of fatal workplace injury among women. Of concern, workplace homicides in which the victim was female were more likely to be committed by relatives (14 per cent for women and 1 per cent for men) or other personal acquaintances (11 per cent for women and 2 per cent for men) than when the victim was male (Rios et al., 2017).

When considering risks and outcomes related to occupational health, Laberge et al. (2020) argue that it is important to consider both sex and gender. This is because sex (biological differences) can be an important factor when physical or physiological components of work are being studied, while gender (social roles) is a factor when social, identity or power dimensions are being considered. Sex and gender can interact to contribute to avoidable morbidity and mortality (World Health Organization, 2010). For example, women are at a higher risk of depression which is influenced by their genetics and hormones; however, gender plays a significant relative risk.

Many studies in occupational health and safety treat sex/gender as a confounding variable, rather than an independent variable of importance, assuming that the underlying mechanisms shaping occupational health and safety outcomes are similar for males and females (Messing & Silverstein, 2009). Messing and Mager-Stellman (2006) argue that studies making simple comparisons between men and women's experiences without considering biological, social and environmental exposure parameters linked to gender can create the impression that female sex alone causes women to be more susceptible (or not) to particular work health or safety outcomes when other mechanisms are at play. This can potentially contribute to stereotyping and reinforce occupational segregation. Similarly, simply controlling for or treating gender as a confounding variable in research into work health and safety outcomes can mask important gender-related differences and reinforce gender-neutral policies. Therefore, it is important to examine in more detail the underlying biological and social mechanisms that contribute to differences in the work injury and illness experiences of men and women.

5.3   Gender as a social determinant of health

Evidence supports the link between people's health and the living and working conditions which form their social environment (Wilkinson & Marmot, 2003). Factors such as socioeconomic position, conditions of employment, power and social support, known collectively as the social determinants of health, act together to strengthen or undermine the health of individuals (Australian Institute of Health and Welfare, 2020). Using the social determinants of health as a framework, there is evidence that health and illness are not distributed equally, and that variations in health status generally follow a gradient, with overall health tending to improve with improvements in socioeconomic position (Australian Institute of Health and Welfare, 2016).

Gender is identified as a determinant of health (World Health Organization, 2010) due to access to and control over resources, power and decision making, and in roles and responsibilities. The socially constructed differences between women and men can lead to discrimination and inequalities for women. A policy or programme is considered gender responsive if it explicitly takes measures to reduce the harmful or discriminatory effects of gender norms, roles and relations (World Health Organization, 2011).

Psychosocial factors at work are increasingly recognised as important contributors to the social gradient of health and have been found to contribute to coronary heart disease, musculoskeletal disorders, and mental ill health (Moure-Eraso et al., 2006). Workplace psychosocial factors such as job demands, job control and an absence of social support are risk factors for high levels of stress in the construction industry. Research indicates that exposure to such psychosocial factors and the resulting psychological stress differ according to gender (Bowen et al., 2014a).

Jain et al. (2018) contend that work organisation and employment need to be considered within the wider context of employment and working conditions across the world. Labour markets and social policies determine employment conditions which heavily influence health inequalities. An example of this is working in hazardous conditions (Jain et al., 2018). However, irrespective of whether they work in an industrialised or developing country, women are identified as a vulnerable group in the workplace (Burton, 2010; Lahiri et al., 2006).

Men and women working in construction face many of the same work hazards; however, women must also contend with additional hazards originating from their sex and gender (Martin & Barnard, 2013; Rosa et al., 2017). For example, Australian research shows that long and inflexible working hours – like those practised in construction – have a greater detrimental effect on the health of women than they do on the health of men (Dinh et al., 2017).

While expectations of presenteeism, total availability, geographical mobility and very long work hours can negatively affect the health and wellbeing of both men and women, Galea et al. (2018) argue that women are more acutely affected because they carry the greatest share of caring responsibilities within families. Rigid working time practices, particularly in project-based roles, have been identified as a source of indirect gender discrimination in construction organisations (Dainty & Lingard, 2006). Galea et al. (2018) also describe construction project work cultures in which employees who arrive late, are perceived to be leaving early or who refuse to take work home if they cannot complete it within their standard work-day, are subjected to verbal and behavioural shaming and sanctioning.

Gender inequality in construction appears to be a global problem. A study of women in civil engineering roles in the UK reported a dominant masculine culture of long work hours in which being available for work at all times was expected and acted as a significant barrier to women's participation (Watts, 2009). Within this culture, working long hours and being visibly present in the workplace was seen as a proxy indicator of commitment and job performance. Importantly, because women are significantly underrepresented in construction workplaces, they tended to adopt similar work styles to their male colleagues. The negative impact of working time practices on gender equality in the construction industry is acknowledged in policy documents and industry initiatives. For example, the Victorian Women in Construction Strategy 2019–2022: Building Gender Equity (Victorian Government, 2019) identifies rigid workplace practices and the expectation to work excessive hours as a major barrier to women entering and staying in construction jobs. However, gender equity initiatives implemented in the construction industry sometimes produce disappointing results. One of the main reasons for this is that these initiatives are undermined by inconsistent application, poor implementation, and mixed messaging on the part of the companies concerned (Galea et al., 2018). They also target women in a vacuum, with no attention paid to the broader context of how masculine cultures operate on site.

There is growing recognition of the need to formally support women in construction through the implementation of diversity and inclusion policies (e.g., Victorian Government, 2019). Case example 5.1 presents an example of a difference in perceptions between senior management and women about the need for women to be formally supported in the construction workplace.

CASE EXAMPLE 5.1 THERE IS "A PROBLEM" WITH DIVERSITY AND INCLUSION

There was a perception by (mostly male) senior management at a large construction organisation in Australia that there was no need for a diversity and inclusion policy because there was "no problem" with the treatment of women. In seeking to provide an evidence base for the need to establish a diversity and inclusion policy at the organisation, women were asked to confidentially outline incidences of inappropriate treatment. Contrary to the perception of senior management that there was "no problem" with the way women working in construction were treated, responses from women indicated otherwise. Thematic analysis of responses from women at the construction organisation identified themes of: assumption of traditional gender-based roles, belittling and intimidating behaviour from male site workers, objectification of women, and uninvited physical contact.

Assumption of traditional gender-based roles

In some instances it was assumed by males that women at the organisation would take on tasks considered to be "women's work." For example, one woman explained: "*I arrived in the morning to dirty plates with pieces of cake that had been placed on my desk. I then approached the person who put them on my desk and asked why he did not put them in the kitchen? [He responded] well, that is your job, you are here to clean up after us.*" Another woman was asked: "*Can you please cut the cake? – that is a girl thing.*" There were occasions when women were assumed to be the partner of a male worker: "*Are you so and so's wife?*" It was also commonplace that men asked women "*When are you having babies?*" Galea et al. (2018) acknowledge the exclusionary nature of the construction industry which functions to remind women both subtlety and overtly of their gender and difference, making women feel like they are intruding in a male-dominated space.

Belittled and intimidated

Women reported being belittled and subjected to intimidatory behaviour by male colleagues. One woman was told: "*Stop nagging me. You're worse than my wife.*" Another woman was reprimanded and belittled for the way she spoke to a subcontractor: "*When I told a subcontractor off for setting up a mobile crane without safety checks, the [organisation] site manager pulled me aside and told me to watch the way I speak to people and asked if I was on my period.*" In another incident, a graduate was discussing her work goals with her manager and mentioned that she planned to find a female mentor working in the construction industry. In response, her manager advised her to: "*take out the 'female' mentor part, you sound like a feminist.*"

Women were often spoken to disrespectfully and called names. For example, one woman was told: "*You're a bitch.*" Other women had experience of threatening behaviour which ranged from subtle to overt. In one instance, a woman was told by her male colleague: "*I am going to f*** you so hard.*" Another woman explained how she was subjected to threatening behaviour at a work function. Her male colleague said: "*Dance with me or I won't help you anymore.*"

Offensive language was identified as an issue by many of the women, and some instances of this have been outlined above. One woman reflected on the language used in her office: "*I have repeatedly walked out of the office because the verbal abuse was that atrocious (not to me – just in an open plan office) – no person should be made to work in an environment where the language is so intolerable and abusive. I have not recorded these individual events because they are too numerous to specify.*"

Aggressive and combative exchanges and swearing are prevalent in the construction industry (Galea et al. 2018). Harassment or aggressive behaviour that creates a fear of violence, such as verbal threats, abuse, yelling and swearing are considered forms of workplace violence (Safe Work Australia, 2020). Safe Work Australia (2020) acknowledge that workplace violence and aggression can result in both physical and/or psychological harm to the person it is directed at and anyone witnessing the behaviour.

Objectification of women

Sexual objectification was experienced by women working on site and in the corporate office, and this finding is consistent with previous research indicating that gendered and sexualised interactions persist in the construction industry, despite laws and regulations to prevent them (Norberg & Johansson, 2021). In this case, women were exposed to a range of problematic behaviours. For example, one woman was told "*I'd pay money for you*" by a male co-worker.

Women were regularly subjected to wolf-whistles while on site. Uninvited and unwelcome comments were also made when women wore a dress or skirt, applied makeup, or did their hair: *"Oh hello, look out"*; *"Who are you trying to impress?"*; and *"Got a date tonight?"* Another woman was told that her appearance was likely to affect the productivity of her male colleagues: *"I once wore a dress to work on a 35-degree day and was told: you shouldn't wear that as it's too distracting and no one will get any work done."*

Women indicated that inappropriate comments came from all levels of the organisation, including subcontractors, peers and managers. For example, one woman explained that during her first week at the organisation she was setting up a colleague's computer and had to get under the desk to plug in the equipment: *"There was a group of four team members having a discussion nearby and the discussion stopped as soon as I bent under the desk. The project manager asked 'Are you OK?' to one of the team members. The team member said, 'Just a little distracted about the view under the desk'. The project manager responded with 'Yes, I know'."* The objectification of women was also prevalent at after-hours work functions. One woman explained that: *"Team functions all ended at the strippers."* Behaviours that reduce women to objects of men's sexual desire are harmful and have negative consequences on women's well-being (Koval et al., 2019).

Uninvited physical contact

According to the Australian Human Rights and Equal Opportunity Commission (2008) unwelcome touching is a form of sexual harassment, and sexual harassment is a legally recognised form of sex discrimination. Some women had experienced uninvited physical contact by their male colleagues. For example, one woman observed *"a subcontractor slapping a receptionist on the ass with a ruler."* Similarly, another woman reported *"being slapped on the ass"* by a male colleague. Women also reported being inappropriately touched on other parts of the body. For example: *"Whilst helping someone carry goods into the office, a person decided to hit me on my breast with some of the items we were carrying."* Women also spoke of the uninvited physical contact they encountered while at organisational events, such as the end-of-year party. Women spoke of *"being inappropriately groped and handled"* by male colleagues. There was a sense that male colleagues crossed the line more often when alcohol was being served: *"hands that wander as people get progressively drunker."*

The case example outlined above highlights that, in some organisations, women are not being protected from inappropriate and harmful behaviour. In lieu of adequate protective support being provided by their organisation, case example 5.2 describes how some women in construction have adapted their behaviour to avert problematic treatment from male co-workers.

CASE EXAMPLE 5.2 STRATEGIES USED BY WOMEN TO AVERT PROBLEMATIC TREATMENT

Women working on construction sites have adapted their behaviour so that inappropriate behaviour by male workers is averted or limited to some degree. For example, one woman explained that, due to lack of support on site, the onus fell on the individual to protect themselves from inappropriate and harmful treatment from male colleagues as much as possible: *"You've got to definitely take steps to protect yourself."* One strategy adopted by women working on site was having one phone for work and a separate phone for personal use to avoid receiving inappropriate and lewd messages and photos from subcontractors. A woman working on site explained: *"We have two phones. Often people will say, well, that's because of business purposes but females, we do it because we don't want to give our numbers out because of what we get sent from [male] subcontractors on site."* Another strategy adopted by women working on site is to remove their surname from their hard hat so that they cannot be traced and contacted by male workers outside of work. A woman who had just started work at a large construction contractor reflected on her experience: *"The first day I started at [company name removed] I was told to remove my second name off my helmet [hard hat] because of harassment online. So I removed that off my helmet and that was like, oh my goodness, what have I stepped into?"*

Emerging evidence suggests that the mental and physical health of women in construction work can be worse than for men. For example, in a survey of construction workers comprised of 2,500 men and 900 women from the United Kingdom, results indicate that 45 per cent of women and 32 per cent of men reported that their mental health was average to poor. The same study found that three-quarters of women respondents had experienced loss of sleep due to poor mental health, compared with 65 per cent of men (Randstad, 2019).

Research indicates that professional women working in construction tend to report higher rates of work-related stress and psychological injuries than men due to the unique challenges women face in the construction industry associated with discrimination, bullying and sexual harassment (Sunindijo & Kamardeen, 2017; Bowen et al., 2014b; Chan et al., 2020).

Women working in direct construction activity such as trades and technical workers can also experience higher levels of mental and physical ill health than males. For example, Curtis et al. (2018) explored the physical and psychosocial exposures faced by tradeswomen and tradesmen. More women reported high perceived stress (31%) than men (18%). Twenty-five per cent of all participants experienced an injury at work in the past year, with women (31%) significantly more likely than men (12%) to report being injured at work. Among those respondents who were injured, 9 per cent of them did not report their injury to others on site. Among those, women were more likely than men to list fear of layoff as the reason for not reporting. For physical exposures, men had higher exposure to dust and welding fumes and working at heights of at least four feet without barriers, compared to women. Women reported higher exposure rates than men for working with chemicals, acids, and solvents. Women in trades (31%) were also more likely than men (9%) to report personal protective equipment (PPE) not fitting them properly. Women reported significantly more bullying and discrimination based on their gender than men. Further, the odds of being injured at work in the past year were increased (>2-fold higher) among those who reported gender discrimination, bullying, or high levels of sexual harassment compared to those not reporting these exposures. For women, experiencing discrimination based on gender and age, bullying, high levels of sexual harassment and isolation, and poor work–life balance were each associated with high perceived stress. Reporting a high safety climate and receiving high levels of social support from their co-workers and supervisors were negatively associated with stress for women.

In contrast to the findings that women in construction can experience poorer health than men, Johansson et al.'s (2019) review of occupational safety in the construction industry found that men are at greater risk of injury than women. Importantly, however, Johansson et al. (2019) acknowledge that studies included in the review neglected to take into consideration what type of tasks women and men performed, and that several studies show that women's roles tend to involve more administrative work than roles taken by men. Johansson et al. (2019) conclude that there is a lack of research which applies a gender perspective on the issue of safety and suggests this may be a consequence of the low number of women employed in trade-based roles in the construction industry. Similarly in their review of research on mental health in construction, Nwaogu et al. (2020) identified the need for a better understanding of the mental health effects of gender-related discrimination in construction.

5.4 Health and minority status

Earlier in the chapter we reported on the low participation rates of women in professional and trade-based roles. It is worth considering, however, that women are in a minority group even before they commence working in construction. Women undertaking STEM-based studies at higher education and vocational educational and training institutions are commonly outnumbered by males. For example, in Australia, of those studying for a post-school qualification in a STEM field in 2018, 73 per cent were male and 27 per cent female (Australian Institute of Health and Welfare, 2019). Oo and Widjaja (2018) report that the percentage

TABLE 5.1 Percentage of women graduating from Australian construction management university degrees

	2016 %	2017 %	2018 %	2019 %
University 1	10.1 (n=9)	21.1 (n=23)	20.0 (n=21)	28.3 (n=41)
University 2	3.2 (n=5)	3.7 (n=6)	2.4 (n=5)	6.6 (n=15)
University 3	9.0 (n=11)	12.8 (n=14)	11.1 (n=11)	9.1 (n=8)

Source: Turner et al. (2021, p.191).

of female construction management enrolments at three Australian universities between 2006 and 2015 ranged from 5 to 20 per cent, and these percentages are consistent with global trends (Oo et al., 2018). Turner et al. (2021) report on the number and percentage of women graduating from three construction management programmes in Australia from 2016 to 2019, as shown in Table 5.1. While the information is not representative of the Australian context, it provides a snapshot from two large urban universities and one regional university. In 2018, University 1 had the largest graduating cohort of women across the three universities during the four-year period from 2016 to 2019 (28.3%, n=41), and University 2 had the lowest graduating cohort of women in 2018 (2.4%, n=5).

The number of women completing vocational training and education in construction trades is very low. For example, in 2017, 1 per cent of apprentices and trainee completions in Australia were women, and in 2018 this percentage decreased to 0.2 per cent (National Centre for Vocational Education Research, 2021). Bridges et al. (2022) outline barriers related to education and training for women:

- Vocational education and training (VET) lacks women in roles of teacher, mentor and role model;
- Manual trade classroom environments in VET institutions have been described as highly masculine;
- Language and behaviour can be disruptive and deliberately exclude women.

Women in male-dominated programmes of study can experience intimidatory behaviour and gender stereotypes as barriers preventing full participation in the classroom (Thurtle et al., 1998; Wilkinson, 2006). The ongoing underrepresentation of women undertaking education and training in construction-related occupations perpetuates risk factors for poor health, i.e., minority status. The stress and health impacts associated with gender and being a woman in construction suggest a critical mass is needed in the classroom for women's health to be improved in the currently male-dominated educational institutions

Case example 5.3 describes the experience of women undertaking vocational training and education and the incidence of psychosocial stressors.

CASE EXAMPLE 5.3 PSYCHOSOCIAL STRESSORS IN VOCATIONAL TRAINING AND EDUCATION

Women working as apprentices in the construction industry participated in research exploring the barriers for wellbeing (Holdsworth et al., 2020). Emerging from the research were incidents of psychosocial stressors, such as hostility, abuse, and incivility. Women were routinely exposed to disrespectful and discriminatory behaviour while undertaking their vocational training and education. Women undertaking apprenticeships had experienced inappropriate language from both male students and teachers while at trade school. For example, an apprentice stated that: "*In class, guys talking about disgusting, inappropriate stuff, yeah, that still happens sometimes.*" One apprentice was able to address this inappropriate behaviour with their trade teachers: "[I was able to] *speak with the teachers at school about that [inappropriate language], and most of them pulled up the students.*" The support from trade teachers is counter to the experience of another apprentice who recalled that: "*On my first day at trade school I was looking for the department, and I came across my trade teacher for the year ... I said I was looking for the construction department and he said, you must be [name removed]. You have me for the year, and if I've got anything to do with it, you won't be here ... by the end of the week.*" The language used by the trade teacher was both threatening and unsupportive. Similarly, another apprentice commented on the poor behaviour she had experienced from her teacher, who consistently used demeaning language to describe her work and commented in front of other teachers and students that it was "*rubbish ... a dog's breakfast.*" This apprentice goes on to describe that the teacher "*made your life miserable*" to the point that she "*decided to go to [Organisation B] in the second year [of her apprenticeship]*" and that this behaviour was in her opinion a result of her being female: "*... it was definitely a female thing.*" These exposures are likely to be detrimental for the health and wellbeing of women in apprentice roles.

Minority stress refers to the excess stress which individuals from stigmatised social categories are exposed to as a result of their social position (Meyer, 2003). Minority stress describes the "chronic stress resulting from experiences or perceptions of unfair treatment or abusive behavior based on belonging to a stigmatized minority group" (Ng et al., 2019, p.49). The minority stress model considers how experiences unique to minority groups, in particular prejudice and discrimination, can lead to chronic psychological stress and heightened physiological responses that affect mental and physical health over time (Pascoe & Smart Richman, 2009). It is possible that the minority status of women in construction contributes to a decrease in their health and wellbeing.

When an individual is a member of a stigmatised minority group, the disharmony between the individual and the dominant culture can be considerable and lead to stress, and this can be seen in the experiences of women in construction. Meyer (2003) contends that negative evaluation by others, such as stereotypes and prejudice directed at minority persons, may lead to adverse psychological outcomes. The minority stress concept is predicated on a number of underlying assumptions.

Minority stress is:

a) unique – that is, minority stress is additive to general stressors that are experienced by all people, and therefore, stigmatized people are required an adaptation effort above that required of similar others who are not stigmatized;

b) chronic – that is, minority stress is related to relatively stable underlying social and cultural structures; and

c) socially based – that is, it stems from social processes, institutions, and structures beyond the individual rather than individual events or conditions that characterize general stressors or biological, genetic, or other nonsocial characteristics of the person or the group.

Meyer, 2003, p.677

Applied to the male-dominated construction industry, the minority stress model contends that gender plays a critical role in women's experience which leads to adverse health outcomes. The model reiterates that the experience of discrimination can be considered to be a stressor that has health impacts for individuals.

5.5   Discrimination–health relationship

Uncontrollable and unpredictable stressors are particularly harmful to health, and these characteristics are common to discrimination experiences (Williams & Mohammed, 2009). In modelling the perceived discrimination–health relationship, Pascoe and Smart Richman (2009, p.533) define perceived discrimination as "a behavioural manifestation of a negative attitude, judgment, or unfair treatment toward members of a group." Perceived discrimination has been linked to specific types of physical health problems, such as hypertension, self-reported poor health, and breast cancer, as well as potential risk factors for disease, such as obesity, high blood pressure, and substance use (Williams & Mohammed, 2009). The harmful health effects of discrimination have also been observed across a range of mental health outcomes that include depression, psychological distress, anxiety, and lack of wellbeing (Williams et al., 2003).

Research on the psychological impacts of perceived discrimination has applied a stress and coping framework to understand the responses of the targets of prejudice and discrimination (e.g., Major et al., 2002). Similarly, physical health outcomes linked to discrimination have also been characterised as a stress response (e.g., Clark et al., 1999). These models conceptualise discrimination as a social stressor that sets into motion a process of physiological responses (e.g., elevated blood pressure, heart rate, cortisol secretions), and these heightened physiological responses over time can have long-term effects on health.

Evidence suggests that repeated exposure to discrimination may prepare the body to be more physically reactive in stressful or potentially stressful social situations (Guyll et al., 2001). Similarly, Gee et al. (2007) have proposed that routine discrimination can become a chronic stressor that may diminish an individual's protective resources and increase vulnerability to physical illness. Pascoe and Smart Richman (2009) contend that, as with other forms of cumulative stress, perceived discrimination may lead to wear and tear on the body because chronic over- or underactivity of allostatic systems produces allostatic load (McEwen, 2005).

There are two conceptual pathways through which discrimination may affect health (Ng et al., 2019):

1. Through activation of an emotional and physiological stress response: discrimination acts as a stressor that adversely affects emotional (e.g., anger) and physiological response (e.g., increased blood pressure) and when activated frequently over time, strains biological systems and increases risk of poor physical and mental health outcomes.
2. By impacting health behaviour: discrimination has an impact on health behaviour in one of two ways. Directly as stress coping, or indirectly, through self-regulation. For example, discrimination may result in unhealthy behaviour (e.g., smoking or drinking as coping mechanisms) or failure to participate in healthy behaviour (e.g., disease screening or management).

Gender minority status and the associated prejudice and discrimination over time can have a cumulative, dose-effect, impact on health (Ng et al., 2019). As previously mentioned, women in construction commence their education and training in a gender minority group and this continues into their working lives. By applying the minority stress model to the experience of women in construction, it is clear that continued exposure to prejudice and discrimination can have serious and long-lasting psychological and physical impacts. Examples of prejudice and discrimination experienced by women are outlined throughout this chapter. Gender minority status can be addressed by attracting and retaining more women into the industry so that numbers reach a critical mass. However, given the consistently low number of women enrolled in university and vocational institutions and employed in construction, this remains a serious challenge for the industry.

5.6   Bullying in the workplace

Bullying is considered a form of harassment and is described as the systematic persecution of a colleague, which if continued, can cause severe social, psychological and psychosomatic problems for the victim (Einarsen, 1999; Nielsen & Einarsen, 2018; Misawa et al., 2019). The effects of bullying can be long-term. For example, Einarsen and Nielsen (2015) showed that exposure to bullying behaviours while at work predicted elevated levels of distress even five years later.

Bullying in an occupational setting can be categorised into five types of behaviour (Zapf, 1999):

1. work-related bullying which may include changing a worker's work tasks or making them difficult to perform;
2. social isolation;
3. personal attacks or attacks on a worker's private life by ridicule, insulting remarks, gossip or the like;
4. verbal threats where the worker is criticised, yelled at or humiliated in public; and
5. physical violence or threats of such violence.

Women working in construction are known to experience bullying, and incidences of exclusion and isolation are common (Galea et al., 2018; Hegewisch et al., 2015). Organisational antecedents of bullying have been identified as organisational culture and climate and leadership (Hoel & Salin, 2003), and these are observed in construction workplaces. For example, Galea et al. (2018, p.4) contend that "there remains a subtle culture of denial and resistance with regards to diversity and equality initiatives."

Throughout the chapter, we have outlined incidences of bullying aligned with the various types of behaviour outlined by Zapf (1999). Table 5.2 focuses on social isolation, a type of bullying, and highlights the experience of trades and semi-skilled women working on site in direct construction activity and how they were made to feel like outsiders (Holdsworth et al., 2020).

Sense of place is focused on community, belonging, and identity and is associated with: "exploring the dimensions of the people-place relationship; reduction of, and recovery from stress; psychological integrity and preventing mental illnesses" (Hausmann et al. 2015, p.121). In Chapter 10 we provide a detailed overview of a sense of place in the workplace and how it can enable positive mental health for construction workers. For many women in construction, however, the exclusionary nature of the construction industry would suggest that women do not always experience a positive, psychologically safe and healthy sense of place in their workplace.

5.7   Perpetuating work hazards for women

While there have been recurring calls over the years to increase the number of women employed in construction, women's participation in professional, trades,

TABLE 5.2 Treated like outsiders

Theme	Participant quotes
Ignored when seeking help and guidance	"I would ask 'Why are you doing that?' or 'How do I do this?' You'd be right next to someone and they would completely just pretend that they hadn't heard you … it really hurt my feelings."
	"I've walked up to someone I didn't know very well and he's kind of a guru. He had more tickets and more qualifications than anybody in our depot. There was this tricky piece of equipment, so I walked up to a small group of them and I said, 'What's this?' I was curious as to this new equipment that we were installing. His response was 'Secret men's business'."
Excluded from decision making	"Whenever I raised issues of health and safety … a better way of solving the problem or delivering the project … it was always disregarded."
Lack of acknowledgement	"Even my supervisor would come in the morning, and he'd shake everyone's hand, but he wouldn't shake my hand."
Excluded from social activities	"My male co-workers would often go off to eat together or leave together, and there was a very, very clear social clique amongst those guys that I was never invited to participate in."
Territorial	"I had one place where the guy, the whole time I was there, he was saying how women are taking jobs off men."
	"What are you doing here? You're taking a job off a fella."
	"Chicks are for cooking and cleaning. They're not supposed to be on site. Get back in your own space."
Being watched	"I had guys hiding in scaffolds, watching me work. To them it may seem harmless, but when there's one of you and a thousand of them, it probably just does put a bit of a crazy thought in the back of your mind."

and technical positions continues to remain very low (Victorian Government, 2019; Williams, 2015). In 1999, the US-based Occupational Safety and Health Administration (OSHA) proposed that the low number of tradeswomen working in construction, along with the safety and health problems unique to women, has a circular effect. That is, safety and health problems in construction create barriers to women entering and remaining in the industry. In turn, the small number of women working on construction sites perpetuates an environment in which these problems arise or continue (OSHA, 1999). More than two decades later, it appears that little has changed in the industry. The safety and health hazards prevalent in construction continue to be reinforced by the prevailing masculine workplace culture (George & Loosemore, 2019) which fails to provide appropriate support and protection for women and offers them limited career pathways.

While males in construction are presumed to be capable, women find that their professional capability is scrutinised, questioned or devalued. If a woman makes a mistake, it is characterised as a "female capability" issue rather than an individual mistake (Galea et al., 2018). Bridges et al. (2020) also identified a culture of targeting and victimising women who raise complaints about incidents of bullying, sexual harassment, and assault. Given the various workplace hazards they must routinely contend with, it is argued that women are exposed to hostile work environments (Curtis et al., 2018). Hostility is described as a form of harassment in which workplace behaviour interferes with a worker's performance on the job and creates an intimidating, offensive, degrading, humiliating or offensive environment (McCann, 2005).

Hostility in the workplace can sometimes be disguised as humour. Humour is defined as consisting of "amusing communications that produce positive emotions and cognitions in the individual, group or organization" (p.59). Given this definition, it is possible for one party to find an exchange of humour funny, while the other party does not (Romera & Cruthirds, 2006). In the workplace, some forms of humour can be positive, reducing stress and enhancing social cohesion (Mesmer-Magnus et al., 2012). However, the use of aggressive humour, i.e., that which victimises, ridicules or belittles others, in a workplace is harmful to mental health and wellbeing (Huo et al., 2012).

Watts (2007) describes how humour is a characteristic of construction work environments, with sarcasm, banter, mocking and irony prevalent in office-based environments and joke-telling (often using crude language, mimicry and innuendo) commonly used on site. Women are in the minority in construction workplaces and Watts (2007) observed them to use humour as a form of resistance and refuge. When used as a form of resistance, women join in with workplace humour in order to "fit in" to the team or site culture and to avoid being seen as humourless or an "outsider." When used as a refuge, women use humour as a coping mechanism, engaging in light-hearted banter with other women in the workplace, typically in secretarial roles. However, as Watts (2007) also observes, the most prevalent way that women experience humour in construction workplaces is when it is used as a form of exclusion. Thus, joking and teasing by the dominant male group is observed to result in "othering" women and sometimes this humour can be excessive, inappropriate and damaging. Watts describes how women are resigned to experiencing this humour, feeling that they can do little to change the situation. However, this acceptance makes it very difficult to establish different standards of conduct in a workplace.

5.8 Neurosexism

Neurosexism refers to "the practice of claiming that there are fixed differences between female and male brains, which can explain women's inferiority or unsuitability for certain roles" (Rippon, 2016). According to Fine (2010), neurosexism reflects and reinforces cultural beliefs about gender, and it may do so in a particularly powerful way. Fine (2010, p.xxviii) further contends that neurosexism is damaging, as "dubious 'brain facts' about the sexes become part of the cultural lore." These beliefs are not substantiated by evidence. For example, Else-Quest et al. (2013) found that male and female adolescents earned similar end-of-year grades in math and science, yet women remain underrepresented in STEM courses and occupations. Neurosexism can perpetuate gender-based stereotypes which specify what is considered "men's" and "women's" work. This belief functions to repress the opportunity of women to enter industries or professions considered as the realm of males. Similarly, it represses the opportunity for men to enter industries or professions considered to be the realm of females.

As recently as 2021, Turner et al. (2021) report that a reviewer [reviewer A] of a high-level construction and engineering journal provided the following feedback on a manuscript related to early career women in construction: "What is considered [gender] underrepresentation in construction? What is the ideal percentage? By thinking that the distribution should be 50–50 (men–women) or any other percentage, one would be undermining or ignoring that the brain by gender could be wired differently" (p.193). It appears that neurosexism emerged in the peer review of the manuscript. The belief that the way women's brains are wired differently renders them less suitable for construction perpetuates the exclusionary nature of the construction industry context, in which women's capabilities and suitability for the work are frequently questioned. As Galea et al. (2018) observe, these unfounded prejudices contribute to women in construction feeling isolated, exhausted and lacking in confidence, all of which have a negative impact on health.

5.9 #MeToo in construction

The #MeToo movement is focused on raising awareness of and addressing violence against women in our society (Bhattacharyya, 2018; Gill & Orgad, 2018). The term "Me Too" was first used by civil rights activist Tarana Burke to empower survivors of sexual abuse and assault, specifically women of colour, to help them understand that they were not alone. As a result of the #MeToo tweet by actress Alyssa Milano in 2017, the "MeToo" hashtag went viral and the issue of violence against women was elevated (Hosterman et al., 2018). Violence against women is defined by the United Nations General Assembly (1993: Article 1) as "any act of gender-based violence that results in, or is likely to result in, physical, sexual or psychological harm or suffering to women, including threats of such acts, coercion or arbitrary deprivation of liberty, whether occurring in public or in private life."

O'Neil et al. (2018) contend that the #MeToo movement has raised awareness of sexual harassment in the workplace, describing sexual harassment as a form of gender-based violence at work that is an organisational, criminal, and ethical issue. Countries in the Organisation for Economic Co-operation and Development, such as Australia, report that as many as 40–60 per cent of women have experienced gender-based violence in the context of employment (O'Neil et al., 2018).

Common to definitions of violence against women is the notion of "harm." It therefore ensues that gender-based violence is a health issue (O'Neil et al., 2018; World Health Organization, 2013). According to the World Health Organization (2013), the experience of gender-based violence by non-partners (as distinct from intimate partners) leads to various health outcomes, including depression, anxiety including post-traumatic stress disorder, obsessive-compulsive disorder, and alcohol use disorder. The Victorian Trades Hall Council (2016) report that the impact of gendered violence at work is significant and can result in physical and psychological illness, and suicide. A 2012 review found sexual harassment doubled the risk of persistent psychological distress after two years for women but not for men (Nielsen & Einarsen, 2012). Importantly, poor organisational responses to sexual harassment in the workplace can revictimise and exacerbate the negative effects on health (O'Neil et al., 2018).

The #MeToo movement has received some, albeit limited, attention in the construction industry. In the United States, a survey conducted by the Engineering News Record found that of the 1,248 respondents, 66 per cent reported experience of sexual harassment or gender bias in the workplace, and nearly 60 per cent indicated they had witnessed it (Rubin et al., 2018). The survey revealed that incidents of harassment were experienced evenly across construction sites and in office settings. Harassment took the form of:

- Inappropriate personal requests, questions, jokes or innuendo;
- Inappropriate physical contact;
- Suggestive text messages/emails;
- Threats of retaliation for non-compliance to inappropriate requests; and
- Gender-different response to an action from a supervisor.

Workplace risk factors enabling gendered violence at work are comprised of the working environment, such as organisational setting and managerial style, as well as the workplace culture and external environment (Cruz & Klinger, 2011). The Australian Human Rights Commission (2020) reports that male-dominated workplace cultures have a higher prevalence of sexual harassment due to an unequal gender ratio (a higher proportion of men than women in the workplace) and identified construction as one of these workplaces. In the Australian construction industry, the proportion of harassers who were male was slightly higher than for industries overall: 81 compared to 79 per cent. The construction industry also had a higher average number of harassers per incident compared to all industries (2.1 compared to 1.7) (Australian Human Rights Commission, 2020).

According to the Australian Human Rights Commission (2004), sexually explicit pictures and posters are defined as forms of sexual harassment. In a study of construction site graffiti, Rawlinson and Farrell (2010) found that the graffiti was often vulgar, possibly a result of the dominant masculinity of the sites. In a blog post at Construction Concrete titled "Me Too" (Construction Concrete, 2017), the author reflected on the construction industry and declared that: "Frankly, I think construction in general has cleaned up its image considerably over the past 30 years. It used to be that crude graffiti in the toilets and girly pictures in the job trailer were the norm, but on professional job sites today, that has become unacceptable." In contrast to the observation that crude graffiti is no longer acceptable on construction sites, a story on #MeToo in Construction by Constructible (2018) observed that crude graffiti is commonplace on sites. The story was informed by interviews with male construction workers in the United States. One of the interviewees commented: "*On the job site we have now I've seen some stuff that would probably touch my soul if I was a woman. They [male colleagues] choose to draw pictures on the wall of the woman and not-so-flattering pictures at that.*" More recently in Australia, crude graffiti was observed in numerous locations across a large commercial construction site in 2020. The site was managed by a large construction contractor. The Learning and Development Team from the contractor organisation took photos of the crude graffiti and used them in cultural awareness training. This training was rolled out at management level; however, it is not known whether the training had an impact on the frequency or acceptance of crude graffiti.

5.10 Workplaces designed for women

5.10.1 Ergonomic design of tools and equipment

The construction workplace has historically been designed by males for males. Tools, equipment and PPE are designed according to the average male body, and females are required to "make do." This is of concern as having to "make do" can have serious impacts on construction women's health. In the context of ergonomics and design, Habib and Messing (2012) acknowledge that treating different populations equally can create inequality and this is considered as a form of systemic discrimination. This has been shown to be the case in the construction industry. The New York Committee for Occupational Safety & Health (2014) report that women carpenters have higher rates of sprains/strains and nerve conditions of the wrist and forearm than men. While the reasons for this were not reported, it is possible that this could be associated with construction site equipment being designed for use by the male body (Criado-Perez, 2019).

Insensitivity to the way in which workplaces are designed could contribute to repetitive strain injury among female workers. For example, the European Agency for Safety and Health at Work (2013, p.33) contends that "many of the musculoskeletal problems experienced by women workers can be exacerbated by work equipment (such as desks, chairs and factory benches) designed to meet the ergonomic needs of the average male."

Tools and equipment designed for men and used by women can problematic, and the Occupational Safety and Health Administration (1999) explain why this is the case:

> handle size and tool weight are designed to accommodate the size and strength of men, yet the average hand length of women is 0.8 inches shorter than the average man's. Their grip strength averages two-thirds the power of a man's grip. The grips of tools are typically too thick. Tools like pliers require a wide grasp which puts inappropriate pressure on the palm, leading to the loss of functional efficiency.

5.10.2 Personal protective equipment (PPE)

Women working in hazardous industries often do not have access to correctly fitting PPE (Ghani, 2017). In the construction industry, women can experience ill-fitting PPE (Kim et al., 2013) which can hinder rather than protect (Onyebeke et al., 2016). The fit of PPE, defined as the relationship of size of the garment or equipment to the size of the wearer, is a key factor in its functionality and durability (Wagner et al., 2013). The use of anthropometric data is an important element in the design of PPE. According to the National Institute for Occupational Safety and Health (2021, p.1), anthropometry is "the science that defines physical measures of a person's size, form, and functional capacities. Applied to occupational injury prevention, anthropometric measurements are used to study the interaction of workers with tasks, tools, machines, vehicles, and personal protective equipment – especially to determine the degree of protection against dangerous exposures."

PPE that is poorly fitting is identified as an occupational hazard for women in many high-risk workplaces, including in construction (Flynn et al., 2017). Importantly, women are not smaller versions of men and so a small size of clothing/equipment designed for the male body does not fit well (Del Castillo, 2015).

Del Castillo (2015) reports on the results of a UK-based survey of women in sectors including construction and utilities which found that 75 per cent of PPE worn by respondents was designed for men, more than half of the respondents indicated their PPE hindered their work, and maternity PPE is not available. The level of protection given by PPE is reduced if the wearer's movement is restricted or where the equipment is too large and loose. Fisher (2020) states that if the PPE fit is not good it can interfere with the use of tools and operation of equipment. The example of a welding glove is provided:

a men's size small welding glove is slightly longer and a bit wider than a similar style of women's size medium welding glove. The thumb also is longer on the men's glove. Downsizing a men's welding glove, rather than using a glove designed specifically for a woman's hand, will likely result in a glove that is too wide, with fingers (and especially the thumb) that are too long. Not only will there be a loss of dexterity and comfort, but the excess glove material can increase hand fatigue (particularly for thicker materials such as leather).

Fisher, 2020, p.1

According to the International Labour Organization & World Health Organization (1995), occupational health is focused on: "the promotion and maintenance of the highest degree of physical, mental and social well-being of workers in all occupations" and incorporates the design of the occupational environment which is adapted for workers' physiological capabilities. In a study of tradeswomen working in the US construction industry, Wagner et al. (2013) found that the availability of PPE that fits well was associated with higher levels of self-efficacy and job satisfaction. The construction industry and suppliers of PPE, tools and equipment can support the occupational health of women by designing products which cater for their physiological capabilities.

In the United States, the Center for Construction Research and Training (2021) emphasises the importance of properly fitting PPE in protecting workers against occupational hazards for all workers. Properly fitting PPE can decrease the risk of illness, injury, and death for workers in construction. On their website, the Center for Construction Research and Training (2021) list examples of commercially available PPE for women in the trades that accommodates female anthropometry, including:

- Construction footwear
- Construction footwear for cold climate and accessories
- Ear protection
- Harnesses for personal fall arrest systems
- Hard hats
- High visibility clothing
- Flame-resistant clothing
- Safety gloves
- Safety glasses

Although many manufacturers of PPE now provide options or size alternatives marketed as suitable for women, Flynn et al. (2017) suggest that ineffective supply networks and employers' lack of awareness of the need for alternative PPE remain as barriers to ensuring that women have access to properly fitting equipment (Flynn et al., 2017). In an analysis of the market availability of PPE designed for women, Flynn et al. (2017) report that, even when alternative sizing is advertised, manufacturers provide little context to explain sizing, e.g., a sizing chart showing dimensions/measurements. Neither is it clear whether PPE marketed as being for women is designed using female anthropometric data.

5.10.3   Reproductive hazards

Reproductive hazards on construction sites, such as lead and other chemicals are an issue for all workers, but especially for pregnant women (Rim, 2017). Controlling exposure to these chemicals is important. Prolonged standing during pregnancy is also associated with premature birth, and strenuous activity such as lifting and climbing can be a hazard during the later stages of pregnancy (National Institute for Occupational Safety and Health, 2019).

5.10.4   Sanitary facilities

The Occupational Safety and Health Administration (1999) noted that on construction sites in the USA the toilet facilities, including the provision of separate ones for women, were poor and could increase disease as well as urinary tract infection. More than two decades later, the lack of separate toilets for women on construction sites remains an issue (Electrical Trades Union, 2021). The lack of adequate sanitary facilities further affects women who are menstruating. On construction sites women are often not provided with separate and/or clean toilets with access to feminine hygiene bins, leading to difficulties in effectively managing their menstruation. Menstruation management requires access to water, sanitation and hygiene facilities, menstrual hygiene materials disposal, and a supportive environment where women can manage menstruation without embarrassment or stigma. Sang et al. (2021) describe the additional burden that is borne by workers who menstruate, particularly in environments that are designed primarily for men and male bodies. This burden comprises the management of a leaky, messy, painful body, the need to access appropriate facilities (which may not be readily available), the need to conceal all aspects of menstruation to avoid embarrassment or stigma, and the workload associated with managing all of these things (Sang et al. 2021).

There have been calls for "period dignity" in the construction industry to support menstruation management (Unite, 2019). A recent article by Rampen (2018) illustrates the experience of a woman who was a crane driver who was not afforded access to sanitary facilities in the workplace and how this affected her while she was menstruating:

> Lucy, a crane operator, took a job on a windfarm, where she was the only woman out of fifteen workers. "I lasted about a month," she told me. First, although she suspected she'd been fired for making a similar request at another job, she asked for a portaloo. But rather than receiving one, she found herself given less and less work. Then she got her period. "I had to

change my tampon in the crane without taking off my coveralls," she said. "That was my last day."

Rampen, 2018, p.1

5.11 Conclusion

While men and women working in construction face many of the same work hazards, this chapter considered the gendered work hazards experienced by women. The chapter identified the characteristics of work and the workplace and how they can be detrimental to women's health. It is evident that change is required in the industry to improve women's experience of work and related health impacts; however, the industry has been slow to change. Limited systemic and structural change has seen women continue to experience harmful work hazards, affecting both their mental and physical health. The experience of women in construction appears to be reflective of broader societal attitudes and treatment of women. However, there appears to be a shift at a societal level, as gender inequity and the treatment of women have received considerable coverage and debate more recently. While change has been slow, there appears to be growing momentum to generate communities which respect, value, and support women and their choices and this is being reflected in calls for change in the workplace.

The occupational health of women in construction has received limited coverage, and this chapter has sought to contribute to an understudied yet important topic. Industry-led innovations which remove gendered work hazards discussed throughout this chapter will enhance the experience of women and support their health outcomes, as well as enabling the industry to meet their occupational health and safety obligations to effectively manage the risks of work-related harm to which workers are exposed. Importantly, sex (biological differences) and gender (social roles) must be considered in the design of work which seeks to reduce or remove harmful work hazards for women and enables them to enjoy a career in construction which does not jeopardise their physical or mental health.

Strategies seeking to support women in construction will be successful only if a whole system approach is taken to implement change. Consistent with the societal level, there appears to be some momentum for systemic and structural change at the industry level, driven by government agencies, peak construction groups, unions, and large construction organisations (e.g., Construction Industry Culture Taskforce, 2021; Victorian Government, 2019). It is acknowledged that major changes are required in construction to facilitate an industry which welcomes, supports, and respects women in the workplace.

5.12 Discussion and review questions

1. Why is it important to consider sex and gender as separate factors when seeking to design work that supports the mental and physical health of women in construction?

2. How is minority status related to health outcomes for workers? How does this affect women and what can be done to improve the situation for women in the construction industry?

3. In taking a systems perspective, what actions can be taken by whom to remove the gendered work hazards experienced by women working in construction?

4. What are the benefits of increasing the participation rates of women in construction?

References

Australian Human Rights and Equal Opportunity Commission. (2008). *Effectively Preventing and Responding to Sexual Harassment in the Workplace: A Code of Practice for Employers.* Australian Human Rights and Equal Opportunity Commission.

Australian Human Rights Commission. (2004). *Sexual Harassment (A Code in Practice)–- What is sexual harassment?* Australian Human Rights Commission. Accessed 8 January 2021 from: https://humanrights.gov.au/our-work/sexual-harassment-code-pract ice-what-sexual-harassment

Australian Human Rights Commission. (2020). *Respect@Work: National Inquiry into Sexual Harassment in Australian Workplaces.* Australian Human Rights Commission.

Australian Institute of Health and Welfare. (2016). *Australia's Health 2016.* Australia's Health Series No. 15. Cat. no. AUS 199.

Australian Institute of Health and Welfare. (2019). *Higher Education and Vocational Education.* Australian Government. Accessed 17 May 2021 from: www.aihw.gov.au/ reports/australias-welfare/higher-education-and-vocational-education

Australian Institute of Health and Welfare. (2020). *Social Determinants of Health.* Australian Government. Accessed 12 May 2021 from: www.aihw.gov.au/reports/australias-hea lth/social-determinants-of-health

Bhattacharyya, R. (2018). # metoo movement: An awareness campaign. *International Journal of Innovation, Creativity and Change,* 3, 1–12.

Bowen, P., Edwards, P., Lingard, H., & Cattell, K. (2014a). Workplace stress, stress effects, and coping mechanisms in the construction industry. *Journal of Construction Engineering and Management,* 140(3), 04013059.

Bowen, P., Govender, R., & Edwards, P. (2014b). Structural equation modeling of occupational stress in the construction industry. *Journal of Construction Engineering and Management,* 140(9), 04014042.

Bridges, D., Bamberry, L., Wulff, E., & Krivokapic-Skoko, B. (2022). "A trade of one's own": The role of social and cultural capital in the success of women in male-dominated occupations. *Gender, Work & Organization,* 29(2), 371–387.

Bridges, D., Wulff, E., Bamberry, L., Krivokapic-Skoko, B., & Jenkins, S. (2020). Negotiating gender in the male-dominated skilled trades: a systematic literature review. Construction Management and Economics, 38(10), 894–916.

Burrowes, K. (2021). *Gender Bias is Still Putting Women's Health at Risk.* Royal Australian College of General Practitioners. Accessed 12 May 2021 from: www1.racgp.org.au/ newsgp/clinical/gender-bias-in-medicine-and-medical-research-is-st

Burton, J. (2010). *WHO Healthy Workplace Framework and Model: Background and Supporting Literature and Practices.* World Health Organization.

Center for Construction Research and Training. (2021). *Personal Protective Equipment for the Female Construction Workforce.* Accessed 14 June 2021 from: www.cpwr.com/ wp-content/uploads/PPE-for-Female-Workforce.pdf

Chan, A. P. C., Nwaogu, J. M., & Naslund, J. A. (2020). Mental ill-health risk factors in the construction industry: Systematic review. *Journal of Construction Engineering and Management*, 146(3), 04020004.

Clark, R., Anderson, N. B., Clark, V. R., & Williams, D. R. (1999). Racism as a stressor for African Americans. A biopsychosocial model. *American Psychologist*, 54(10), 805–816.

Constructible. (2018). *Construction Workers Respond to the Women's #MeToo Movement.* Accessed 6 January 2021 from: https://constructible.trimble.com/construction-indus try/construction-workers-respond-to-the-womens-metoo-movement

Construction Concrete. (2017). *Me Too.* Bill's Blog. Construction Concrete. Accessed 5 January 2021 from: www.concreteconstruction.net/business/management/me-too_o

Construction Industry Culture Taskforce (2021). *Culture Standard.* Accessed 24 November 2021 from: www.cultureinconstruction.com.au/culture-standard/

Criado-Perez, C. (2019). The deadly truth about a world built for men – from stab vests to car crashes. *The Guardian.* Accessed 8 January 2021 from: www.theguardian.com/ lifeandstyle/2019/feb/23/truth-world-built-for-men-car-crashes

Cruz, A., & Klinger, S. (2011). *Gender-based violence in the world of work: Overview and selected annotated bibliography.* International Labour Organization. Accessed 9 December 2020 from: www.ilo.org/wcmsp5/groups/public/---dgreports/---gender/documents/publ ication/wcms_155763.pdf

Curtis, H. M., Meischke, H., Stover, B., Simcox, N. J., & Seixas, N. S. (2018). Gendered safety and health risks in the construction trades. *Annals of Work Exposures and Health*, 62(4), 404–415.

Dainty, A. R., & Lingard, H. (2006). Indirect discrimination in construction organizations and the impact on women's careers. *Journal of Management in Engineering*, 22(3), 108–118.

Del Castillo, A. P. (2015). Personal protective equipment: Getting the right fit for women. *HesaMag*, 12, 34–37.

Dinh, H., Strazdins, L., & Welsh, J. (2017). Hour-glass ceilings: Work-hour thresholds, gendered health inequities. *Social Science & Medicine*, 176, 42–51.

Dusenbery, M. (2018). *Doing Harm: The Truth About How Bad Medicine and Lazy Science Leave Women Dismissed, Misdiagnosed, and Sick.* HarperOne.

Einarsen, S. (1999). The nature and causes of bullying at work. *International Journal of Manpower*, 20(1/2), 16–27.

Einarsen, S., & Nielsen, M. B. (2015). Workplace bullying as an antecedent of mental health problems: a five-year prospective and representative study. *International Archives of Occupational and Environmental Health*, 88(2), 131–142.

Electrical Trades Union. (2021). *Nowhere To Go.* Accessed 22 November 2021 from: www. etunational.asn.au/women_have_nowhere_to_go

Else-Quest, N., Mineo, C., & Higgins, A. (2013). Math and science attitudes and achievement at the intersection of gender and ethnicity. *Psychology of Women Quarterly*, 37, 293–309.

European Agency for Safety and Health at Work. (2013). *New Risks and Trends in the Safety and Health of Women at Work.* European Agency for Safety and Health at Work.

European Commission. (n.d.). *Gender-Based Violence (GBV) by Definition.* European Commission. Accessed 8 December 2020 from: https://ec.europa.eu/info/policies/ justice-and-fundamental-rights/gender-equality/gender-based-violence_en

Fairweather, D., & Rose, N. R. (2004). Women and autoimmune diseases. *Emerging Infectious Diseases*, 10(11), 2005–2011.

Fine, C. (2010). *Delusions of Gender: The Real Science Behind Sex Differences*. Icon: London.

Fisher, R. (2020). The need for unique women's PPE. *Safety and Health*. Accessed 7 January 2021 from: www.safetyandhealthmagazine.com/articles/19752-the-need-for-uni que-womens-ppe

Flynn, M. A., Keller, B., & DeLaney, S. C. (2017). Promotion of alternative-sized personal protective equipment. *Journal of Safety Research*, 63, 43–46.

French, E., & Strachan, G. (2017). Women in the Construction Industry: Still the Outsiders. In F. Emuze and J. Smallwood (Eds.), *Valuing People in Construction*, Taylor & Francis (pp.151–171).

Galea, N., Powell, A., Loosemore, M., & Chappell, L. (2018). *Demolishing Gender Structures*. University of New South Wales.

Gee, G. C., Spencer, M., Chen, J., Yip, T., & Takeuchi, D. T. (2007). The association between self-reported racial discrimination and 12-month DSM-IV mental disorders among Asian Americans nationwide. *Social Science Medicine*, 64(10), 1984–1996.

George, M., & Loosemore, **M**. (2019). Site operatives' attitudes towards traditional masculinity ideology in the Australian construction industry. Construction Management and Economics, 37(8), 419–432.

Ghani, R. (2017). Is PPE working for women? *Occupational Health at Work*, 3(6): 32–35.

Gill, R., & Orgad, S. (2018). The shifting terrain of sex and power: From the 'sexualization of culture' to #MeToo. *Sexualities,* 21(8), 1313–1324.

Guyll, M., Matthews, K. A., & Bromberger, J. T. (2001). Discrimination and unfair treatment: relationship to cardiovascular reactivity among African American and European *American women*. Health Psychology, 20(5), 315–325.

Habib, R. R., & Messing, K. (2012). Gender, women's work and ergonomics. *Ergonomics,* 55(2), 129–132.

Hasan, A., Ghosh, A., Mahmood Muhammad, N., & Thaheem Muhammad, J. (2021). Scientometric review of the twenty-first century research on women in construction. *Journal of Management in Engineering*, 37(3), 04021004.

Hausmann, A., Slotow, R. O. B., Burns, J. K., & Di Minin, E. (2015). The ecosystem service of sense of place: benefits for human well-being and biodiversity conservation. *Environmental Conservation,* 43(2), 117–127.

Hegewisch, A., & O'Farrell, B. (2015). *Women in the Construction Trades: Earnings, Workplace Discrimination, and the Promise of Green Jobs*. Institute for Women's Policy Research. Accessed 11 January 2021 from: https://iwpr.org/wp-content/uploads/2020/10/ C428-Women-in-Construction-Trades.pdf

Hoel, H., & Salin, D. (2003). Organisational antecedents of workplace bullying. In S. Einarsen, H. Hoel, D. Zapf, and C. Cooper (Eds.), *Bullying and Emotional Abuse in the Workplace: International Perspectives in Research and Practice*. Taylor & Francis/Balkema (pp. 203–218).

Holdcroft, A. (2007). Gender bias in research: How does it affect evidence based medicine? *Journal of the Royal Society of Medicine*, 100(1), 2–3.

Holdsworth, S., Turner, M., Scott-Young, C.M., & Sandri, K. (2020). *Women in Construction: Exploring the Barriers and Supportive Enablers of Wellbeing in the Workplace*. RMIT University.

Hosterman, A. R., Johnson, N. R., Stouffer, R., & Herring, S. (2018). Twitter, social support messages, and the #MeToo Movement. *Journal of Social Media in Society*, 7(2), 69–91.

Huo, Y., Lam, W., & Chen, Z. (2012). Am I the only one this supervisor is laughing at? Effects of aggressive humor on employee strain and addictive behaviors. *Personnel Psychology*, 65, 859–885.

International Labour Office. (2009). *Gender Equality at the Heart of Decent Work*. International Labour Office. Accessed 7 January 2021 from: www.ilo.org/wcm sp5/groups/public/@ed_norm/@relconf/documents/meetingdocument/wcms_105 119.pdf

International Labour Organization & World Health Organization. (1995). *Joint International Labour Organization (ILO)/World Health Organization (WHO) Committee on Occupational Health 12th session*.

Jain, A., Leka, S., & Zwetsloot, G. I. J. M. (2018). Work, health, safety and well-being: current state of the Art. In A. Jain, S. Leka, and G. Zwetsloot (Eds.), *Managing Health, Safety and Well-Being: Ethics, Responsibility and Sustainability*. Springer (pp. 1–31).

Johansson, J., Berglund, L., Johansson, M., Nygren, M., Rask, K., Samuelson, B., & Stenberg, M. (2019). Occupational safety in the construction industry. *Work*, 64, 21–32.

Kim, A., Wagner, H., & Griffin, L. (2013). Relationship between personal protective equipment, self-efficacy, and job satisfaction of women in the building trades. *Journal of Construction Engineering and Management*, 139, 1–7.

Koval, P., Holland, E., Zyphur, M. J., Stratemeyer, M., Knight, J. M., Bailen, N. H., Thompson, R. J., Roberts, T.-A., & Haslam, N. (2019). How does it feel to be treated like an object? Direct and indirect effects of exposure to sexual objectification on women's emotions in daily life. *Journal of Personality and Social Psychology*, 116(6), 885–898.

Laberge, M., Blanchette-Luong, V., Blanchard, A., Sultan-Taïeb, H., Riel, J., Lederer, V.,... & Messing, K. (2020). Impacts of considering sex and gender during intervention studies in occupational health: Researchers' perspectives. *Applied Ergonomics*, 82, 102960.

Lahiri, S., Moure-Eraso, R., Flum, M., Tilly, C., Karasek, R., & Massawe, E. (2006). Employment conditions as social determinants of health part I: the external domain. *New Solutions*, 16(3), 267–288.

Lyons, A. (2018). *Same Disease, Different Outcomes: Heart Attack and Gender*. Royal Australian College of General Practitioner. Accessed 12 May 2021 from: www1. racgp.org.au/newsgp/clinical/same-disease,-different-outcomes-heart-attack-and

Maas, A., & Appelman, Y. (2010). Gender differences in coronary heart disease. *Netherlands Heart Journal*, 18(12), 598–603.

Major, B., Quinton, W. J., & McCoy, S. K. (2002). Antecedents and consequences of attributions to discrimination: Theoretical and empirical advances. In M. P. Zanna (Ed.), *Advances in Experimental Social Psychology*. Academic Press (pp. 251–300).

Martin, P., & Barnard, A. (2013). The experience of women in male-dominated occupations: A constructivist grounded theory inquiry. SA *Journal of Industrial Psychology*, 39, 01–12.

Master Builders Association. (2021). *Women Building Australia*. Accessed 13 May 2021 from: www.masterbuilders.com.au/Resources/Career-Centre/Women-Building-Australia

McCann, D. (2005). *Sexual Harassment at Work: National and International Responses*. Project Report. International Labour Organization.

McEwen, B. S. (2005). Stressed or stressed out: What is the difference? *Journal of Psychiatry & Neuroscience*, 30(5), 315–318.

Mesmer-Magnus, J., Glew, D. J., & Viswesvaran, C. (2012). A meta-analysis of positive humor in the workplace. *Journal of Managerial Psychology*, 27(2), 155–190.

Messing, K., & Silverstein, B. A. (2009). Gender and occupational health. *Scandinavian Journal of Work, Environment & Health*, 35(2), 81–83.

Messing, K., & Stellman, J. M. (2006). Sex, gender and women's occupational health: The importance of considering mechanism. *Environmental Research*, 101(2), 149–162.

Meyer, I. H. (2003). Prejudice, social stress, and mental health in lesbian, gay, and bisexual populations: conceptual issues and research evidence. *Psychological Bulletin*, 129(5), 674–697.

Misawa, M., Andrews, J. L., & Jenkins, K. M. (2019). Women's experiences of workplace bullying: A content analysis of peer-reviewed journal articles between 2000 and 2017. *New Horizons in Adult Education and Human Resource Development*, 31(4), 36–50.

Moure-Eraso, R., Flum, M., Lahiri, S., Tilly, C., & Massawe, E. (2006). A review of employment conditions as social determinants of health. Part II: The workplace. *New Solutions*, 16(4), 429–448.

National Centre for Vocational Education Research. (2021). *Apprentices and Trainees*. Accessed 17 May 2021 from: www.ncver.edu.au/research-and-statistics/collections/apprentices-and-trainees-collection

National Institute for Occupational Safety and Health. (2019). *Reproductive Health and The Workplace*. Accessed 12 November 2021 from: www.cdc.gov/niosh/topics/repro/specificexposures.html

National Institute for Occupational Safety and Health. (2021). *Anthropometry*. Accessed 22 November 2021 from: www.cdc.gov/niosh/topics/anthropometry/default.html

New York Committee for Occupational Safety & Health. (2014). *Risks Facing Women in Construction*. Accessed 8 January 2021 from: https://nycosh.org/wp-content/uploads/2014/09/Women-in-Construction-final-11-8-13-2.pdf

Ng, J. H., Ward, L. M., Shea, M., Hart, L., Guerino, P., & Scholle, S. H. (2019). Explaining the relationship between minority group status and health disparities: A review of selected concepts. *Health Equity*, 3(1), 47–60.

Nielsen, M. B., & Einarsen, S. V. (2018). What we know, what we do not know, and what we should and could have known about workplace bullying: An overview of the literature and agenda for future research. *Aggression and Violent Behavior*, 42, 71–83.

Nielsen, M., & Einarsen, S. (2012). Prospective relationships between workplace sexual harassment and psychological distress. *Occupational Medicine*, 62, 226–228.

Norberg, C., & Johansson, M. (2021). "Women and "ideal" women": the representation of women in the construction industry. *Gender Issues*, 38(1), 1–24.

Nwaogu, J. M., Chan, A. P. C., Hon, C. K. H., & Darko, A. (2020). Review of global mental health research in the construction industry. *Engineering, Construction and Architectural Management*, 27(2), 385–410.

O'Neil, A., Sojo, V., Fileborn, B., Scovelle, A. J., & Milner, A. (2018). The #MeToo movement: an opportunity in public health? *The Lancet*, 391(10140), 2587–2589.

Occupational Safety and Health Administration (OSHA). (1999). *Women in the Construction Workplace: Providing Equitable Safety and Health Protection*. Health and Safety of Women in Construction (HASWIC) Workgroup, OSHA, and the Advisory Committee on Construction Safety and Health (ACCH), Department of Labor. Accessed on 9 November 2020 from: www.osha.gov/advisorycommittee/accsh/products/1999-06-01#acknowledgments

Onyebeke, L. C., Papazaharias, D. M., Freund, A., Dropkin, J., McCann, M., Sanchez, S. Hashim, D., Meyer, J. D., Lucchini, R. G., & Zuckerman, N. C. (2016). Access to properly fitting personal protective equipment for female construction workers. *American Journal of Industrial Medicine*, 59(11), 1032–1040.

Oo, B. L., & Widjaja, E. C. (2018). *Female Student Enrolments in Construction Management Programs.* Paper presented at the Proceedings of the 21st International Symposium on Advancement of Construction Management and Real Estate, Singapore.

Oo, B. L., Li, S., & Zhang, L. (2018). Understanding female students' choice of a construction management undergraduate degree program: Case study at an Australian university. *Journal of Professional Issues in Engineering Education and Practice,* 144(3), 05018004.

Pascoe, E. A., & Smart Richman, L. (2009). Perceived discrimination and health: a meta-analytic review. *Psychological Bulletin,* 135(4), 531–554.

Rampen, J. (2018). Want More Women in Construction? Then Give Them Proper Toilets. DiversityQ. Accessed 20 May 2021 from: https://diversityq.com/want-more-women-in-construction-then-give-them-proper-toilets-1004378/

Randstad. (2019). *Taking Down the Walls Around Mental Health in Construction.* Accessed 13 January 2021 from: www.randstad.co.uk/s3fs-media/uk/public/2019-11/r-006-randstad-white-paper-digital-version_0.pdf

Rawlinson, F., & Farrell, P. (2010). *Construction Site Graffiti: Discourse Analysis as a Window Into Construction Site Culture.* In C. Egbu (Ed.), Proceedings of the 26th Annual ARCOM Conference, 6–8 September 2010, Leeds, UK, Association of Researchers in Construction Management (pp. 361–370).

Rim, K. T. (2017). Reproductive toxic chemicals at work and efforts to protect workers' health: a literature review. *Safety and Health at Work,* 8(2), 143–150.

Rios, F. C., Chong, W. K., & Grau, D. (2017). The need for detailed gender-specific occupational safety analysis. *Journal of Safety Research,* 62, 53–62.

Rippon, G. (2016). *How 'Neurosexism' is Holding Back Gender Equality – And Science Itself.* The Conversation. Accessed 16 March 2021from: https://theconversation.com/how-neurosexism-is-holding-back-gender-equality-andscience-itself-67597

Romero, E. J., & Cruthirds, K. W. (2006). The use of humor in the workplace, *Academy of Management Perspectives,* 20(2), 58–69.

Rosa, J., Hon, C., & Lamari, F. (2017). Challenges, success factors and strategies for women's career development in the Australian construction industry. *Construction Economics and Building,* 17, 27–46.

Rubin, D., Tuchman, J., Powers, M., Cubarrubia, E., & Shaw, M. (2018). #MeToo in Construction: 66% Report Sexual Harassment in ENR Survey. *Engineering News Record.* Accessed on 5 January 2021 from: www.enr.com/articles/45452-metoo-in-construction-66-report-sexual-harassment-in-enr-survey

Safe Work Australia. (2020). *Building & Construction: Work-Related Violence.* Accessed 24 May 2021 from: www.safeworkaustralia.gov.au/covid-19-information-workplaces/industry-information/building-and-construction/work-related

Sang, K., Remnant, J., Calvard, T., & Myhill, K. (2021). Blood work: Managing menstruation, menopause and gynaecological health conditions in the workplace. *International Journal of Environmental Research and Public Health,* 18(4), 1951.

Sinyai, C., & Choi, S. (2020). Fifteen years of American construction occupational safety and health research. *Safety Science,* 131, 104915.

Slowey, K. (2019). By the numbers: Women in construction. *Construction Dive.* Accessed 13 May 2021 from: www.constructiondive.com/news/by-the-numbers-women-in-construction/549359/#:~:text=The%20percentage%20of%20women%20in,%2C%20only%203.4%25%20were%20women

Stocks, S. J., McNamee, R., Carder, M., & Agius, R. M. (2010). The incidence of medically reported work-related ill health in the UK construction industry. *Journal of Occupational and Environmental Medicine,* 67, 574–576.

Sunindijo, Y., & Kamardeen, I. (2017). Work stress is a threat to gender diversity in the construction industry. *Journal of Construction Engineering and Management*, 143(10), 0401707.

Thurtle, V., Hammond, S., & Jennings, P. (1998). The experience of students in a gender minority on courses at a college of higher and further education. *Journal of Vocational Education & Training*, 50(4), 629–645.

Turner, M., Zhang, R. P., Holdsworth, S., & Andamon, M. M. (2021). Taking a broader approach to women's retention in construction: Incorporating the university domain. In: Scott, L and Neilson, C. J. (Eds.) *Proceedings of the 37th Annual ARCOM Conference*, 6–7 September 2021, UK, Association of Researchers in Construction Management (pp. 188–197).

Unite. (2019). *Construction Period Dignity*. Accessed 12 January 2021 from: https://unitet heunion.org/campaigns/construction-period-dignity/

United Nations General Assembly. (1993). *Declaration on the Elimination of Violence against Women*. United Nations General Assembly (A/RES/48/104): New York, 20 December 1993.

van Vollenhoven, R. F. (2009). Sex differences in rheumatoid arthritis: more than meets the eye. *BMC Medicine*, 7, 12–12.

Victorian Government. (2019). *Victoria's Women in Construction Strategy*. Accessed 6 January 2021 from: www.vic.gov.au/victorias-women-construction-strategy

Victorian Trades Hall Council. (2016). *Stop Gendered Violence at Work: Women's Rights at Work Report*. Victorian Trades Hall Council.

Wagner, H., Kim Angella, J., & Gordon, L. (2013). Relationship between Personal Protective Equipment, Self-Efficacy, and Job Satisfaction of Women in the Building Trades. *Journal of Construction Engineering and Management*, 139(10), 1–7.

Watts, J. (2007). IV. Can't take a joke? Humour as resistance, refuge and exclusion in a highly gendered workplace. *Feminism & Psychology*, 17(2), 259–266.

Watts, J. H. (2009). "Allowed into a Man's World" Meanings of Work–Life Balance: Perspectives of Women Civil Engineers as "Minority" Workers in Construction. *Gender, Work, Organisation*, 16 (1), 37–57.

Weikle, B. (2019). Women are making inroads in the trades but still have a ways to go. CBC News. Accessed 12 May 2021 from: www.cbc.ca/news/business/women-in-tra des-1.5215384

Wilkinson, R., & Marmot, M. (2003). *The Social Determinants of Health: The Solid Facts* (2nd edn). World Health Organization.

Wilkinson, S. (2006). Women in civil engineering. In A.W. Gale and M. Davidson (Eds.), *Managing Diversity and Equality in Construction: Initiatives and Practice*. Taylor & Francis (pp. 113–127).

Williams, D. R., & Mohammed, S. A. (2009). Discrimination and racial disparities in health: evidence and needed research. *Journal of Behavioral Medicine*, 32(1), 20–47.

Williams, D. R., Neighbors, H. W., & Jackson, J. S. (2003). Racial/ethnic discrimination and health: findings from community studies. *American Journal of Public Health*, 93(2), 200–208.

Williams, M. (2015). Where are all the women? Why 99% of construction site workers are male. *The Guardian*. Accessed 24 November 2020 from: www.theguardian.com/ careers/careers-blog/2015/may/19/where-are-all-the-women-why-99-of-construct ion-site-workers-are-male

World Health Organization. (2010). *Gender, Women and Primary Health Care Renewal: A Discussion Paper*. World Health Organization.

World Health Organization. (2011). *Gender Mainstreaming for Health Managers: A Practical Approach*. World Health Organization.

World Health Organization. (2013). *Global and Regional Estimates of Violence Against Women: Prevalence and Health Effects of Intimate Partner Violence and Non-Partner Sexual Violence*. World Health Organization.

Zapf, D. (1999). Mobbing in Organisationen – Überblick zum Stand der Forschung (Mobbing in organisations. A state of the art review). *Zeitschrift für Arbeits- und Organisationspsychologie A&O*, 43(1), 1–25.

6

EMPLOYEE RESILIENCE

6.1 Introduction

Resilience has gained much attention as we grapple with ways to manage increasing levels of workplace stress. This is particularly relevant in construction as it is known as a demanding and stressful industry in which its workers experience high levels of mental ill health. In Chapter 10, we consider resilience as a strengths-based capability which can contribute to a sense of place and support mental health. In this chapter, we take a broader approach to resilience beyond its relationship to a sense of place. We consider what resilience means in a work setting using an interactionist lens, describe a resilience framework, and outline the antecedents and outcomes of resilience at both the individual and team levels. Strategies supporting resilience at both the individual and team levels are examined and described. The chapter finishes with a case study illustrating how resilience can be used to navigate difficult work environments.

6.2 What is resilience?

Before we consider resilience in the workplace, it is helpful to consider how resilience is understood more broadly, how it can impact on human functioning, and how this is reflected in occupational research. Conceptual reviews (e.g., Herrman et al., 2011; Shaikh & Kauppi, 2010; Tusaie & Dyer, 2004; Windle, 2011) acknowledge the breadth and scope of definitions of resilience and the lack of conceptual clarity. Among the various definitions, the *person-centred approach* holds that resilience represents a set of personal characteristics which enable the individual to thrive in the face of adversity (Connor & Davidson, 2003; Greve & Staudinger, 2006). Consistent with this focus on the individual is another view contending that resilience is a relatively stable personality trait (Bartone, 2007;

DOI: 10.1201/9780367814236-6

Kirkwood et al., 2008) characterised by the ability to overcome, steer through and bounce back from adversity (Ong et al., 2006). Arguably, frameworks which conceptualise resilience as a set of personal characteristics are limited as they do not consider the impact of the environment on the individual.

Across disciplines, resilience is often understood as a process rather than the static trait of a system (Ungar, 2018). The *process-centred approach* considers how aspects of the person and environment are connected with consequences to adversities (Greve & Staudinger, 2006). Masten (2018, p.16) aptly asserts that "resilience should not be construed as a singular or stable trait, as it arises from dynamic interactions involving many processes across and between systems."

Masten (2018) argues that definitions and models of resilience have changed in response to the broad shift to systems thinking, and highlights four key attributes of a systems framework (p.15):

- Many interacting systems at multiple levels shape the function and development of living systems;
- The capacity for adaptation of a system and its development are dynamic (always changing);
- Because of interconnections and interactions inherent to living systems, change can spread across domains and levels of function;
- Systems are interdependent.

Masten (2018) contends that the attributes of complex adaptive systems have critical implications for an individual's resilience, as individuals are embedded within multiple systems. In recognition that resilience is an interplay between an individual and their environment, alternative views of resilience have emerged which position resilience as a process that encompasses the individual and the wider environment (American Psychological Association, 2020; Bryan et al., 2018; Windle, 2011; World Health Organization, 2017). Resilience may change over time as a function of development and one's interaction with their environment (Southwick et al., 2014). Central to definitions which view resilience as a process is the notion that resilience is contextual and will differ over the life course. For example:

- "A dynamic process wherein individuals display positive adaptation despite experiences of significant adversity or trauma. This term does not represent a personality trait or an attribute of the individual. Rather, it is a two-dimensional construct that implies exposure to adversity and the manifestation of positive adjustment" (Luthar & Cicchetti, 2000, p.858).
- "The process of adapting well in the face of adversity, trauma, tragedy, threats or significant sources of stress – such as family and relationship problems, serious health problems or workplace and financial stressors. It means 'bouncing back' from difficult experiences" (American Psychological Association, 2020).

- "The process of effectively negotiating, adapting to, or managing significant sources of stress or trauma. Assets and resources within the individual, their life and environment facilitate this capacity for adaptation and 'bouncing back' in the face of adversity. Across the life course, the experience of resilience will vary" (Windle, 2011, p, 163).

Resilience has also been conceptualised as a response in circumstances where an individual: 1) has been exposed to a stressor; 2) adapts positively; and 3) does not lose normal functioning (Bonanno, 2004).

Consistent with the myriad resilience definitions and the apparent lack of conceptual clarity, case example 6.1 illustrates how participants differ in their understanding of resilience.

CASE EXAMPLE 6.1 CONCEPTUALISING RESILIENCE

As previously mentioned, resilience has been conceptualised in various ways. For example, resilience is represented as a set of personal qualities that enable the individual to thrive in the face of adversity; resilience is a relatively stable personality trait characterised by the ability to overcome, steer through and bounce back from adversity; and resilience is viewed as a personality factor that protects against life's adversities and negative emotions by resourceful adaptation, flexibility and inventiveness (Fletcher & Sarkar, 2013; Hartmann et al., 2020; Windle, 2011). To explore the diversity of views on resilience, students undertaking postgraduate studies in project management were asked about their understanding of resilience. There was no consensus around the meaning of resilience. Instead, resilience was understood as a personality factor, a result of environmental factors, or as an individual capability that can be developed. Responses are reflective of the various conceptualisations outlined in the literature.

Personality	"If you are optimistic then you are more inclined to push through, it is those personal characteristics, it's those innate things that make up your character."
Environmental	"The way a child is raised directly reflects on how they interact in the world. They are either raised in a way where they have self-esteem and self-confidence and do learn tenacity and all of that. It (resilience) is definitely how they are raised."
	"Being due to one's background, like upbringing and what sort of environment they have grown up in."
	"Someone that grows up in a developed country would have a totally different resiliency then someone who grows up in a non-developed country."

> Capability "I think experiences and how you deal with it and your personal experience on those experiences support resilience."
> "Through life experience."

Case example 6.1 illustrates that resilience is understood in different ways by different people. This is crucial to acknowledge, as the way a person understands resilience has implications for how they may seek to develop their own resilience to overcome adversity. It also has implications for the way individuals may seek to support the resilience of others. An important aspect raised by participants is the influence of context and culture on resilience. Culture has a critical impact on resilience through the availability and accessibility of resources, and the meaningfulness of the resources provided (Ungar, 2013). For example, developing and accessing social support networks is considered as a key resource underpinning resilience capability (Windle, 2011; APA, 2020; Shatté et al., 2017). Social support is described as a network of family, friends, neighbours, and community members that are available in times of need to give psychological, physical, and financial help (Lin et al., 1979; Ozbay et al., 2007). In times of stress and adversity, the capacity to seek help and support may be shaped by cultural norms. For example, in Australia, seeking help for mental health and adversity is actively encouraged (Productivity Commission, 2020). In contrast to Australia, cultural shame and stigma about mental health problems may present as a barrier for seeking help in other countries (O'Brien et al., 2008). This may also be the case in cultures where help-seeking behaviours can be associated with shame and losing face (Tse & Haslam, 2021). It is therefore important to consider that cultural attributes and values originating from their context and environment will contribute to an individual's resilience capability (APA, 2020).

6.3   Team resilience

Resilience in the workplace has been considered at both the individual and team levels. While often referred to as separate concepts in the extant literature, Hartmann et al. (2020) contend that individual resilience and team resilience are interdependent and can mutually influence each other. While much of the research into resilience at work has occurred at the individual level, emerging research has sought to better understand team resilience; however, it remains in the early stages of conceptual development. Given its stage of conceptual development, there is little consensus about definitions of team resilience (Bowers et al., 2017; Gucciardi et al., 2018; Hartmann et al., 2020; Hartwig et al., 2020; Chapman et al., 2020). For example, in a review of definitional descriptions of team resilience attributes, Hartwig et al. (2020) identified three key themes: the dynamic nature of resilience, resilience as a positive adaptation to adversity, and resilience as sustained team viability. In contrast, Chapman et al. (2020) identified commonalities of definitions of team resilience as: the presence of stressors, setbacks, pressure, challenge or adversity; the nature of team functioning in the midst of demands; team resilience is either an ability or capacity.

Gucciardi et al. (2018) draws on the dynamic nature of team resilience and positions it within an interactionist framework: "team resilience is best viewed as an outcome that emerges over time via dynamic person–situation interactions, rather than a trait, capacity, or process. Formally, team resilience as an emergent outcome characterizes the trajectory of a team's functioning, following adversity exposure, as one that is largely unaffected or returns to normal levels after some degree of deterioration in functioning" (p.735). Gucciardi et al. (2018) raise two important issues in relation to team resilience: (i) team resilience emerges over time and fluctuates through the interaction of individual-, contextual-, and team-level factors; and (ii) a group of resilient individuals does not always result in a resilient team. This is because resilient individuals may cope with adversity and risk in ways that are effective for their individual performance and functioning but are detrimental to the structures and processes of the team. Three broad possible trajectories for teams following exposure to an adverse event are proposed by Gucciardi et al. (2018):

- *Resistance trajectory:* team functioning remains relatively unaffected (i.e., disruption to the system is minimal) in that there is little variability in team functioning post-adversity relative to baseline levels.
- *Bounce back trajectory:* characterized by initial negative effects of the adverse event (e.g., substantial decrease in performance indices), followed quickly by recovery to competent functioning within a timeframe that is salient with regard to key contextual factors (e.g., nature of the task, type of objective).
- *Recovery trajectory:* deterioration in functioning lasts for some period of time (e.g., several weeks or months) and is followed by a return to competent functioning gradually over time.

p.735

Throughout this book, we have referred to construction as an ecosystem with various inter-related parts; therefore, it is helpful to consider resilience within an interactionist perspective. However, given that team resilience is in its early stages of conceptual development and lacks a valid and reliable measure through which to understand and evaluate resilience-building strategies, we focus in this chapter on individual resilience in the workplace. At this early stage of conceptual development, outcomes of team resilience appear to be aligned with team performance (Meneghel et al., 2016) and team attitude and behaviour (West et al., 2009). More research is required to better understand whether team resilience may interact with individual resilience to support the health outcomes of employees. Furthermore, one of the key characteristics of construction is the projectised nature of the industry. Construction teams are temporary coalitions comprised of members from multiple organisations whose membership is dependent on undertaking specific tasks at a specific time during the construction process (Berggren et al., 2001; Engebø et al., 2022). Research has yet to consider how the temporary nature of teams comprised of transient membership can affect the resilience of a team.

6.4 Employee resilience

Unlike broad definitions of resilience which often focus on experiences of adversity and trauma, resilience in the work environment describes the ability of an individual worker to respond to everyday problems and challenges associated with work (McEwan, 2018; Cooper et al., 2013). For example, Cooper et al. (2013, p.1) describe resilience in the workplace as: "being able to bounce back from setbacks and to stay effective in the face of tough demands and difficult circumstances." Beyond merely bouncing back, Cooper et al. (2013, p.1) go on to emphasise that resilience in the work environment "goes beyond recovery from stressful or potentially stressful events, to include the sustainability of that recovery and the lasting benefit – the strength that builds through coping well with such situations." Similarly, McEwan (2018, p. 4) describes resilience at work as the ability to "manage the everyday stress of work while staying healthy, adapting and learning from setbacks and preparing for future challenges proactively."

Other definitions of resilience focus on the experience of "significant adversity" in the workplace. Britt et al. (2016) argue that many of the traditional work stressors, such as role ambiguity and work overload, may not always constitute significant adversity, especially if these stressors are judged as not being present at a high intensity and/or for a long duration. Britt et al. (2016) consider significant adversity in the workplace in relation to intensity, frequency, duration, and predictability of a stressor, and recommend that the presence of stressors in the workplace that constitute significant adversity can occur through an analysis of objective features of the work environment (e.g., the presence of traumatic events, documented long work hours over an extended period of time, high levels of noise, crowded work conditions) or through consistent employee reports of demands in the work environment that are judged to be of high intensity and/ or of a long duration (e.g., multiple employee reports of sustained harassment/abusive supervisor behaviour).

Windle (2011, p.158) cautions that "it is misleading to use the term resilience if a stressor, under normal circumstances with a majority of people, would not ordinarily pressure adaptation and lead to negative outcomes." Similarly, Vanderbilt-Adriance & Shaw (2008) contend that not all risks are equivalent in severity. Some risks may be acute and others chronic and persistent. Vanderbilt-Adriance and Shaw (2008) underscore that any findings for the occurrence of resilience can only be considered within the context of that specific adversity.

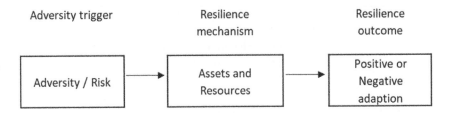

FIGURE 6.1 Process of resilience
Source: Adapted from Fisher et al., 2019.

Such an approach to resilience reinforces the interactionist perspective of resilience which considers the individual within their environment.

Using a process-based definition of employee resilience embedded with an interactionist framework, resilience is premised on the three requirements of: (1) the need for an adversity/risk; (2) the presence of assets or resources to offset the effects of the adversity; and (3) the positive adaptation or the avoidance of a negative outcome (Windle, 2011). This process is outlined in Figure 6.1. Positive adaptation, or demonstration of resilience, has been predicated on the employee's performance of competence-related tasks, low symptoms of mental and physical ill health, high wellbeing, and healthy relationships (Britt et al., 2016).

In relation to employee resilience, there exist definitional constraints in the literature whereby resilience, recovery, and coping are used interchangeably. However, all are argued to be distinct concepts. For example, Bonanno (2008) raises the issue of resilience and recovery, and questions how the two concepts may differ. When an individual experiences recovery from adversity, there is a period in which normal functioning is suspended. In contrast, resilience involves the maintenance of equilibrium in which no loss of normal functioning occurs (Bonanno, 2008).

In addition to positioning resilience within an interactionist model, resilience has also been positioned in an occupational stress model. Occupational stress is influenced by work organisation and work design and occurs when the demands of the job do not match or exceed the capabilities, resources, or needs of the worker, or when the abilities of an individual worker or group to cope are not matched with the expectations of the organisational culture (International Labour Organization, 2016). Models of occupational stress contend that interventions to reduce stress can take place at three levels (Cooper & Cartwright, 1997; Tetrick & Winslow, 2015):

> *Primary:* Focus on changing the workplace by either reducing or removing the risk factors or changing the nature of the job stressors.
>
> *Secondary:* Focus on the management of experienced stress by increasing awareness and improving the stress management skills of the individual through training and educational activities. Individual factors can alter or

modify the way employees exposed to workplace risk factors perceive and react to this environment.

Tertiary: Focus on treatment, rehabilitation, and recovery process of those individuals who have suffered or are suffering from serious ill health as a result of stress.

The Productivity Commission (2020) refers to workplace interventions as programmes or initiatives which improve mental health in the workplace, and resilience development is positioned at both the primary intervention and secondary intervention levels:

- Primary interventions are delivered to all workers irrespective of their current mental health or exposure to risks. Primary interventions include strategies to improve job design and control, and to build organisational resilience though manager and leadership training.
- Secondary interventions target specific employees often at greater risk of mental ill health through *resilience training* and workplace activity programmes.
- Tertiary interventions are aimed at those who are already unwell, either currently at work or absent from work, and focus on their return to work. Resilience is not included in this category of intervention.

In contrast to the Productivity Commission (2020), some authors position resilience solely as a secondary intervention focused on the worker's ability to respond to and manage stress (Nwaogu et al., 2022a). Resilience as a secondary intervention has been criticised for an over-reliance on the individual to manage workplace stress and thereby absolving the workplace of responsibility (van Breda, 2018). As will be discussed in a later stage of this chapter, contemporary models of employee resilience recognise the interplay between the organisation and the individual and move away from the over-reliance on the individual to be resilient.

Individual resilience in the workplace is linked to various positive effects such as individual job performance and organisational commitment (Luthans et al., 2007a), mental health (Kinman & Grant, 2011), physical health (Ferris et al., 2005), job satisfaction (Badran & Youssef-Morgan, 2015), and openness to organisational change (Wanberg & Banas, 2000). Robertson et al. (2015) examined the effect of resilience training on personal resilience and four broad categories of dependent variables relating to mental health and subjective well-being outcomes (e.g., depression, anxiety, stress, happiness, purpose), physical/biological outcomes (e.g., fasting blood glucose, heart rate, systolic blood pressure, indigestion), psychosocial outcomes (e.g., job satisfaction, morale, optimism), and performance outcomes (e.g., product sold, observed performance, productivity). Findings of Robertson et al. (2015) indicated that resilience training can improve personal resilience and is a useful means for developing mental health and subjective wellbeing in employees. It was also found that resilience training has a number of wider benefits that include enhanced psychosocial functioning and improved performance.

Hartmann et al. (2020) undertook a review of the workplace literature and identified a wide range of positive outcomes associated with resilience, many of which are similar to those identified by Robertson et al. (2015):

- *Performance:* job performance, career success, organisational citizenship behaviours;
- *Mental and physical health:* reduction in burnout, depression, emotional exhaustion, strain, biopsychosocial distress;
- *Work-related attitudes:* career/job satisfaction, happiness, reduced cynicism about work, organisational commitment, work engagement;
- *Change-related attitudes:* openness/commitment to organisational change, career change intentions, entrepreneurial intentions.

6.5   Protective factors, assets and resources

A key concept informing models of resilience is the centrality of protective factors to manage stressful events more effectively to either mitigate or eliminate risk. According to Windle (2011), protective factors are the defining attributes of resilience. Within the literature, however, the terms used to describe protective factors vary and include "assets," "resources," "capacities," "capabilities," "strengths," or "antecedents."

Some studies distinguish the individual-level protective factors as assets, while resources are regarded as external to the individual (Fergus & Zimmerman, 2005; Sacker & Schoon, 2007):

Internal protective factors are individual qualities or characteristics/capabilities that are responsible for fostering resilience and are specific to the individual. For example, these may be optimism, self-efficacy (Johnson, 2011), emotional intelligence, reflective ability, aspects of empathy and social confidence (Grant & Kinman, 2012), vision, composure, reasoning, tenacity, collaboration (Rossouw & Rossouw, 2016), network leveraging, learning, and adaptability (Kuntz et al., 2017).

External protective factors are positive environmental support structures from the environment in which the individual is situated. For example, these may be caring relationships, high expectations, and opportunities for meaningful contributions (Johnson, 2011).

Internal and external protective factors that contribute to the development of employee resilience are wide-ranging. For example, Hartmann et al. (2020) contend that antecedents (protective factors) comprise five broad categories:

- personality traits and cultural value orientation
- personal resources (e.g., expertise, self-efficacy, self-reflection)

- personal perceptions/attitudes (e.g., sense of purpose and meaning, calling, self-direction)
- personal emotions (e.g., positive emotions)
- work resources (e.g., social support and feedback, positive organisational context, learning/knowledge sharing culture, leadership styles)

Models of workplace resilience draw from both internal and external protective factors. For example, the Resilience at Work (RAW) framework (Winwood et al., 2013) conceptualises workplace resilience as a skill that can be taught, practised, and developed and is associated with behaviours that reliably facilitate recovery from work stress experiences. Winwood et al. (2013) developed a measure of resilience based on the RAW framework that is recommended as a suitable measure of employee resilience (Hartmann et al., 2020; Robertson et al., 2015). In the RAW framework (Winwood et al., 2013), employee resilience is said to comprise seven elements which draw on various antecedent categories outlined by Hartmann et al. (2020):

- *Living authentically:* knowing and holding onto personal values, deploying personal strengths, and having a good level of emotional awareness and regulation.
- *Finding your calling:* seeking work that has purpose, a sense of belonging and a fit with core values and beliefs.
- *Maintaining perspective:* having the capacity to reframe setbacks, maintain a solution focus, and manage negativity.
- *Managing stress:* using work and life routines that help manage everyday stressors, maintain work–life balance, and ensure time for relaxation.
- *Interacting cooperatively:* a workplace work style that includes seeking feedback, advice, and support as well as providing support to others.
- *Staying healthy:* maintaining a good level of physical fitness and a healthy diet.
- *Building networks:* developing and maintaining personal support networks (which might be both within and outside the workplace).

In order to be work-ready, Turner et al. (2017a) contend that built environment graduates require the capacity to bounce back and recover from stressful circumstances. Building the resilience of students is a critical skill that can assist them in their transition into professional life and support their mental health and wellbeing in the high-demands construction industry. Turner et al. (2017b) adapted the RAW scale for use in a university setting and found that students undertaking studies in the built environment scored highest on building networks, staying healthy, interacting cooperatively, and living authentically, and lowest in maintaining perspective. Maintaining perspective is associated with an ability to reframe challenging experiences, maintain a solution focus and manage negativity, all of which are essential in managing the stressors workers in construction experience on a regular basis.

6.6   Occupational approach to resilience

Kossek and Perrigino (2016) took an occupational approach to resilience, seeking to understand specific demands (conditions of adversity) associated with particular occupations. This has particular relevance to the construction workforce which consists of people who perform a wide variety of job roles and who experience occupation-specific demands. For example, occupations engaged in direct construction activity have a level of physicality associated with their job which is not experienced by office-based occupations. In their study, Kossek and Perrigino (2016) contend that "resilience, the ability to bounce back from adversity and endure demands, in one form or another, is critical to all occupations; but it can be critical in different ways" (p.739). The types of demands experienced by occupations can be considered according to three broad categories: cognitive, emotional, and physical. Across the study of 11 occupations (dancers; elementary school teachers; child, family, and school social workers; police patrol officers; doctors; fine artists; nurse practitioners; municipal firefighters; accountants; mechanical engineers; models), four themes emerged as generic occupational facilitators (protective factors) to reduce occupational risk and impede resilience or conversely foster an occupational work context supportive of resilience (Kossek & Perrigino, 2016). All of these themes are relevant to work characteristics and contexts in construction:

- Designing workplaces to increase the ability to control hours as a facilitator for, and ensure work schedules and workload do not present a barrier to, occupational resilience;
- Strengthening the work context to foster open access and use of positive workplace social supports to help workers perform job tasks, and alleviate work cultures that demand the sacrifice of personal and family wellbeing in order to progress one's career;
- Implementing organisational preventative and stress management initiatives to reduce the resiliency depletion for jobs that have high exposures to work-related risks (e.g., stigma due to demographic minority status; constant contact with pain; physical injury);
- Implementing integrated professional initiatives to promote lifelong learning and skills currency to reduce the risk of job obsolescence, particularly for occupations with high demands.

When considering occupational resilience, work context factors are important. Work context factors can be understood as resources originating from the organisation and are critical for positive adaptation. Many of these work context factors have been considered throughout this book as having an impact on health outcomes. For example, Chapter 4 discusses the different approaches to working time and associated effects on the health and wellbeing of workers in the Australian construction industry.

6.7   Employee resilience in construction

In the construction industry, emerging research has identified that resilience is associated with workers' wellbeing. For example, in the Canadian construction industry, individual resilience has been shown to have a significant negative impact on psychological stress and is considered as a secondary preventer of job stress for trade workers (Chen et al., 2017a). In another study conducted by Chen et al. (2017b) with construction trade workers in Canada, individual resilience was shown to have a significant negative correlation with workplace interpersonal conflict with supervisors and co-workers, which in turn could decrease the frequency of physical safety outcomes and job stress. Resilience was identified as a protective factor for mental health in a study of construction tradesmen in Nigeria (Nwaogu et al., 2022b). Nwaogu et al. (2022b) found that tradesmen with increased resilience were less likely to experience depressive and anxiety symptoms as well as suicide ideation. Level of resilience was also associated with the use of positive reappraisal coping behaviours which refer to efforts to create positive meaning by focusing on personal growth. As resilience level increased from normal to high, the likelihood to engage in positive reappraisal behaviour increased. He et al. (2019) explored the resilience of Chinese construction workers in the context of safety behaviour (safety compliance and safety participation). In the study, resilience was positioned as an element of psychological capital. Results suggested that resilience was significantly and positively related to safety participation but not to safety compliance. In considering this finding, He et al. (2019) note that, in China, a very high proportion of construction workers come from the agricultural industry as temporary or seasonal workers and often face unforeseen problems, such as skill learning, communication with others, and isolation from their family.

Despite the emerging body of knowledge on employee resilience in construction, research has largely been non-cumulative, owing to varying conceptualisations of individual and employee resilience and the use of assorted measures which either directly or indirectly measure resilience. For example:

Chen et al. (2017a, 2017b) draw on the definition of Stewart et al. (1997) to conceptualise individual resilience in their study. Resilience is defined as "the capacity of individuals to cope successfully in the face of significant change, adversity, or risk. This capacity changes over time and is enhanced by protective factors in the individual and environment" (Stewart et al., 1997, p.22). Chen et al. (2017a) measured individual resilience using six statements. Three statements were adapted from a self-efficacy scale (Schwarzer & Jerusalem, 1995), and three statements were taken from the Connor-Davidson Resilience Scale (Connor & Davidson, 2003) which focus on a person's tolerance of negative impacts and positive acceptance of change.

He et al. (2019) draw on the psychological capital model (Luthans et al., 2004) to conceptualise and measure resilience (Luthans et al., 2007a). Luthans et al. (2004) describe psychological capital as a multidimensional construct consisting of four variables, one of which is resilience. Drawing on Luthans et al. (2004), He et al. (2019, p.232) conceptualise resilience as reflecting "one's ability to recover from adversity, failure, or irreversible change. Resilience can be developed using strategies of focusing on the asset, risk, and process."

Nwaogu et al. (2022b) measured resilience using the Brief Resilience Scale (BRS) (Smith et al., 2008). The BRS assesses the ability to bounce back or recover from stress.

In contrast to other studies, Turner et al. (2021) used the nine-item Employee Resilience Scale (Näswall et al., 2015) which conceptualises resilience as an adaptable employee capability, facilitated and supported by the organisation. Employee resilience is focused on behaviours which address everyday challenges at work (Näswall et al., 2019).

The non-cumulative nature of resilience research in construction is reflective of a broader limitation in the extant literature. Hartmann et al. (2020) conducted a critical review of research on resilience in the workplace and concluded that there is no consensus among researchers on how to define resilience at the individual level in the workplace. Furthermore, numerous scales of resilience have been used and developed and they rely on different conceptualisations of resilience. This is problematic for the advancement of the field (Hartmann et al., 2020).

There have been calls to use contextually relevant measures of resilience (Robertson et al., 2015) which are practical and enable results to be translated into the settings for which they are intended (Winwood et al., 2013). Context-specific measures can guide resilience development within a specific population and measure the effectiveness of resilience-building strategies in that setting. Various measures of resilience are used in the workplace, and authors such as Hartmann et al. (2020), Robertson et al. (2015), and Windle et al. (2011) provide useful overviews of the breadth and varying quality of measures.

6.8   Navigating difficult work environments

Resilience has been identified as a strategy for surviving and thriving in the face of workplace risk and adversity (Jackson et al., 2007), and has been identified as a capability that can help workers to navigate difficult work environments. For example, Shatté et al. (2017) found that workers with high resilience have better outcomes in difficult work environments and that, for depression, resilience has a more protective effect when job strain is high. Mealer et al. (2012) found that highly resilient intensive care nurses utilised positive coping skills and psychological characteristics that allowed them to continue working in a stressful work environment. Grant and Kinman (2014) suggest that resilience can enhance wellbeing for workers in helping professions such as nurses and social workers. Kossek et al. (2016) found that resilience was deemed a critical capability for those occupations with high job demands including police, firefighters, teachers, doctors, and nurses. Resilience has also been identified as a key resource for women in male-dominated professions (Richman, 2011). Kossek et al. (2016)

suggest that underrepresented groups in certain occupations, such as women in male-dominated professions, may need to be more resilient to avoid leaving the profession.

It is possible that resilience may be a critical resource that can help women to navigate the work hazards they experience in the male-dominated construction industry and thereby facilitate retention (Bridges et al., 2020). Case example 6.2 illustrates how women in construction utilise resilience to manage work stressors.

CASE EXAMPLE 6.2 RESILIENCE OF WOMEN ON CONSTRUCTION SITES

Turner et al. (2021) used the Employee Resilience Scale (EmpRes) (Näswall et al., 2015) to measure the resilience of trade and semi-skilled women working on site in construction. A total of 168 women completed the EmpRes. The age of participants ranged from 20 to 64 years; the mean age was 36 years. Years working in construction ranged from 1 to 42, with a mean of 9 years. The mean score of resilience was 6.0 (SD=.81) and the median score was 6.2, where 7.0 was the highest possible score. To provide some context to the findings, Turner et al. (2021) contrasted their results with other industries and groups that had used the EmpRes to measure employee resilience. Table 6.1 shows that the mean score for employee resilience ranged from 6.0 for women in our study, through to 4.03 for white-collar workers from finance, healthcare and education industries. Apart from the Turner et al. (2021) study, only one other study incorporated workers from the construction industry (Lin & Liao, 2020); however, the proportion of responses from construction workers was very small (0.9%) and results were not reported at the industry level. It is therefore not possible to consider the results outlined by Turner et al. (2021) in relation to other studies in construction. Furthermore, none of the studies using the EmpRes reported on employee resilience using a gender lens; therefore, it is not clear how the findings of Turner et al. (2021) compare with women in other occupational groups or industries.

TABLE 6.1 Studies using the EmpRes to measure employee resilience

Industry/Group	Mean	Study
Australian trade and semi-skilled women in construction	6.0	Turner et al. (2021)
Leaders from various organisations and industries in Taiwan	5.80	Lin and Liao (2020)
Frontline hotel employees in Ethiopia	5.80	Senbeto and Hon (2020)
Employees from a financial organisation in New Zealand	5.76	Näswall et al. (2019)

Employees from various organisations and industries in Taiwan	5.49	Lin and Liao (2020)
Employees from various organisations in China	4.91	Zhu and Li (2021)
Employees from a government department and tertiary education provider in New Zealand	4.14	Tonkin et al. (2018)
White-collar workers from finance, healthcare and education industries in New Zealand	4.03	Nguyen et al. (2016)

Source: Adapted from Turner et al. (2021).

Turner et al. (2021) interviewed 43 of the 168 survey respondents to explore why women working on site had a high level of employee resilience. Analysis of the survey data revealed that resilience was considered an essential capability for women to overcome workplace challenges and to survive and thrive in the construction industry.

Women considered that resilience was a critical capability for managing the challenges and hazards they experienced in their workplace. Resilience also assisted women to stay focused on work tasks. For example, one woman commented: *"I think resilience is having the determination and focus on what I need to do to get where I have to go, and that's not always easy. But it's also recognising my limitations and trying to work out other ways to reach my goal – and recognising that you can't fix everything."* Another woman explained how resilience enabled her to bounce back from challenging or difficult circumstances: *"Being able to keep just coming back. Getting up the next day and saying, 'okay, that day is done, let's move on', get up and do it all again kind of thing. Being able to come back, get knocked down and get back up again."* Being able to proactively manage challenges was also considered an important aspect of resilience. For example, a woman commented: *"I think resilience to me is putting up with unusual circumstances and being able to manage that in a way that's suitable for you … being able to put your own coping mechanism into place and managing the situation where you feel, you know, safe and comfortable."*

Resilience was recognised by women as integral for succeeding in the male-dominated construction industry. This belief was captured by a participant who commented that resilience is *"a strong adjective required for women in a male-dominated industry."* Many women experienced lack of support in achieving their work goals and thereby relied on resilience to succeed in the industry. For example, one participant commented: *"Nobody's going to help you achieve what you want. So, I think having that resilience there so that you can always bounce back, it's almost your number one necessity in trades."* Similarly, another participant explained: *"Because there's a lot of old school mentality, the culture is restrictive. So, if you want to succeed, or you want to progress and grow in the industry, resilience or sticking with what you're doing and pushing through is something that I think most definitely is part of the deal."*

While women acknowledged that resilience was a requirement to enable women in construction to manage setbacks, overcome challenges, and attain career goals, it was also acknowledged that cultural change needed to occur in the industry. For example, one woman commented: *"People always tell you 'Oh, you've got to be resilient. Yeah, you are resilient. Wow, you're really tough'. Being told you're resilient doesn't stop the s**t things happening to you that require you to be resilient. I think all of us would like to be in a position where being told that you're resilient is not necessarily something that you have to celebrate, because you don't need to do it anymore."*

6.9 Resilience training in the workplace

While there is emerging literature on employee resilience in construction, there appears to be very little literature on the implementation or evaluation of resilience-building activities. This is an important area of future research in construction. Notwithstanding that, a range of systematic reviews and meta-analysis studies have considered the vast array of workplace resilience-building measures more broadly. See for example: Robertson et al. (2015), Vanhove et al. (2016), Ijntema et al. (2019), Bryan et al. (2019).

Resilience training programmes in the workplace vary considerably in content, length, and delivery mode. For example, Robertson et al. (2015) reported on examples of divergence in resilience training programmes. Programmes varied considerably in their content, length and delivery mode. These variations are summarised as follows:

- *Content:* skills-based coaching approach; mindfulness- and compassion-based practice; biopsychospiritual enrichment programme designed to improve mental and spiritual health.
- *Length:* single 90-minute session; two-and-a-half-day retreat; programme delivered over 12 weeks.
- *Delivery mode:* online training; one-to-one sessions; group-based sessions; group-based sessions with one-to-one training.

Vanhove et al. (2016) report that the overall effect of resilience-building programmes is small, and that programme effects diminish over time. Vanhove et al. (2016) contend that programmes utilising a one-on-one delivery format (e.g., coaching) were most effective, followed by the classroom-based group delivery format. Programmes utilising train-the-trainer and computer-based delivery formats were least effective. Robertson et al. (2015) caution that there is a shortage of studies evaluating work-based resilience training: "the research that is available is not methodologically strong, limiting the possibility of drawing clear conclusions about the efficacy of resilience training and further supporting the need for researchers to execute well-designed studies that minimize threats to external validity" (p.556). Ijntema et al. (2019) note the growing interest in developing resilience-building programmes in the work context, and concur with Robertson et al. (2015) that the resilience literature provides no clear answer about what constitutes an effective resilience-building programme.

Kuntz et al. (2017) identify that interventions aimed at developing employee resilience focus primarily on individual rehabilitation or the development of personal resources, and argue that interventions should also consider the development of organisational resources that ensure both the inherent and adaptive resilience of employees. As such, Kuntz et al. (2017) emphasise the importance of resilience-building initiatives originating from the organisation, and outline four areas in which interventions should focus:

- valuing employees;
- human-capital development;
- support for challenges at work;
- fostering learning and collaboration.

To support the development of resilience-building programmes, Ijntema et al. (2019) present a set of criteria, developed systematically by reviewing studies published between 2009 and 2018. Table 6.2 outlines the criteria that should be met in a programme for building employee psychological resilience.

6.10   Conclusion

In recognition of the increasing damage created by occupational stress (International Labour Organization, 2016), resilience has been identified as an important capability which can support individual workers and work teams to positively adapt to stressors originating from the workplace. This chapter identified the various ways in which employee resilience can have a positive impact on health and wellbeing. Central to interactionist models of resilience is the integral role an organisation plays in providing employees with access to resources which can assist with adaptation to risk and adversity. Positioning employee resilience within an interactionist framework is critical as it takes the emphasis away from resilience as relying solely on the individual. Research on resilience in construction has received some attention, albeit limited. Furthermore, resilience to date has largely been non-cumulative in construction and this is reflective of the broader study of resilience which has been limited by inconsistent definitions and measures. A further limitation is the lack of empirical evidence as to the

TABLE 6.2 Criteria guiding resilience-building programs in the workplace

Criteria	Guiding remarks
1. The topic of interest is psychological resilience.	Psychological resilience does not include biological types of resilience.
2. The working population for whom the program is intended is specified.	The population can be general (e.g., employees) or specific (e.g., apprentices).
3. The work context in which the program is provided is specified.	e.g., construction
4. Resilience is defined, incorporating the terms dynamic process, adversity, and positive adaptation.	An example definition is "a dynamic process representing positive adaptation to adversity."
5. The characteristics of the adversity that trigger the need for resilience are specified.	e.g., unemployment, change, characteristics of adversity concern a single event or multiple events, the nature, intensity, duration, predictability, and frequency
6. An explanation is provided as to how positive adaptation is understood.	e.g., recovery, sustainability, growth
7. The process by which people adapt to adversity is displayed and explained.	Basic elements of a resilience process model are: pre-adversity adjustment, adversity, resilience mechanism, resources, outcomes.
8. The timing of the program is explained in relation to the adversity.	Before, during, or after the adversity
9. A general program aim and a specific program aim are provided. The general aim is to enhance resilience. The specific aim concerns which element(s) in the process of resilience is (are) targeted.	e.g., to enhance pre-adversity adjustment, to enhance resilience mechanisms, to enhance resources, to facilitate positive adaptation, to manage the amount and duration of adversity
10. An explanation is provided for how resilience is measured:	
a. which element(s) in the process of resilience is (are) measured, and	
b. at which time points so that change in resilience can be observed.	b. The time points can be determined in relation to the timescale of the program and of the adversity.
11. Specify whether there is a baseline level of a specific element of resilience at which people are eligible for the program.	
12. An explanation is provided for how the program enhances resilience	
a. by which approach,	a. e.g., cognitive-behavioural, scenario-, mindfulness-, skills-based
b. which mode of delivery, and	b. e.g., individual, group, electronic
c. in which time period (duration).	

Source: Adapted from Ijntema et al. (2019).

effectiveness of resilience-building interventions. Evaluating resilience-building interventions is an important area for future research. A resilience-based approach emphasises the building of skills and capacities that facilitate successful adaptation to risk and adversity. In contrast, a risk-reduction approach emphasises the removal of factors or processes considered harmful (Olsson et al., 2003), as has been addressed in other chapters. These two approaches are not mutually exclusive. For sustained effect, Olsson et al. (2003) recommend that both approaches are essential to support workers' wellbeing.

6.11   Discussion and review questions

1. How does employee resilience differ from team resilience?
2. Identify some examples of internal and external protective factors against risk and adversity. What can organisations do to ensure protective factors are present in the workplace?
3. What resources can an organisation provide to enhance employee resilience? What resources might be particularly important or helpful in a construction work environment?
4. What are the positive outcomes of employee resilience?

References

American Psychological Association (APA). (2020). *Building Your Resilience*. American Psychological Association. Accessed 17 August 2022 from www.apa.org/topics/resilie nce/building-your-resilience

Badran, M. A., & Youssef-Morgan, C. M. (2015). Psychological capital and job satisfaction in Egypt. *Journal of Managerial Psychology,* 30(3), 354–370.

Bartone, P. T. (2007). Test-retest reliability of the dispositional resilience scale-15, a brief hardiness scale. *Psychological Reports*, 101(3), 943–944.

Berggren, C., Söderlund, J., & Anderson, C. (2001). Clients, contractors, and consultants: the consequences of organizational fragmentation in contemporary project environments. *Project Management Journal*, 32(3), 39–48.

Bonanno, G. A. (2004). Loss, trauma, and human resilience: have we underestimated the human capacity to thrive after extremely aversive events? *American Psychologist,* 59(1), 20–28.

Bonanno, G. A. (2008). Loss, trauma, and human resilience: Have we underestimated the human capacity to thrive after extremely aversive events? *Psychological Trauma: Theory, Research, Practice, and Policy*, S(1), 101–113.

Bowers, C., Kreutzer, C., Cannon-Bowers, J., & Lamb, J. (2017). Team resilience as a second-order emergent state: A theoretical model and research directions. *Frontiers in Psychology*, 8, 1360–1360.

Bridges, D., Wulff, E., Bamberry, L., Krivokapic-Skoko, B., & Jenkins, S. (2020). Negotiating gender in the male-dominated skilled trades: a systematic literature review. *Construction Management and Economics*, 38(10), 894–916.

Britt, T. W., Shen, W., Sinclair, R. R., Grossman, M. R., & Klieger, D. M. (2016). How much do we really know about employee resilience? *Industrial and Organizational Psychology*, 9(2), 378–404.

Bryan, C., O'Shea, D., & Macintyre, T. (2019). Stressing the relevance of resilience: A systematic review of resilience across the domains of sport and work. *International Review of Sport and Exercise Psychology*, 12, 70–111.

Bryan, C., O'Shea, D., & MacIntyre, T. E. (2018). The what, how, where and when of resilience as a dynamic, episodic, self-regulating system: A response to Hill et al. (2018). *Sport, Exercise, and Performance Psychology*, 7(4), 355–362.

Chapman, M. T., Lines, R. L. J., Crane, M., Ducker, K. J., Ntoumanis, N., Peeling, P. Parker, S.K., Quested, E., Temby, P., Thøgersen-Ntoumani, C., & Gucciardi, D. F. (2020). Team resilience: A scoping review of conceptual and empirical work. *Work & Stress*, 34(1), 57–81.

Chen, Y., McCabe, B., & Hyatt, D. (2017a). Impact of individual resilience and safety climate on safety performance and psychological stress of construction workers: A case study of the Ontario construction industry. *Journal of Safety Research*, 61, 167–176.

Chen, Y., McCabe, B., & Hyatt, D. (2017b). Relationship between individual resilience, interpersonal conflicts at work, and safety outcomes of construction workers. *Journal of Construction Engineering and Management*, 143(8), 04017042.

Connor, K. M., & Davidson, J. R. (2003). Development of a new resilience scale: the Connor-Davidson Resilience Scale (CD-RISC). *Depression and Anxiety*, 18(2), 76–82.

Cooper, C. L., & Cartwright, S. (1997). An intervention strategy for workplace stress. *Journal of Psychosomatic Research*, 43(1), 7–16.

Cooper, C., Flint-Taylor, J., & Pearn, M. (2013). *Building Resilience for Success: A Resource for Managers and Organizations*. Palgrave Macmillan.

Engebø, A., Klakegg, O. J., Lohne, J., Bohne, R. A., Fyhn, H., & Lædre, O. (2022). High-performance building projects: how to build trust in the team. *Architectural Engineering and Design Management*, 8(6), 774–790.

Fergus, S., & Zimmerman, M. A. (2005). Adolescent resilience: a framework for understanding healthy development in the face of risk. *Annual Review of Public Health*, 26, 399–419.

Ferris, P. A., Sinclair, C., & Kline, T. J. (2005). It takes two to tango: Personal and organizational resilience as predictors of strain and cardiovascular disease risk in a work sample. *Journal of Occupational Health Psychology*, 10(3), 225–238.

Fisher, D. M., Ragsdale, J. M., & Fisher, E. C. S. (2019). The importance of definitional and temporal issues in the study of resilience. *Applied Psychology*, 68(4), 583–620.

Fletcher, D., & Sarkar, M. (2012). A grounded theory of psychological resilience in Olympic champions. *Psychology of Sport and Exercise*, 13(5), 669–678.

Fletcher, D., & Sarkar, M. (2013). Psychological resilience: A review and critique of definitions, concepts, and theory. *European Psychologist*, 18(1), 12–23.

Grant, L., & Kinman, G. (2012). Enhancing wellbeing in social work students: Building resilience in the next generation. *Social Work Education: The International Journal*, 31(5), 605–621.

Grant, L., & Kinman, G. (2014). Emotional resilience in the helping professions and how it can be enhanced. *Health and Social Care Education*, 3(1), 23–34.

Greve, W., & Staudinger, U. M. (2006). Resilience in later adulthood and old age: Resources and potentials for successful aging. In D. Cicchetti and D. J. Cohen (Eds.), *Developmental Psychopathology, Volume 3: Risk, Disorder, and Adaptation*. John Wiley & Sons (pp. 796–840).

Gucciardi, D. F., Crane, M., Ntoumanis, N., Parker, S. K., Thøgersen-Ntoumani, C., Ducker, K. J., Peeling, P., Chapman, M.T., Quested, E., & Temby, P. (2018). The emergence of team resilience: A multilevel conceptual model of facilitating factors. *Journal of Occupational and Organizational Psychology*, 91(4), 729–768.

Hartmann, S., Weiss, M., Newman, A., & Hoegl, M. (2020). Resilience in the workplace: A multilevel review and synthesis. *Applied Psychology*, 69(3), 913–959.

Hartwig, A., Clarke, S., Johnson, S., & Willis, S. (2020). Workplace team resilience: A systematic review and conceptual development. *Organizational Psychology Review*, 10(3–4), 169–200.

He, C., Jia, G., McCabe, B., Chen, Y., & Sun, J. (2019). Impact of psychological capital on construction worker safety behavior: Communication competence as a mediator. *Journal of Safety Research*, 71, 231–241.

Herrman, H., Stewart, D., Diaz-Granados, N., Berger, E., Jackson, B, & Yuen, T. (2011). What is resilience? *Canadian Journal of Psychiatry*, 56(5), 258–265.

Ijntema, R. C., Burger, Y. D., & Schaufeli, W. B. (2019). Reviewing the labyrinth of psychological resilience: Establishing criteria for resilience-building programs. *Consulting Psychology Journal: Practice and Research*, 71(4), 288–304.

International Labour Organization. (2016). *Workplace Stress: A Collective Challenge*. International Labour Organization.

Jackson, D., Firtko, A., & Edenborough, M. (2007). Personal resilience as a strategy for surviving and thriving in the face of workplace adversity: A literature review. *Journal of Advanced Nursing*, 60(1), 1–9.

Johnson, E. (2011). *Protective Factors and Levels of Resilience Among College Students*. PhD Thesis, Department of Educational Studies in Psychology, Research Methodology, and Counselling. University of Alabama.

Kinman, G., & Grant, L. (2011). Exploring stress resilience in trainee social workers: The role of emotional and social competencies. *British Journal of Social Work*, 41(2), 261–275.

Kirkwood, T., Bond, J., May, C., McKeith, I., & Teh, M.-M. (2008). *Mental Capital and Wellbeing: Making the Most of Ourselves in the 21st Century. Mental Capital Through Life: Future Challenges*. Government Office for Science, Foresight (Program), Mental Capital and Wellbeing Project.

Kossek, E. E., & Perrigino, M. B. (2016). Resilience: A review using a grounded integrated occupational approach. *Academy of Management Annals*, 10(1), 729–797.

Kuntz, J. R. C., Malinen, S., & Näswall, K. (2017). Employee resilience: Directions for resilience development. *Consulting Psychology Journal: Practice and Research*, 69(3), 223–242.

Leung, C. H. (2017). University support, adjustment, and mental health in tertiary education students in Hong Kong. *Asia Pacific Education Review*, 18(1), 115–122.

Lin, N., Simeone, R. S., Ensel, W. M., & Kuo, W. (1979). Social support, stressful life events, and illness: a model and an empirical test. *Journal of Health and Social Behaviour*, 20(2), 108–119.

Lin, T.T., & Liao, Y. (2020). Future temporal focus in resilience research: When leader resilience provides a role model. *Leadership & Organization Development Journal*, 41(7), 897–907.

Luthans, F., Avolio, B. J., Avey, J. B., & Norman, S. M. (2007a). Positive psychological capital: Measurement and relationship with performance and satisfaction. *Personnel Psychology*, 60(3), 541–572.

Luthans, F., Luthans, K. W., & Luthans, B. C. (2004). Positive psychological capital: beyond human and social capital. *Business Horizons*, 47(1), 45–50.

Luthar, S. S., & Cicchetti, D. (2000). The construct of resilience: Implications for interventions and social policies. *Development and Psychopathology*, 12(4), 857–885.

Masten, A. S. (2018). Resilience theory and research on children and families: Past, present, and promise. *Journal of Family Theory & Review,* 10(1), 12–31.

McEwan, K. (2018). *Resilience at Work: A Framework for Coaching and Interventions.* Accessed 18 August 2022: https://workingwithresilience.com.au/wp-content/uplo ads/2018/09/Whitepaper-Sept18.pdf

McLarnon, M. J. W., & Rothstein, M. G. (2013). Development and initial validation of the workplace resilience inventory. *Journal of Personnel Psychology,* 12(2), 63–73.

Mealer, M., Jones, J., & Moss, M. (2012). A qualitative study of resilience and post-traumatic stress disorder in United States ICU nurses. *Intensive Care Medicine,* 38(9), 1445–1451.

Meneghel, I., Martínez, I. M., & Salanova, M. (2016). Job-related antecedents of team resilience and improved team performance. *Personnel Review,* 45(3), 505–522.

Näswall, K., Kuntz, J.R.C., & Malinen, S. (2015). *Employee resilience scale (EmpRes): Measurement properties.* Resilient Organisations research report 2015/04.

Näswall, K., Malinen, S., Kuntz, J., & Hodliffe, M. (2019). Employee resilience: development and validation of a measure. *Journal of Managerial Psychology,* 34(5), 353–367.

Nguyen, Q., Kuntz, J., Näswall, K., & Malinen, S. (2016). Employee resilience and leadership styles: The moderating role of proactive personality and optimism. *New Zealand Journal of Psychology,* 45(2), 13–21.

Nwaogu, J. M., Chan, A. P. C., & Tetteh, M. O. (2022b). Staff resilience and coping behavior as protective factors for mental health among construction tradesmen. *Journal of Engineering, Design and Technology,* 20(3), 671–695.

Nwaogu, J., Chan, A., & Naslund, J. (2022a). Measures to improve the mental health of construction personnel based on expert opinions. *Journal of Management in Engineering,* 38(4), 04022019.

O'Brien, A. P., Cho, M. A. A., Lew, A.-M., Creedy, D., Ho Chun Man, R., Chan, M. F., & Gordon, A. D. (2008). The Need for Mental Health Promotion and Early Intervention Services for Higher Education Students in Singapore. *International Journal of Mental Health Promotion,* 10(3), 42–48.

Olsson, C., Bond, L., Burns, J., Vella-Brodrick, D., & Sawyer, S. (2003). Adolescent resilience: A concept analysis. *Journal of Adolescence,* 26(1), 1–11.

Ong, A. D., Bergeman, C. S., Bisconti, T. L., & Wallace, K. A. (2006). Psychological resilience, positive emotions, and successful adaptation to stress in later life. *Journal of Personality and Social Psychology,* 91(4), 730–749.

Ozbay, F., Johnson, D. C., Dimoulas, E., Morgan, C. A., Charney, D., & Southwick, S. (2007). Social support and resilience to stress: from neurobiology to clinical practice. *Psychiatry,* 4(5), 35–40.

Productivity Commission. (2020). *Mental Health, Report No. 95,* Australian Government.

Richman, L. S., van Dellen, M., & Wood, W. (2011). How women cope: Being a numerical minority in a male-dominated profession. *Journal of Social Issues,* 67(3), 492–509.

Robertson, I. T., Cooper, C. L., Sarkar, M., & Curran, T. (2015). Resilience training in the workplace from 2003 to 2014: A systematic review. *Journal of Occupational and Organizational Psychology,* 88(3), 533–562.

Rossouw, P., & Rossouw, J. (2016). The Predictive 6-Factor Resilience Scale: Neurobiological Fundamentals and Organizational Application. *International Journal of Neuropsychotherapy,* 4, 31–45.

Sacker, A., & Schoon, I. (2007). Educational resilience in later life: Resources and assets in adolescence and return to education after leaving school at age 16. *Social Science Research,* 36(3), 873–896.

Schwarzer, R., & Jerusalem, M. (1995). Generalized self-efficacy scale. In J. Weinman, S. Wright, and M. Johnston (Eds.), *Measures in Health Psychology: A User's Portfolio.* NFER-NELSON (pp. 35–37).

Senbeto, D. L., & Hon, A. H. Y. (2020). Market turbulence and service innovation in hospitality: examining the underlying mechanisms of employee and organizational resilience. *Service Industries Journal,* 40(15–16), 1119–1139.

Shaikh, A., & Kauppi, C. (2010). Deconstructing resilience: Myriad conceptualizations and interpretations. *International Journal of Arts and Sciences,* 3, 155–176.

Shatté, A., Perlman, A., Smith, B., & Lynch, W. D. (2017). The positive effect of resilience on stress and business outcomes in difficult work environments. *Journal of Occupational and Environmental Medicine,* 59(2), 135–140.

Smith, B., Dalen, J., Wiggins, K., Tooley, E., Christopher, P., & Bernard, J. (2008). The Brief Resilience Scale: Assessing the ability to bounce back. *International Journal of Behavioural Medicine,* 15, 194–200.

Southwick, S. M., Bonanno, G. A., Masten, A. S., Panter-Brick, C., & Yehuda, R. (2014). Resilience definitions, theory, and challenges: Interdisciplinary perspectives. *European Journal of Psychotraumatology,* 5(1), 25338.

Stewart, M., Reid, G., & Mangham, C. (1997). Fostering children's resilience. *Journal of Pediatric Nursing: Nursing Care of Children and Families,* 12(1), 21–31.

Tetrick, L. E., & Winslow, C. J. (2015). Workplace stress management interventions and health promotion. *Annual Review of Organizational Psychology and Organizational Behavior,* 2(1), 583–603.

Tonkin, K., Malinen, S., Näswall, K., & Kuntz, J. C. (2018). Building employee resilience through wellbeing in organizations. *Human Resource Development Quarterly,* 29(2), 107–124.

Tse, J. S. Y., & Haslam, N. (2021). Inclusiveness of the concept of mental disorder and differences in help-seeking between Asian and White Americans. *Frontiers in Psychology,* 12, article 699750.

Turner, M., Holdsworth, S., & Scott-Young, C. M. (2017b). Resilience at University: the development and testing of a new measure. *Higher Education Research & Development,* 36(2), 386–400.

Turner, M., Holdsworth, S., Scott-Young, C. M., & Sandri, K. (2021). Resilience in a hostile workplace: The experience of women onsite in construction. *Construction Management and Economics,* 39(10), 839–852.

Turner, M., Scott-Young, C. M., & Holdsworth, S. (2017a). Promoting wellbeing at university: The role of resilience for students of the built environment. *Construction Management and Economics,* 35(11–12), 707–718.

Tusaie, K., & Dyer, J. (2004). Resilience: A historical review of the construct. *Holistic Nursing Practice,* 18(1), 3–10.

Ungar, M. (2013). Resilience, trauma, context, and culture. *Trauma, Violence, & Abuse,* 14(3), 255–266.

Ungar, M. (2018). Systemic resilience: principles and processes for a science of change in contexts of adversity. *Ecology and Society,* 23(4), article 34.

van Breda, A. D. (2018). A critical review of resilience theory and its relevance for social work. *Social Work,* 54(1), 1–18.

Vanderbilt-Adriance, E., & Shaw, D. S. (2008). Conceptualizing and re-evaluating resilience across levels of risk, time, and domains of competence. *Clinical Child and Family Psychology Review,* 11(1–2), 30–58.

Vanhove, A. J., Herian, M. N., Perez, A. L. U., Harms, P. D., & Lester, P. B. (2016). Can resilience be developed at work? A meta-analytic review of resilience-building programme effectiveness. *Journal of Occupational and Organizational Psychology,* 89(2), 278–307.

Wanberg, C. R., & Banas, J. T. (2000). Predictors and outcomes of openness to changes in a reorganizing workplace. *Journal of Applied Psychology,* 85(1), 132–142.

West, B. J., Patera, J. L., & Carsten, M. K. (2009). Team level positivity: Investigating positive psychological capacities and team level outcomes. *Journal of Organizational Behavior,* 30(2), 249–267.

Windle, G. (2011). What is resilience? A review and concept analysis. *Reviews in Clinical Gerontology,* 21(02), 152–169.

Winwood, P. C., Colon, R., & McEwen, K. (2013). A Practical Measure of Workplace Resilience: Developing the Resilience at Work Scale. *Journal of Occupational and Environmental Medicine,* 55(10), 1205–1212.

World Health Organization. (2017). *Building Resilience: A Key Pillar of Health 2020 and the Sustainable Development Goals.* World Health Organization.

Zhu, Y., & Li, W. (2021). Proactive personality triggers employee resilience: A dual-pathway model. *Social Behavior and Personality,* 49(2), 1–11.

7

HEALTH ISSUES IN THE CONSTRUCTION INDUSTRY IN DEVELOPING COUNTRIES

The case of Sub-Saharan Africa

Peter J. Edwards[1] and Paul A. Bowen[2]

[1]School of Property, Construction & Project Management, RMIT University, Melbourne, Australia

[2]Department of Construction Economics and Management, University of Cape Town, Private Bag, Rondebosch, Cape Town, South Africa

7.1 Introduction

Our chapter first deals with development generally in the Sub-Saharan region of Africa and the economic and social issues that pertain to it. We then examine the construction industry in relation to some of these issues. This provides sufficient contextualisation to explore factors that affect the occupational health and wellbeing of workers in the construction industry in Southern Africa, covering matters such as morbidity, infections and diseases. A separate section of the chapter is devoted to the scourge of HIV/AIDS. We then explore construction industry health testing; and family and lifestyle factors relating to occupational health and wellbeing. Readers will find that we have made extensive use of statistics throughout this chapter, and we make no apologies for this. They are essential for communicating the extent and importance of occupational health issues for construction industries in the nations of Sub-Saharan Africa (SSA).

7.2 Occupational wellbeing

Occupational wellbeing embraces the physical, mental, emotional and social health of people in their work (see, for example, Faragher et al., 2004). While physical health can be medically established, the other three components of wellbeing are less easy to assess. They are usually measured through worker self-perception surveys of the degree to which influencing factors are seen to contribute positively or negatively to their health. Leung et al. (2015) have summarised over 40 such studies relating to the construction industry, categorising them in terms

DOI: 10.1201/9780367814236-7

of foci such as sources and strain effects (performance and job satisfaction) and coping behaviours. Failure to promote positive worker wellbeing may eventually lead to lower productivity (e.g., through work tedium and de-motivation), while failure to address negative wellbeing may exacerbate existing impaired performance of workers. Either outcome brings costs to national economies and to society if occupational health issues are not dealt with effectively.

Research using validated and replicable data-gathering instruments and administration may be aimed at the general working population of a country, through the accretion of data from different industry segments (e.g., Faragher et al., 2004; Donald et al., 2005; Robertson Cooper, 2012) or at workers engaged in particular occupations or industries, such as professionals working in the construction industry (e.g., Cattell et al., 2017). The research findings expose, support or contradict the nature and extent of health issues relating to any or all of the four wellbeing states noted above. For example, the Cattell et al. (2017) survey of 790 professionals in the construction industry found that, compared to the general working population, while their overall wellbeing (measured across eight scales) was typical, in two respects (balanced workload and work relationships) they should be considered atypical and at high risk, and in two others (job conditions and resources & communication) they were approaching high-risk status. These research findings thus supported other evidence of industry issues relating to mental stress (workload) and social and emotional stress (work relationships). Additional findings were that wellbeing was significantly higher among self-employed or very senior construction professionals than among salaried workers, suggesting that job autonomy plays an important part in wellbeing. Also, female construction professionals felt less confident (and correspondingly displayed less resilience) than their male counterparts. The latter finding points towards a cultural issue in the construction industry that is discussed in detail in Chapter 5 of this book.

Why is it important to explore wellbeing in the construction industry? Construction is known for being dirty, difficult and dangerous (Lingard & Francis, 2009), and to that we might add a fourth "d" – disjointed. It is a dirty industry because of the largely hands-on nature of the tasks involved for the majority of workers it employs, the types of materials used, the task environments (below and high above ground level), exposure to extremes of weather, and the green-field (undeveloped) or brown-field (redevelopment) sites on which construction takes place. It is difficult because of the multiplicity of tasks to be performed, the task schedule interdependencies that arise, and the uncertainty associated with their inputs and outputs. To this difficulty must also be added the temporary management structures associated with almost all projects and the adversarial nature of many building contracts. Construction is dangerous because of the risks involved in carrying out physical tasks under often severe conditions (e.g., at height from ladders or in confined spaces); the technologies required (e.g., heavy machinery and equipment, welding, cutting, or even explosives); and the time constraints (e.g., the inevitable pressure to complete every project to tight deadlines) that exacerbate all these factors. Finally, construction is disjointed because of the structural complexity of the industry itself, with public-sector and private-sector projects driven by different objectives, a wide variety of project types, manifold building codes and regulations, budgetary constraints that have stop/go effects, quality assurance expectations, professional discipline separation and trades and specialist fragmentation. In the case of Sub-Saharan Africa (SSA), distinction is also found between formal and informal sectors of the industry, and in terms of what and how construction is carried out and by whom.

7.3   The Sub-Saharan region

The World Bank identifies 48 countries regarded as being in the SSA region. These nations range alphabetically from Angola to Zimbabwe (see: https://data. worldbank.org/country/sub-saharan-africa?display=). Given their number, it is not possible to cover every country in a single chapter and thus, where we go beyond the general, we have been selective.

"Development" is commonly understood to be an ongoing process, with the 48 Sub-Saharan nations regarded as "developing" or "emerging" in stark contrast to the "developed" status of the advanced economies of most Western nations. The development process is seen as positive when measured in terms of improvements taking place in economic performance, living standards, sustainability and equality, but outcomes in these areas are not always consistent. Progress in some areas may stagnate or even decline – the latter outcome most often occurring as a result of natural disasters or human malfeasance. The United Nations Human Development Index assesses the effects of development on people (relative to other countries) in terms of life expectancy, level of education, and income. Developing countries are usually found to have transitional economies, an under-developed industrial base, weak financial borrowing capacity, poor levels of governance, and inadequate provision of housing and education for their populations. They can be vulnerable to exploitation of valuable resources by foreign entrepreneurs, and are highly vulnerable to corruption.

Across the SSA region, the United Nations Development Programme (UNDP) indicators have been generally positive over the six decades from 1960 to 2018, although it is still too early to consider in any depth the potential impacts and longer-term effects of the novel-coronavirus (COVID-19) global pandemic which emerged in late 2019, other than to note that the supply and administration of effective vaccines across Africa has lagged behind that of more developed nations. Adverse impacts of COVID-19 are thus likely to be later and longer in SSA.

Using the World Bank data (see World Bank URL above), gross domestic product across the region increased from US$30 billion to US$1.7 trillion over the period 1960–2018. Life expectancy at birth rose from about 41 years in 1960 to just over 61 years in 2018. Primary school enrolments, as a percentage of age eligibility for enrolment, have risen from 54 to 98 per cent over the same period.

Gross national income (GNI) per capita increased from the equivalent of US$121 per annum in 1962 to US$1,520 in 2018.

In terms of sustainability, however, carbon dioxide (CO_2) emissions have increased gradually from 0.55 metric tonnes per capita in 1960 to 0.85 tonnes in 2014, reflecting the slowly growing trend of industrialisation in the region and the use of fossil-based fuels for electricity generation and transport vehicles.

These statistics must also be seen against the background of population growth (227 million in 1960 to just over 1.7 billion in 2018). Of all the World Bank data, population growth is the only one to display a completely smooth upward exponential trend; all the others reveal short-term volatility, probably ascribable to national or international events.

On an inter-nation basis there is wide disparity between these data; for example, GNI in South Africa was equivalent to US$5,750 in 2018 – nearly four times that for the region as a whole, despite sharing a similar ratio at the start of the 1968–2018 period, indicating a far more volatile curve over time.

7.4   Development issues

That population growth in SSA has increased exponentially is the underlying key to development issues for the whole region. If large families are no longer required to overcome high infant mortality and to ensure support for elderly parents, the economic "cake" available to individuals can grow as the cost of raising a smaller family is decreased and discretionary spending and saving capacity are increased. The impacts of this economic "lever," however, are only experienced in the long term and, as the contemporary situations of many westernised developed nations show, if birth rates decline too far they can exert a reverse effect on productivity and the economic prosperity of countries.

Better development levers are found in increasing education opportunities and standards, providing adequate and affordable housing, improving living and social standards, health and health facilities, employment opportunities, training and re-training, raising productivity and, through all of these, thereby increasing all-round prosperity. Of all these, the provision of adequate housing has proved the most intractable problem in SSA.

There is a circularity about all this that is vexing, since exacerbating a downward spiral is easier than encouraging and facilitating an upward trend. For example, the effect of HIV/AIDS in this region has been distressing and devastating for families, especially where primary family breadwinners have died, leaving child-headed families struggling for survival or young children in the care of elderly grandparents ill-equipped for the role. Anti-retroviral (ARV) medication may now extend the working lives of HIV+ infectees but this requires long-term compliance with treatment programmes and a commitment to healthier lifestyles. It does not address the immediate legacy effects of HIV/AIDS-related deaths, especially in countries where public health and welfare systems are already stretched beyond sustainable limits.

Uniform and simultaneous emphasis on, and response to, all these economic and social factors is impossible, of course, and politics and internally related sub-influences may come into play, but common to all of them, and to development itself, is the role of the construction industry. Anything that affects this industry has an onward positive or negative impact upon development. Worker health and wellbeing is clearly one such factor. Poor management, corruption and lack of strong democratic government are others, but the latter three are beyond the remit of this chapter.

7.5   The construction industry

The economic role of the construction industry in a country is to increase the amount of gross domestic fixed investment (GDFI) – the value of fixed assets in the form of buildings and physical infrastructure, and the machinery for manufacturing. This "stock" may range from housing to facilities for manufacturing, assembly and storage of products, education, health, justice, administration, food production and processing, for social, sports, cultural, religious observance and leisure activities, and for many other purposes. Infrastructure assets include facilities for power generation and distribution, water treatment, effluent and waste treatment, pipelines, roads, railways, ports and airports. Maintenance, repair and alteration work also adds to the output of the industry. Increases in GDFI may lead or lag behind movements in other sectors of a nation's economy, and are largely driven by the availability of investment capital and the capacity of the construction industry to respond to the demands placed upon it. Economic and social issues come into play.

7.5.1   Construction industry economic issues

Across SSA, the construction industry accounts for about 5–6 per cent of gross domestic product (GDP) but accounts for 8–12 per cent of employment (about 85 per cent of that being male). It is thus a significant contributor to national economies and employment everywhere in the region. It also acts as a stepping stone for workers wanting to exploit the opportunity to transition from unskilled to better skilled status. At the same time, however, it is vulnerable to changes taking place in other sectors and to global events. Clearly, it also offers little by way of redressing the issues of female disadvantage.

In the third quarter of 2018 construction industry output growth forecasts for the SSA region over the period 2018–2022 ranged from 1.2 per cent (South Africa) to 12.7 per cent (Ethiopia) (see: https://globaldata.com/construction). In the light of the COVID-19 pandemic, however, others now suggest that these rates are likely to be at least halved (see: https://bakermackenzie.com and https://infrast ructurenews.co.za/2020/04/03/sub-saharan-africa-construction-sector-highly-vulnerable-to-coronavirus-impact/). This is due to weakened local economies, the effects of lockdown virus suppression policies and containment measures, the slowdown in China's geographically targeted global development programme (its "Belt and Road Initiative"), decreases in Chinese demand for the region's exportable mineral resources as the Chinese economy itself continues to slow down, and reduction in the ready and rapid availability of Chinese-manufactured building materials and components. The globaldata.com source is even more pessimistic, reducing its growth forecast for SSA from 6 per cent (Q4 2019) down to 3.6 per cent, and for South Africa to -4.1 per cent for 2018–2022. The same sources note that these rates are likely to be accompanied by higher national debt and lowered spending on infrastructure, with economies going into recession in many SSA countries. All this will inevitably affect the capacity and willingness of construction organisations to increase spending upon worker wellbeing.

Throughout SSA, employment-seeking migration brings large numbers of mainly young males from rural into urban areas. Often the only job opportunities available to them are as unskilled workers in the construction industry. This distorts the skills-development and training structure of the industry, as the low levels of education usually associated with migrant workers, together with their inability to afford further education, inhibit their capacity to engage more effectively in the workforce. Productivity thus becomes a major issue as, for many workers, skills are learned only partially on the job. Also, given their lack of education, migrant workers' learning curves are likely to be slow and erratic.

The economic recessions occurring in countries globally as a result of COVID-19 impacts have already begun to affect employment levels in the construction industry worldwide as growth slows down. Unskilled or semi-skilled workers are among the first to be retrenched, and the last to be re-engaged. The employment structures of the construction industries in SSA nations are likely to exacerbate this situation, since casually focused recruitment (for the project duration; and weekly or even daily hiring) generally predominates over other structural arrangements that deliver greater job security.

All this has added further volatility to an industry that is already cyclical as it responds to changes occurring in national economies, and as it is used by governments as an economic regulator through monetary and fiscal policies. Ideally, governments should act counter-cyclically, increasing spending on public projects and infrastructure when their national economies are in decline, and encouraging greater private-sector investment when upturns occur. Nowadays, however, this rarely occurs. Almost all jurisdictions have been attracted by the public-private partnership (PPP) route to physical infrastructure development and service delivery in the public sector, largely to avoid public borrowing for finance and the consequent appearance of large amounts of debt on public balance sheets (thereby attracting the wrath of central government auditors). This route, however, is highly susceptible to shifting appetites for risk among global entrepreneurs and financiers. Nevertheless, PPP procurement is still attractive, as costs can be recovered (and private-sector returns on investment achieved) through user-pays approaches (e.g., toll roads) or availability charges (e.g., hospitals, correctional facilities) over decades-long concession periods, which can be further extended to encourage private financing for improvements or additions to the PPP "assets." The "acquire now/pay later" approach is as tempting for governments as "never-never" hire purchase is for individuals. At the same time, however, it affects governments' desire and capacity to engage in counter-cyclical spending activities. Furthermore, for the construction industry, PPP highs and lows create a "feast or famine" scenario for major industry players and transnational construction companies. This has a cascading effect on the resources and opportunities available for smaller and micro-firms – not only for construction companies but also for the suppliers, subcontractors and professional firms that service the industry.

How do all these economic issues affect health and wellbeing in the construction workforce? By and large their effects are indirect, through the stresses of job insecurity, the need to travel long distances for work, and long working days that affect work–life balances. More directly, when the industry is in a downturn, market competition for construction work increases and forces down prices. Construction companies then try to cut costs and increase productivity through longer working hours, or by bidding for work in more remote locations, thus exacerbating the work–life imbalance. More seriously, greater competition and the pursuit of increased productivity may lead to compromises in construction safety and environmental precautions, putting the health of construction workers at greater risk. For a largely ill-educated construction workforce, this may occur complicitly (willingness to work long hours in dangerous conditions) or in ignorance (lack of knowledge about safety regulations and health requirements) on the workers' part. Even for well-educated construction professionals, high-pressure work demands at one extreme, and job insecurity at the other, adversely affect work–life balance, health and wellbeing.

7.5.2   Construction industry social issues

Beyond what we may describe as the structural economic issues for the SSA construction industries lie social issues relating to the industry that can affect worker health and wellbeing. These include the legacy effects of European colonialism; remote working and rural migration and their effects on family life; and the lack of comprehensive medical insurance across the SSA construction industries.

The effects of historical European colonialism linger on to a marked degree in SSA. Whether emanating from Great Britain, France, Portugal, Germany, the Netherlands or Belgium, the colonial powers all treated construction in a "master–servant" manner in terms of Indigenous workers. Artisan trades would be carried out by the more qualified European immigrants, and Indigenous workers were employed only as cheap unskilled, or at best semi-skilled, labour. Vestiges of this still remain, and nowhere more so than in South Africa, where the former apartheid regime legislated the racial segregation of trade skills when it came to power after the Second World War. Apart from the mixed-race coloured population of the Western Cape, artisan trades were reserved for white workers, and Indigenous Black African workers were limited to employment as unskilled or semi-skilled labourers in the construction industry. Little or no security of employment was available to them. Despite the racial de-segregation and Black employment opportunity enhancement measures (eg., affirmative action and bid preferment for public-sector projects) introduced after the 1994 transition to a post-apartheid democratic regime, the South African construction industry has largely been slow to respond to change. Skills transfer and training opportunities for skills improvement have been inadequate, since most Black African construction workers have first needed more education, and education at all levels has inevitably proved a vexing problem to address.

Contemporary lifestyle influences of dormitory living, alcoholism and substance abuse all affect construction workers. Some will be considered later in our discussion about HIV/AIDS, as also will be the issue of transactional sex.

The extent of job security is highly related to the availability of employer-provided medical health insurance benefits. The absence of such benefits, for workers employed under more precarious casual hiring arrangements, leads to masking effects as workers underplay illnesses and injuries in order to remain at work, and also to social unease within families.

7.6 Occupational health and wellbeing in the construction industry in Southern Africa

In this section we consider morbidity factors that more directly affect the health and wellbeing of construction workers in SSA, noting, however, that many are not exclusive to this region. We have narrowed our focus here to Southern Africa, and for the most part to South Africa since information is more readily available for this nation.

Aside from accidents on site, morbidity in the construction industry is largely attributable to disease and opportunistic infection. The more important ones from our perspective are the recent novel-coronavirus (COVID-19) pandemic, malaria, tuberculosis, and HIV/AIDS.

7.6.1 COVID-19

Emergence of the novel-coronavirus global pandemic in late 2019 (officially termed COVID-19 by the World Health Organization) has left few industries and organisations, public or private, free of its risks to health and its effects upon everyday living.

After exposure to the virus, and infection has occurred, morbidity may occur when oxygenation of the body's essential blood supply is compromised, and vital organs shut down. Re-oxygenation, through the use of mechanical ventilators to assist patients with breathing, may assist in recovery, but shortages of such equipment in hospital intensive care units (ICUs) and in aged-care homes, together with the concomitant pressure placed upon the bed-spaces and staff in such places, has been a matter of great concern worldwide. Supply shortages for personal protective equipment (PPE), in the face of rapid increases in demand, are an aggravating factor in a pandemic that, in just a few years since its arrival, has already seen more than 1 million deaths worldwide – the majority of these among the elderly and infirm. This number is not accurate, since many disease-related deaths have been under-reported or not reported at all. Many countries are now experiencing "second wave" effects, and "third waves" may occur in parallel with the roll-out of effective vaccines.

While countries have differed in terms of adopting suppression or eradication strategies, many have introduced restrictions and limitations on normal day-to-day activities, either nationally or for areas with higher infection rates.

COVID-19 work restrictions generally limit construction workers in terms of where and how they can work, and how far they are permitted to travel to work. For jurisdictions where tighter restrictions are in place, this may affect whether construction work can be carried out at all and, if so, how many workers can be employed on each site, what "social distancing" (mandatory physical separation spacing between individuals – usually from 1.5 to 2.0 metres) measures must be continuously maintained and whether or not appropriate face masks must be worn at all times. Clearly this has a direct and adverse bearing on work planning, supervision, productivity and not least upon worker morale.

To date, no severe restrictions have been placed upon the construction industries in any of the countries in the SSA region, compared to those enforced in developed countries.

7.6.2 Malaria

With a global prevalence of over 219 million reported cases in 2017 (WHO, 2018) the parasitic disease of malaria is a major health concern, across almost all continents, ages and genders. The SSA region alone accounted for nearly 200 million cases. While malaria has declined globally and in a few African countries from 2016–17, increases have occurred in many more. About 400,000 deaths from malaria occurred in 2017 in the SSA region, but the further south of the equator you travel, the greater the decline found in the prevalence statistics.

Since malaria is transmitted into the human bloodstream by disease-bearing female mosquitoes, prevention and eradication campaigns (strongly urged by the World Health Organization) have largely focused upon the reduction of areas holding stagnant water (the insects' typical breeding grounds) in urban environments, the localised use of insecticides, and upon curtailing or destroying the capacity of mosquitoes to breed and carry the disease.

Dichlorodiphenyltrichloroethane (DDT), the chemical compound insecticide used for many years as an insect control, is now almost universally banned due to its harmful side effects upon humans and its increasing ineffectiveness as mosquitoes have developed resistance to its properties.

Clearly, "wet" sites or those close to large areas of stagnant water pose health risks for workers in SSA construction industry organisations. Since these conditions can make work more difficult, they tend to be avoided or the wet locations minimised. Consequently, malaria is not considered a critical concern for the construction industry in much of SSA.

7.6.3 Tuberculosis

According to Churchyard et al. (2014), tuberculosis (TB) remains a global threat to health. Although successfully treatable for many years, and exhibiting a slow global decline, the 2006 emergence of drug-resistant strains of TB was a cause for major concern.

TB is one of several opportunistic infections that are driven by HIV/AIDS and thus acts as a frequent cause of death (almost 13%) among people living with HIV (PLWH). In South Africa, prevalence of TB is almost four times higher among PLWH than among those who have tested negative. South Africa is included among the top few of high-burden countries for TB identified by the World Health Organization.

The exact prevalence of TB in the construction industries in SSA is not known. It is likely to arise through aerosol transmissions of sputum, in the exhalations from infectees, falling upon other people working in close proximity, especially in closely confined spaces. Since these conditions constitute much of the outdoor and indoor working environments for construction sites, the presence of TB there is not surprising. High labour intensity and the comparative lack of on-site mechanised processes and prefabrication technologies in SSA, together with poor on-site sanitary facilities and the cramped and crowded living environments of workers, serve to exacerbate the situation.

Given its prevalence and importance in SSA, we now turn separately to the issue of HIV/AIDS and its significance in the construction industry, focusing upon South Africa.

7.7 HIV/AIDS and the construction industry

This section is structured in several parts. Firstly, the anatomy and treatment of the disease is described. Secondly, an overview of HIV/AIDS in SSA is given, with Kharsany and Karim (2016), UNAIDS, and the World Health Organization (WHO) being the primary sources of information. Thirdly, an overview of the pandemic in South Africa is documented, based on the latest report of the Human Sciences Research Council in 2019 (Simbayi et al., 2019). Fourthly, HIV/AIDS and the South African construction industry is discussed.

7.7.1 Disease anatomy and treatment

For this section we draw on an explanatory document entitled "The Science of HIV and AIDS – overview" (see www.avert.org/professionals/hiv-science/overview) by Avert (n.d.) (www.avert.org), and a comprehensive guide to HIV/

AIDS provided by Pietrangelo (2018) and available at: www.healthline.com/hea lth/hiv-aids.

HIV is the human immunodeficiency virus, a pathogen that attacks the human immune system and belongs to a class of viruses called retroviruses. This means that it works in a reverse way. Unlike other viruses, retroviruses store their genetic information using RNA instead of DNA, and need to "make" DNA when they enter a human cell in order to make new copies of themselves. HIV cannot replicate on its own so, to make copies of itself, it infects cells of the human immune system (CD4 cells). CD4 cells are white blood cells that are pivotal in responding to infections. They are destroyed by HIV and the body's ability to recognise and fight certain types of infection begins to decline. Loss of CD4 cells resulting from lack of treatment leads to vulnerability to "opportunistic infections," such as pneumonia, tuberculosis, oral thrush, cytomegalovirus (CMV – a type of herpes virus), and cryptococcal meningitis (a fungal infection in the brain). The most advanced stage of HIV is when someone has a collection of these infections and is then said to have developed AIDS (acquired immunodeficiency syndrome). Effective testing and treatment of HIV is crucial for HIV-infected persons to avoid reaching this advanced stage.

The clinical stages of infection comprise the primary or acute stage and the chronic stage. In the primary stage, HIV enters the human body by infecting CD4 cells in the mucous membranes of the vagina or rectum, or by direct infection of CD4 t-cells in the bloodstream. In essence, HIV is transmitted through bodily fluids such as blood, semen, vaginal and rectal fluids, breast milk, and to a baby *in-utero* during pregnancy. Common symptoms of HIV infection include fever, body rash, swollen glands, fatigue, headaches, and weight loss. Not everyone will experience fever and body rash. Symptoms of acute infection can last for up to two weeks. Within a further four to eight days, HIV antibody-only tests using blood will show a positive result. After about six months the viral load and CD4 cell count levels will stabilise at a level known as the "set point."

In the chronic infection phase, HIV infection may not cause further illness for some years (the asymptomatic phase). During this period, HIV gradually reduces the number of CD4 cells in the body until the CD4 cell count falls below 200 cells/mm^3. Once the count falls below this level, the risk of developing AIDS-related opportunistic infections greatly increases. This phase lasts for about ten years, depending upon the rate of decline of the CD4 cell count. If the infectee has a very high viral load (above 100,000 copies/ml), CD4 cell loss is more rapid. During the asymptomatic phase, CD4 cell counts and viral load blood tests are used clinically to monitor the progression of HIV disease.

Treatment should begin as soon as possible after an HIV-positive diagnosis, irrespective of viral load. The primary treatment is antiretroviral therapy (ART), a combination of daily medications that prevent the HIV virus from reproducing – thereby protecting the CD4 cells and sufficiently maintaining the strength of the immune system to fight disease. ART suppresses HIV to undetectable levels, restores the CD4 cell count to normal levels, and prevents opportunistic disease – as long as treatment is started in time during the asymptomatic phase and taken daily. Compliance with the treatment regimen is critical, and is not compatible with high alcohol intake or drug abuse. We return to this later when we discuss lifestyle issues. If the infectee stops taking ART, the viral load will increase again and the HIV pathogen can recommence attacking the CD4 cells.

More than 25 ART preparations are clinically approved to treat HIV, with medications grouped into six classes of inhibitors (see Pietrangelo, 2018). Recommended treatment utilises a commencing regimen of three HIV medications from at least two of the drug classes. This combination helps to prevent HIV from developing drug resistance. In practice, many of the ART medications are combined so that a person with HIV typically takes only one or two pills daily. Blood tests will determine if the regimen is appropriate to suppress the viral load and promote the CD4 count. If an ART regimen is not performing satisfactorily, it should be switched to a more effective combination.

Prevention is better than cure, especially given that there is currently no vaccine available for the prevention of HIV transmission. Appropriate prevention strategies comprise practising safe sex (including regular testing for HIV and other sexually transmitted infections (STIs), condom use, and not engaging in risky sexual behaviours such as concurrent partners or engaging in transactional sex); avoidance of sharing needles and other drug-related equipment; and employing pre-exposure prophylaxis (PrEP) when at high risk of contracting HIV.

7.7.2 HIV/AIDS in Sub-Saharan Africa – an overview

We draw here on the work of Kharsany and Karim (2016), available at: https://openaidsjournal.com/VOLUME/10/PAGE/34/. Additional material is drawn from UNAIDS and WHO sources.

SSA remains the continental region most affected by the HIV pandemic. Kharsany and Karim (2016) report an estimated 35 million people were living with HIV (PLWH) worldwide in 2013 and that, whilst SSA accounts for only 12 per cent of the global population, it accounts for 71 per cent (nearly 25 million people) of the global burden of HIV infection. According to UNAIDS (2014), ten countries, mostly in southern and eastern Africa, account for almost 80 per cent of all people living with HIV. These are: South Africa (25%), Nigeria (13%), Mozambique (6%), Uganda (6%), Tanzania (6%), Zambia (4%), Zimbabwe (6%), Kenya (6%), Malawi (4%) and Ethiopia (3%).

In the SSA region the primary mode of HIV transmission is through heterosexual sex with an HIV+ partner. There is a concomitant epidemic in children through vertical transmission. Consequently, women are disproportionately affected; accounting for 58 per cent of the total number of persons living with HIV, they have the highest number of children living with HIV, and indicate the highest number of AIDS-related deaths.

The costs of ART treatment have been a constant issue for nations in SSA, but increased access to ART has led to a steady decline in the number of AIDS-related deaths, and in SSA these decreased by 39 per cent between 2005 and 2013 (UNAIDS, 2014). In South Africa the decline was 51 per cent, in Ethiopia 37 per cent and in Kenya 32 per cent. Empirical studies in South Africa, Uganda, Tanzania, Rwanda and Malawi have demonstrated the positive impact of modest ART coverage (at CD4 cell counts <200 to 500 cell/mm3) with significant declines in mortality and with increased life expectancy (see, for example, Reniers et al., 2014). These studies provide evidence for the benefits of early ART initiation to HIV+ persons.

This is important for the construction industry to grasp and consider. Many construction organisations invest large sums in equipment operator training and licensing for selected employees. If these operators become HIV+, there is a strong business case for employers to encourage them to be compliant with treatment regimes, especially as their working lives can thereby be extended to up to 70 years of age or beyond.

However, despite the benefits of ART, in 2013 the SSA region still accounted for 74 per cent of deaths from AIDS-related illnesses (Kharsany & Karim, 2016).

Regarding HIV prevention interventions, comprehensive and effective public health strategies include programming for behaviour change, condom use, HIV testing and knowledge of HIV status, harm reduction efforts for injecting substance use, medical male circumcision, and provision of post-exposure prophylaxis. However, these have not been implemented and utilised in direct ratio to the magnitude of HIV burden (Kharsany & Karim, 2016). Smith et al. (2014) report that, notwithstanding the combination of these HIV prevention packages having the potential to prevent more than 90 per cent of HIV transmission via vaginal and anal sexual intercourse, their use is mainly influenced by tribal custom, relationship type and by the form of partnerships. Research indicates that gendered power relations mean that the majority of women are unable to negotiate consistent condom use which is largely dependent on male co-operation. Moreover, despite voluntary counselling and testing (VCT) efforts to enhance knowledge of HIV status, access HIV prevention and treatment programmes, and minimise stigma and discrimination in association with HIV, knowledge of HIV status remains low (Kharsany & Karim, 2016). A major challenge to the use of more promising interventions such as ARV-based vaginal microbicides, oral pre-exposure prophylaxis (PrEP) and early ART initiation, is that they are not yet licensed in SSA for public sector use. These interventions would fill an important gap as HIV prevention options for young women and bring down the rate of new HIV infections.

In the SSA region, AIDS-related deaths have declined by 39 per cent in the period 2005 to 2013, most notably in Rwanda (76%), Eritrea (67%), Ethiopia (63%), Kenya (60%), Botswana (58%), Burkina Faso (58%), Zimbabwe (57%), Malawi (51%), South Africa (48%) and Tanzania (44%) – all attributable to the rapid increase in the number of people undergoing ART. Approximately 75 per cent of all people receiving ART worldwide live in SSA, yet many more need it and are eligible for it. However, UNAIDS (2014) notes that, despite the successes in the region in scaling up ART, there is significant variability between countries. For example, Botswana, South Africa, Zambia, Zimbabwe and Malawi are providing better treatment access compared to countries such as Nigeria and the Central African Republic where less than 25 per cent of the adult population have access to treatment.

Aside from the awful human toll of the pandemic, the high HIV/AIDS burden has had, and continues to have, a negative effect on total gross domestic product (GDP) in the most affected countries – the very countries requiring the most significant increases in healthcare expenditure to meet their treatment goals (Over, 2004). High rates of HIV-related sickness and premature adult deaths severely compromise household stability and investment in children. They put stress on extended family and broader social networks; and diminish labour supply and productivity while increasing costs for households, public institutions, and private-sector companies (Institute of Medicine (US), 2011). Issues germane to such negative effects include household-level impacts (poverty triggers, food insecurity, inadequate family-coping to support orphaned and vulnerable children, scarcity of alternative care options for orphans and vulnerable children, and family-care policy implications with a long-term perspective); economic performance (issues of labour and productivity, and economic growth); and the influence of treatment on household and economic wellbeing (for example, improvements in physical health, improvements in subjective wellbeing, and positive outcomes relating to depression, dementia, and anxiety).

Booysen (2004) comments on the positive effects of social grants in mitigating the socioeconomic impact of HIV/AIDS at a household level, but notes that the magnitude of the epidemic in South Africa necessitates consideration of the fiscal affordability and longer-term sustainability of such a system. The US Institute of Medicine (2011) also draws attention to the impact of the pandemic in SSA on the state (security and conflict; state capacity and governance, including effects on electoral processes and outcomes; government responses; and civil society participation and governance practices) and on education and skills development (training doctors and nurses; training for HIV/AIDS professional support staff; training for less specialised workers; and technical and vocational education and training). The link between the HIV/AIDS pandemic and the issues noted above is clear, with profound implications for economic growth and wellbeing in the whole SSA region.

There is far less information available concerning the impact of HIV/AIDS on the construction industry, and what can be found relates almost entirely to the situation in South Africa.

7.7.3 HIV/AIDS in South Africa – an overview

In 2017, the overall estimated HIV prevalence for people of all ages living in South Africa was 14 per cent (Simbayi et al., 2019). This prevalence estimate is higher than the HSRC 2012 estimate of 12.2 per cent (Shisana et al., 2014) and the HSRC 2008 estimate of 10.3 per cent (Shisana et al., 2010). The 2017 estimate translates to an estimated 7.9 million people living with HIV (PLWH), representing an increase of approximately 1.6 million more PLWH compared to the 2012 survey estimate. Excluding children under the age of 2 years, the prevalence estimate was 14.6 per cent, higher than the 12.6 per cent reported in 2012. This points to a consistent trend increase of HIV prevalence over time. Venkatesh et al. (2011) report that HIV prevalence among South African youth is among the highest in the world, likely driven by a range of sexual behaviours, including low levels of condom use, multiple sex partners, and densely connected sexual networks in which few HIV-positive individuals are aware of their infection (see also Pettifor et al., 2005).

Within South Africa, HIV prevalence varies considerably across the nation's nine provinces: from 8.3 per cent in the Northern Cape to 18.1 per cent in KwaZulu-Natal. The Western Cape has indicated 8.9 per cent prevalence. The highest national prevalence (26.4%) occurred among people aged 25–49 years. Within this age group, HIV prevalence was significantly higher among females (33.3%) than males (19.4%). In all the adult age categories, females indicate a disproportionately higher burden of HIV infection than do males. Specifically, significant differences by gender were indicated from the 20–24-years age group right through to the 40–44-years age group.

In terms of exposure to ARV treatment, 62.3 per cent of infectees were receiving ART (as determined by a blood test for the presence of ART drugs), which translates to an estimated 4.4 million PLWH who were receiving ART in South Africa in 2017. KwaZulu-Natal had the highest ARV exposure (69.8%; 1.2 million people), followed closely by the Eastern Cape (68.2%; 653,000 people). Gauteng had the lowest exposure to ARV treatment (53.7%; 896,000 people), marginally lower than the Western Cape (53.9%; 284,000 people).

Key drivers of the HIV pandemic in South Africa are sex-related behaviours, specifically early age sex, age-disparate relationships, multiple sexual partners, transactional sex, condom misuse or non-use, lack of awareness of HIV status, poor HIV risk perception, poor knowledge of HIV and tuberculosis risk factors, and sensitivity about HIV stigma.

High-risk groups were identified (in terms of prevalence) as: "black" African women aged 20–34 years, people who were cohabiting, "black" African men aged 25–49 years, recreational drug users, high-risk alcohol drinkers, and persons with disabilities who were aged 15 years or older. In terms of multiple sex partners amongst the high-risk groups, hazardous drinkers reported the highest proportion of multiple sex partners (22.4%), followed by recreational drug users (18.2%), "black" African men aged 25–49 years (16.3%), and persons with disabilities (12.1%). The lowest proportion of multiple sex partners in the previous 12 months was indicated by unmarried people living together aged 15–49 years (8.6%) and "black" African women aged 20–34 years (7.1%).

Within high-risk groups, consistent condom use with the most recent partner and during the last 12 months was highest among "black" African men aged

25–49 years (37.5%), followed by "black" African women aged 20–34 years (35.6%). The lowest level of consistent condom use was reported by cohabiting people aged 15–49 years (15.4%). Notably, a large proportion of people (45.6%) reported never having used a condom with their most recent sexual partner. Disturbingly, most people (73% to 80%) in all high-risk groups believed themselves to be at *low* risk for HIV infection. In respect of HIV transmission knowledge within high-risk groups, despite an improvement over time, the level of accurate knowledge about HIV transmission remained comparatively low among all high-risk groups in 2017.

7.7.4 HIV/AIDS and the South African construction industry

The construction industry has been identified as one of the economic sectors in South Africa most adversely affected by HIV/AIDS, third only to the mining and transportation sectors. It has also been found by the Department of Public Works (DPW), the Bureau for Economic Research (BER) and the South African Business Coalition on HIV/AIDS (SABCOHA) to be one of the least responsive to the disease (DPW, 2004; BER/SABCOHA, 2004).

Few studies involving large sample sizes have been undertaken in South Africa to establish the situation regarding HIV/AIDS in the construction industry, with even fewer focusing on the degree of association between risk factors and the prevalence of HIV/AIDS. Documented studies have focused on: the relationship between age and worker perceptions, knowledge, beliefs, attitudes and behaviours (Haupt & Smallwood, 2004; Haupt et al., 2005); awareness of HIV/AIDS among older workers (Haupt & Smallwood, 2003a); and awareness of HIV/AIDS among construction workers (Haupt & Smallwood, 2003b). These surveys were all based on quite small sample sizes with a maximum of 300 interviewees. Bowen et al. (2008), in a national study of 10,243 construction workers, report an estimated infection of 13.9 per cent – compared to the 2012 prevalence of 12.2 per cent identified by the HSRC (Shisana et al., 2014). In a more recent study, Bowen et al. (2017), in a site-based study of 512 construction workers in the Western Cape, report an estimated infection of 10 per cent – lower than the previous estimate of 13.9 per cent, but still higher than the 8.9 per cent prevalence in the Western Cape identified by the HSRC (Simbayi et al., 2019). Another national study by Bowen et al. (2018), involving 52,113 construction workers, indicates an estimated HIV infection of 10.1 per cent – again lower than the earlier estimate of 13.9 per cent, but still higher than the 8.9 per cent prevalence noted earlier.

The level of infection in the construction industry is most likely attributable to the industry's fragmented nature, the predominance of small firms and the diversity of construction work in terms of its nature and location, the comparatively low levels of worker education and literacy (especially among older workers), and the widespread use of "informal" labour in the construction workforce (Meintjes et al., 2007). The migratory employment pattern (rural to urban) typically found in the South African construction industry may exacerbate HIV infection as workers engage in unprotected sexual activity in between infrequent visits to their rural homes.

General impacts of AIDS are reported by the United Nations Department of Economic and Social Affairs – Population Division (United Nations, 2004). These include:

- Worker absenteeism, especially as more frequent clinic attendance is needed, or for longer periods of rest and recovery at home;
- Loss of worker skills and tacit knowledge which may be difficult to replace;
- Increased cost burden to firms (estimated to add between 1 and 6 per cent to labour costs), especially where public health services are inadequate, through increased administration costs and premium costs of medical insurance schemes, and assistance with funeral costs (especially where repatriation of bodies for burial in distant tribal family homes is entailed);
- Productivity decline;
- Lowering of worker morale and organisational cohesion through the effects of stigmatisation.

It is easy to see how these impacts can affect the construction industries (and hence the developing economies) of countries in the SSA region.

Businesses most seriously affected by HIV/AIDS will be those dependent on migrant labour (Whiteside & Sunter, 2000) as HIV prevalence rates are considerably higher in those who travel for employment. The migratory employment of construction employees thereby substantially increases their vulnerability. The nature of migrant employment increases the risk of contracting HIV while simultaneously often removing workers' proximity to appropriate healthcare facilities. Aspects of risk and vulnerability for migrant construction workers include sub-standard living environments, high rates of alcohol abuse and unsafe sexual practices. In some cases, migrant workers who become HIV-positive are reported to spread the virus in their home communities when they return home (Fourie & Schonteich, 2002).

Barnett and Whiteside (2002) note that the more unregulated and "informal" an industry is, the greater its vulnerability to HIV/AIDS because workers whose employment is transient and insecure are particularly vulnerable to the disease. In construction, almost 60 per cent of the construction workforce is engaged on an informal basis. Risk of infection is increased among these workers by low levels of education, lack of knowledge, adherence to custom and unsafe sexual practices.

In developing countries, with high unemployment and inadequate social security, socioeconomic dislocation results in a burgeoning informal industry. Unlicensed and unregulated businesses enjoy the benefits of engaging in this industry through casualised employment structures. Statistics South Africa (Stats SA) indicate that this has been a significant trend in the construction industry with permanent and fixed-period contract employment decreasing as a percentage of total employment from 54.6 per cent (September 2002) to 50.9 per cent (September 2006). Moreover, the situation is compounded by low barriers to entry into construction jobs.

Another factor contributing to the high rates of disease prevalence in the construction industry is the ageing of the skilled workforce. A decline in interest in careers in the construction industry (a common phenomenon in many countries) has meant that the construction industry attracts fewer young recruits, particularly into the skilled and professional occupations, leading to an increase in the average age of skilled workers and the narrowing of the skills base. Older workers carry the "institutional memory" of the industry, a repository of skills and acquired tacit knowledge that only time and experience can accumulate. These older workers (those over the age of 40) comprise more than half the skilled workforce, 69 per cent of specialised plant and machine operators and 60 per cent of skilled workers (Haupt et al., 2005).

Additionally, older workers are vulnerable to myriad health threats within a harsh and dangerous working environment. As a large portion of unskilled and semi-skilled labourers come from poor socioeconomic backgrounds, they may be more vulnerable to infectious diseases such as HIV (Deacon & Smallwood, 2003). In addition, they appear to be more susceptible to poverty-related diseases, such as TB, hypertension and ischaemic strokes. This combination between vulnerability to poverty-related diseases and age means that the time between HIV infection and the onset of AIDS will be much shorter for older workers. This is partly because of lower levels of education and literacy which in turn have implications for health education initiatives since they reduce older workers' access to information, leaving them less well equipped to protect themselves and more prone to believe the myths engendered by fear and uncertainty surrounding the pandemic (Haupt et al., 2005).

Lost days of work among construction workers are a major concern for the industry (Haupt et al., 2005). Studies indicate that South African businesses in general lose up to a month's work per employee per year due to HIV-related absenteeism (see Moodley, 2005). This equates to a loss of over ZAR2 billion (nearly US$135 million per annum) (Moodley, 2005). Ellis et al. (2003) estimated that the private industry would experience a 40 per cent reduction in the productivity of both skilled and unskilled workers over the next two decades, due to AIDS. At the time of writing, it is not known whether this prediction has become a reality.

As noted above, the construction industry has been one of the slowest sectors to respond to HIV/AIDS (Meintjes et al., 2007), thus placing greater strain on other institutions and stakeholders to compensate for this inaction. Given the already overburdened public sector's difficulties in providing support for prevention and for care of people infected by HIV/AIDS, it is argued that civil society and the private sector have an increasingly greater role to play. Historically, the focus of the construction industry has been on safety rather than on health, though more recently the focus has widened among a few companies to include the need to reduce work-related illnesses, and, to a lesser extent, provide primary healthcare and management.

Central to HIV prevention is voluntary counselling and HIV antibody testing. HIV testing benefits those who test positive, permitting them to receive appropriate and timely treatment and monitoring. HIV testing has been shown to be an effective measure in reducing the spread of HIV by making people aware of their status and promoting safer sex (Scott-Sheldon et al., 2013). An important aspect of testing is thus the provision of HIV/AIDS prevention information, currently often delivered by peer educators in workplace awareness campaigns. Bowen et al. (2010) report that most construction organisations have HIV awareness policies in place, but that prevention and treatment policies are less common. Treatment programmes are the least implemented measure of all due to employer misperceptions, insufficient resource capacity, fears about confidentiality and the potential stigmatisation of infected persons, and low take-up rates of such programmes by workers reluctant to disclose their status. Despite acknowledging the benefits flowing from providing workplace-based treatment programmes, doubt exists among construction firms as to their financial viability.

Other related studies of construction workers in South Africa have focused on matters such as: guidelines for effective workplace HIV/AIDS intervention management by construction firms (Bowen et al., 2014); factors determining South African construction workers' prejudice towards and discrimination against HIV+ persons (Bowen et al., 2015); attitudinal fear of HIV testing (Bowen et al., 2016); AIDS-related knowledge, stigma and customary beliefs of South African construction workers (Govender et al., 2017); and determinants of condom use (Bowen et al., 2017).

Bowen et al. (2014) have explored the nature of, and extent to which, construction firms in Cape Town are addressing the issue of HIV/AIDS. They report that the presence within firms of a formal HIV/AIDS policy is important for the provision of effective intervention management. In this survey, whilst firms' responses varied considerably, HIV/AIDS policies (where they existed) provided a framework for interventions, including support for the families of workers and non- discrimination in terms of access. In terms of awareness campaigns, these include "toolbox talks," informal talks and other discussions, an annual AIDS Day, workplace posters, pamphlets, teaching sessions, peer education, voluntary testing and counselling courses, and medical clearance assessments. Regarding prevention measures, these include precautionary discussions, training in the importance of correct and consistent condom use, and the provision of free condoms on site. Assistance with workers' treatment focuses on ensuring confidentiality, providing time off to obtain medication, providing transportation to clinics, providing access to the company doctor, and providing ART medication and patient counselling. Some firms have used external service providers for the provision of HIV testing and even the provision of ART medication. Lastly, the more proactive firms have increased funding for HIV awareness, prevention, and treatment in their annual budgets, whilst other firms have introduced medical aid coverage, although this is typically limited. However, a few firms continue to deny the existence of HIV/AIDS among their employees and have offered little or no proactive intervention measures.

7.8 Industry health testing in South Africa

South Africa is probably a leader in SSA with regard to industry health testing. However, while medical surveillance is a welcome development in the SA construction industry, there remain several shortcomings about it in practice.

The South African Occupational Health and Safety Act (No. 85 of 1993) (RSA, 1993) sets out the legal requirements for employers to undertake risk assessments in terms of hazards and their associated risks encountered in the workplace, including dangerous tasks (e.g., working at height), dangerous locations (e.g., working in confined spaces) and other environments (e.g., extremes of heat or cold), and dangerous materials (e.g., toxic or noxious substances). Specific Construction Regulations (established under the South African Occupational Health and Safety Act in 2014) require that periodic health examinations for workers exposed to particular hazardous activities be conducted by registered occupational health practitioners.

The examinations cover medical history, physical examination (weight, height), eyesight, hearing, lung function and capacity for working at heights. Most examinations will also include urine tests for diabetes. More specialised tests are required for operators of heavy equipment such as heavy goods vehicles, cranes (fixed and mobile), excavators, bulldozers, forklifts and other construction plant.

Where indicated by the initial examination, workers may be referred for more specialised follow-up tests (e.g., chest x-rays) and treatment. If the reference and treatment are for tuberculosis (TB) or malaria, the treating healthcare professional is responsible for notifying the presence of these infections to relevant authorities.

Currently, there is no mandatory testing for HIV/AIDS. Nor is this infection legally notifiable. Political sensitivities have so far prevented HIV/AIDS from being made a legally notifiable disease in South Africa.

Similarly, there are currently no requirements for testing for any of the strains of hepatitis or bilharzia (attributable to parasitic worm infection and found in freshwater river systems throughout the region). Consequently, the prevalence of these illnesses is unknown.

Data privacy and confidentiality laws mean that the availability of medical surveillance information is limited to the three parties involved (examining practitioner, employer and worker) and workers may not be fully informed. There are currently no requirements in place (other than for TB and malaria as noted above) for reporting to other authorities. Reporting requirements for many serious occupational illnesses do not exist for construction workers. This contrasts with requirements relating to mining workers who are covered by different legislation in SA. Consequently, data pertaining to the occupational health of construction workers in SA is not available.

Finally, the frequency of medical surveillance is also somewhat loosely controlled. Other than for heavy equipment operators, who are required to undergo annual examinations after the age of 52, the currency of medical certificates of fitness may last for up to three years unless more frequent conditions for surveillance are imposed by the examining practitioner or any follow-up treatment authority.

Regular medical surveillance clearly has an important role to play in promoting a healthy construction industry workforce in SSA. However, appropriate legislation is required across all the nations in the region, backed up by effective regulatory and enforcement environments and by efficient approaches to data capture and management.

7.9 Family and lifestyle issues

Unskilled or semi-skilled workers in SSA rarely earn sufficient money to satisfy their family needs. For migrant workers seeking to remit money back to their rural families, the situation is exacerbated as they also have to pay for their urban accommodation and subsistence. This stretches their resources to the point where they can only afford cheap, often shared, rental properties. Limited availability of accommodation forces rental seekers further towards the outer fringes of cities, adding further to transport costs.

Low wages mean that family members of construction workers need to work to subsist and it is common for children to work in paid employment, affecting their education and contributing to the cycle of poverty. Inadequate parental supervision (with both parents working all day) aggravates the situation, even where grandparents are called in to help, thus endangering family cohesion and contributing to rising levels of youth crime and drug taking.

Family problems and community disadvantages are made worse by the use of alcohol and drugs as maladaptive coping strategies. According to the World Health Organization (WHO, 2014), alcohol abuse and illicit drug use are increasing across SSA, and are associated with increased risk for diseases such as HIV/AIDS, tuberculosis and hepatitis, and for death by suicide, overdose and cardiovascular disease.

Alcohol consumption in African-style shebeens is also linked to transactional (often unsafe) sex. Alcohol dependency also contributes to financial disadvantage and poverty, and contributes to domestic violence and a reliance on prostitution (among women) to earn a living. Transactional sex that is engaged in unsafely greatly increases the risk of sexually transmitted infections, including HIV/AIDS.

7.10 Organisational support for workers

The construction industries of SSA countries typically provide little support for workers' health or wellbeing.

Construction employment structures mean that few workers, other than those with monthly-paid permanent employment status, are provided with subsidised or employer-paid medical insurance protection. Even fewer are eligible for employer-subsidised accommodation or transport benefits. Opportunities for skills upgrading or further education are rare, and few education or training grants are available except from major national or transnational construction companies. Indeed, practical help with housing, family education needs and employee self-development is largely found only among the smallest micro-level construction companies where a more paternal family-centric management employer-employee relationship approach may be practised by owners and principals.

Corporate social responsibility (CSR), where it is found in the construction industry, is often more outwardly than inwardly focused, whereby employees are encouraged to participate in volunteering activities.

7.11 Conclusion

In this chapter, we have explored development in the SSA region, the economic and social issues pertaining to it, and their effects on worker wellbeing. Factors that affect occupational health include disease causes of morbidity, the influence of toxic materials used in the construction industry, and industry health surveillance, together with issues relating to low income, insecure work and the need to live and work away from the family home. We pay particular attention to the issue of HIV/AIDS due to the prevalence and effect of this disease in SSA. The construction industry has been slower than other sectors to address issues of workers' health and wellbeing in SSA. However, the importance of sustaining a healthy workforce is such that construction companies should consider ways in which they can better support workers to live healthy and productive lives.

7.12 Discussion and review questions

For readers, we pose three topics for potential discussion:

1. What are some of the challenges to construction workers' health experienced in Sub-Saharan Africa? How do these differ in their nature and cause compared to issues experienced by construction workers in developed economies?
2. Why are construction workers in Sub-Saharan Africa susceptible to HIV/AIDS infection? To what extent should construction organisations implement strategies to prevent infection or support the treatment of infected workers?
3. With reference to social determinants of health, consider how employment conditions experienced by construction workers in Sub-Saharan Africa

contribute to poor health. What job/employment characteristics contribute to poor health and how could these be addressed?

References

Avert. (n.d.) *The Science of HIV and AIDS – Overview*. Global Information and Education on HIV and AIDS, Avert. Available at: www.avert.org/professionals/hiv-science/overview (accessed 14 September 2020).

Barnett, T., & Whiteside, A. (2002). *AIDS in the Twenty-First Century: Disease and Globalisation*. Palgrave Macmillan.

Booysen, F. (2004). Social grants as safety net for HIV/AIDS-affected households in South Africa. *Journal of Social Aspects of HIV/AIDS Research Alliance/SAHARA/Human Sciences Research Council*, 1(1), 45–56.

Bowen, P., Allen, Y., Edwards, P. J., Cattell, K., & Simbayi, L. (2014). Guidelines for effective workplace HIV/AIDS intervention management by construction firms. *Construction Management and Economics*, 32(4), 362–381.

Bowen, P., Cattell, K., Edwards, P.J., & Marks, J. (2010). Perceptions of HIV/AIDS policies and treatment programmes by Western Cape construction firms. *Construction Management and Economics*, 28(9), 997–1006.

Bowen, P., Dorrington, R., Distiller, G., Lake, H., & Besesar, S. (2008). HIV/AIDS in the South African construction industry: an empirical study. *Construction Management and Economics*, 26(8), 827–839.

Bowen, P., Govender, R., & Edwards, P. (2017). Condom use by South African construction workers. *Construction Management and Economics*, 35(7), 432–444.

Bowen, P., Govender, R., Edwards, P., & Cattell. K. (2016). An explanatory model of attitudinal fear of HIV/AIDS testing in the construction industry. *Engineering, Construction and Architectural Management*, 23(1), 92–112.

Bowen, P., Govender, R., Edwards, P., & Lake, A. (2018) HIV infection in the South African construction industry. *Psychology, Health & Medicine*, 23(5), 612–618.

Bowen, P., Govender, R., Edwards, P., Cattell, K., & Street, A. (2015) Factors determining South African construction workers' prejudice towards and discrimination against HIV+ Persons. *Journal of Construction Engineering and Management*, 141(7), 04015014.

Bureau for Economic Research (BER), & South African Business Coalition on HIV/AIDS (SABCOHA). (2004). *The Economic Impact of HIV/AIDS on Business in South Africa, 2003*. Bureau for Economic Research.

Cattell, K. S, Bowen, P. A., Cooper, C. L., & Edwards, P. J. (2017). *The State of Well-being in the Construction Industry*. Chartered Institute of Building (CIOB).

Churchyard, G. J., Mametja, L. D., Mvusi, L., Ndeka, N., Hesseling, A. C., Reid, A., Babatunde, S., & Pillay, Y. (2014). Tuberculosis control in South Africa: Successes, challenges and recommendations. *South African Medical Journal*, 114(3), 244–248.

Deacon, C., & Smallwood, J. (2003). Health promotion in South African construction. *Journal of Construction Research*, 4(2), 129–140.

Department of Public Works (DPW). (2004). *HIV/AIDS Awareness Programme: Training Manual*. Accessed 2 September 2022 from: http://bit.ly/1croHIP

Donald, I., Taylor, P., Johnson, S., Cooper, C., Cartwright, S., & Robertson, S. (2005). Work Environments, Stress, and Productivity: An Examination Using ASSET. *International Journal of Stress Management*, 12(4), 409–423.

Ellis, L. L., Smit, B. W., & Laubscher, P. (2003). The macroeconomic impact of HIV/AIDS in South Africa. *Journal for Studies in Economics and Econometrics*, 27(2), 1–28.

Faragher, E. B., Cooper, C. L., & Cartwright, S. (2004). A shortened stress evaluation tool (ASSET). *Stress & Health: Journal of the International Society for the Investigation of Stress*, 20(4), 189–201.

Fourie, P., & Schonteich, M. (2002). Die, the beloved countries: Human security and HIV/AIDS in Africa. *Politeia*, 21(2), 6–30.

Govender, R., Bowen, P., Edwards, P., & Cattell, K. (2017). AIDS-related knowledge, stigma and customary beliefs of South African construction workers. *AIDS Care*, 29(6), 711–717.

Haupt, T. C., & Smallwood, J. (2003a). HIV and AIDS in construction: are older workers aware? *Journal of Engineering, Design and Technology*, 1(1), 42–53.

Haupt, T. C., & Smallwood, J. (2003b). HIV and AIDS in construction: Are contractors aware? *Construction Information Quarterly*, 5(3), 3–6.

Haupt, T. C., & Smallwood, J. (2004). HIV/AIDS in SA construction: Attitudes and perceptions of workers. *Journal of Construction Research*, 5(2), 311–327.

Haupt, T.C., Munshi, M., & Smallwood, J. (2005). HIV and AIDS in South African construction: Is age nothing but a number? *Construction Management and Economics*, 23(1), 107–120.

Institute of Medicine (US). (2011). *Preparing for the Future of HIV/AIDS in Africa: A Shared Responsibility*. Committee on Envisioning a Strategy for the Long-Term Burden of HIV/AIDS: African Needs and U.S. Interests. National Academies Press.

Kharsany, A. B. M., & Karim, Q. A. (2016). HIV Infection and AIDS in Sub-Saharan Africa: Current Status, Challenges and Opportunities. *The Open AIDS Journal*, 3, 34–48

Leung, M-Y., Chan, I. S. A, & Cooper, Sir C. L. (2015) *Stress Management in the Construction Industry*. Wiley Blackwell.

Lingard, H., & Francis, V. (2009). *Managing Work–Life Balance in Construction*. Spon Press.

Meintjes, I., Bowen, P. A., & Root, D. (2007). HIV/AIDS in the South African construction industry: Understanding the HIV/AIDS discourse for a sector specific response. *Construction Management and Economics*, 25(3), 255–266.

Moodley, N. (2005). *Absenteeism costs R12bn a year, with up to R2.2bn due to Aids*. Accessed 19 August 2022 from: www.busrep.co.za

Over, M. (2004). Impact of the HIV/AIDS epidemic on the health sectors of developing countries. In M. Haacker (Ed.), *The Macroeconomics of HIV/AIDS*. The International Monetary Fund (pp. 311–344).

Pettifor, A., Rees, H.V., Kleinschmidt. I., Steffenson, A. E., MacPhail. C., Hlongwa-Madikizela, L., Vermaak, K., & Padian, N. S. (2005). Young people's sexual health in South Africa: HIV prevalence and sexual behaviors from a nationally representative household survey. *AIDS*, 19(4), 1525–1534.

Pietrangelo, A. (2018). *A Comprehensive Guide to HIV and AIDS*. Accessed 14t September 2020 from: www.healthline.com/health/hiv-aids ()

Reniers, G., Slaymaker, E., Nakiyingi-Miiro, J., et al. (2014). Mortality trends in the era of antiretroviral therapy: Evidence from the network for analysing longitudinal population based HIV/AIDS data on Africa (ALPHA). *AIDS*, 28(Supplement 4), S533–542.

Republic of South Africa (RSA). (1993). *Occupational Health and Safety Act (No. 85 of 1993)*. Government Printer.

Republic of South Africa (RSA). (1994). *Construction Regulations, No. R184*. Government Printer.

Robertson Cooper. (2012). *Work-related resilience questionnaire: Technical Manual*. Robertson Cooper Ltd.

Scott-Sheldon, L. A. J., Carey, M. P., Carey, K. B., Cain, D., Simbayi, L. C., Mehlomakhulu, V., & Kalichman, S. C. (2013). HIV testing is associated with increased knowledge and reductions in sexual risk behaviours among men in Cape Town, South Africa. *African Journal of AIDS Research*, 12(4), 195–201.

Shisana, O., Rehle, T., Simbayi, L. C., Zuma, K., Jooste, S., Zungu, N., Labadarios, D., Onoya, D., et al. (2014). *South African National HIV Prevalence, Incidence and Behaviour Survey, 2012*. HSRC Press.

Shisana, O., Simbayi, L. C., Rehle, T., Zungu, N. P., Zuma, K., Ngogo, N., Jooste, S., Pillay-van Wyk, V., Parker, W., Pezi, S., Davids, A., Nwanyanwu, O., Dinh, T. H., & the SABSSM III Implementation Team. (2010). *South African National HIV Prevalence, Incidence, Behaviour and Communication Survey, 2008: The Health of Our Children*. HSRC Press.

Simbayi, L. C., Zuma, K., Zungu, N., Moyo, S., Marinda, E., Jooste, S., Mabaso, M., Ramlagan, S., North, A., van Zyl, J., Mohlabane, N., Dietrich, C., Naidoo, I., & the SABSSM V Team. (2019). *South African National HIV Prevalence, Incidence, Behaviour and Communication Survey, 2017*. HSRC Press.

Smith, J., Nyamukapa, C., Gregson, S., et al. (2014). The distribution of sex acts and condom use within partnerships in a rural sub-Saharan African population. *PLoS One*, 9(2), e88378.

UNAIDS. (2014). *The Gap Report 2014*. UNAIDS.

United Nations. (2004). *The impact of AIDS*. United Nations Department of Economic and Social Affairs/Population Division. United Nations. (Document Reference: ST/ESA/SER.A/229).

Venkatesh, K. K., Madiba, P., De Bruyn, G., Lurie, M. N., Coates, T. J., & Gray, G. E. (2011). Who gets tested for HIV in a South African urban township? Implications for test and treat and gender-based interventions. *Journal of Acquired Immune Deficiency Syndrome*, 56(2), 151–165.

Whiteside, A., & Sunter, C. (2000). *AIDS: The Challenge for South Africa*. Human & Rousseau.

World Health Organization (WHO). (2014). *The Health of the People: What Works. The African Regional Health Report 2014*. World Health Organization.

World Health Organization (WHO). (2018). *World Malaria Report*. World Health Organization.

8

YOUNG CONSTRUCTION WORKERS' HEALTH AND WELLBEING

Helen Lingard, Rita Peihua Zhang and Michelle Turner

SCHOOL OF PROPERTY, CONSTRUCTION & PROJECT MANAGEMENT, RMIT UNIVERSITY, MELBOURNE, AUSTRALIA

8.1 Introduction

In this chapter, we examine the health and wellbeing of young construction workers. We consider wellbeing to include experiences of physical and bodily health as well as psychological and social health. Included in this broad understanding of wellbeing is the extent to which people are happy and embedded in supportive social networks in life (i.e., with friends and relatives) and at work (i.e, with co-workers and supervisors) (Burke, 2017).

Young workers (including those in the construction industry) are known to be a vulnerable group for work-related injury and mental ill health. Young workers' disproportionately high involvement in workplace accidents is often attributed to risk-taking behaviour and/or vulnerabilities implicit in being young. Mental ill health is similarly linked to unhealthy "lifestyle" behaviours, such as problem drinking, gambling or substance misuse. However, health behaviours and experiences are increasingly understood as being influenced by the social environment within which people live and work (see Chapter 1).

We begin this chapter by describing the apprenticeship model which is the pathway through which many young workers enter the construction industry. This sets the scene for the subsequent discussion of the work health and wellbeing experiences of young construction workers, in particular the reasons why young construction workers may be particularly at risk of work-related injuries and/or mental ill health.

We explore ways in which young workers' behaviours and experiences can be shaped by the workplace social and cultural context, and present examples from a study of the experiences of young workers (apprentices) in the Australian construction industry.

DOI: 10.1201/9780367814236-8

The importance of supportive and effective communication, particularly between young workers and their supervisors, is examined. Finally, we discuss opportunities to design targeted interventions to help protect the health and wellbeing of young construction workers.

8.2 The apprenticeship model

Apprenticeships are a core feature of the approach to skills development in Australia and many other countries (Couldrey & Loveder, 2016). Apprenticeships are an important pathway for young people to transition from school to full-time work (Bednarz, 2014) and from adolescence into adulthood (Buchanan et al., 2016). The Australian Government describes an Australian apprentice as someone who is:

- employed under a training contract that has been registered with, and validated by, their state/territory training authority; and
- undertaking paid work and structured training which commonly comprises both on and off the job training; and
- undertaking a negotiated training programme that involves obtaining a nationally recognised qualification (Australian Government, 2021).

Apprenticeships supplement the acquisition of abstract knowledge (often learned away from the workplace) with the learning of applied skills via experienced practitioners (Buchanan et al., 2016). But apprenticeships involve a great deal more than learning technical knowledge. Because they are immersed in workplaces, apprentices also acquire the occupational values and skills that denote membership and status in a trade (Marchand, 2008; Fisher, 1986) and gain first-hand understanding of labour market policy and practices (Buchanan et al., 2016). Apprenticeship is therefore a critical phase in a young worker's socialisation into work in general and to their profession in particular (Bakkevig Dagsland et al., 2015). Gherardi and Nicolini (2002) describe how construction apprentices are socialised into a workplace community of practices through which they develop competencies relating to safety and danger.

Despite their importance, the numbers of young Australian workers commencing apprenticeships and those currently in training are reported to be the lowest for a decade (Australian Industry Group, 2016). The National Centre for Vocational Education Research data also shows completion rates for apprenticeships in construction steadily declined between the years 2012 and 2017 (National Centre for Vocational Education Research, 2018). Poor retention is a particular problem among women apprentices. In Queensland, completion rates in construction trade apprenticeships are reported to be 12 per cent lower for women than for men (CSQ, 2018).

On commencement, apprentices usually hold positive expectations towards the apprenticeship, with a strong focus on learning and professional development

(Dagsland et al., 2011). However, in the three-way partnership between the apprentice, a training organisation and the training employer, apprentices' expectations towards their learning and development are sometimes unmet. This can occur if apprentices' learning expectations are not respected and if apprentices are insufficiently supported, and not allowed enough time to develop and try out new skills in the workplace.

Bednarz (2014) identifies the workplace-based training experience as a key factor influencing apprentices' satisfaction and the likelihood that Australian apprentices will complete their training. The majority of apprentices who complete their training (80 per cent) were satisfied with their employment experience, whereas just 42 per cent of non-completers were satisfied. Experiencing interpersonal difficulties with employers or colleagues, or not liking the work, are common reasons for leaving an apprenticeship (Einboden et al., 2021; Bednarz, 2014). This is consistent with the finding that (male) apprentices' relationships with their boss/supervisor and their co-workers are the most significant predictors of intention to quit (Gow et al., 2008). Lopata et al. (2015) identified further barriers affecting apprentices finishing their apprenticeships and found that a poor job fit, a lack of support or not being able to adhere to or follow work policies or rules contribute to non-completion. Apprentices note that having a work supervisor who is willing to teach them is one of the most important factors for them and not having a supportive supervisor or a mentor may discourage them from completing their apprenticeship (Lopata et al., 2015).

The experience of women apprentices entering male-dominated occupations may be different from that of males. For example, Jones et al. (2017) identified gendered stereotyping of trade-based work and biased perceptions of women's suitability for this work to be significant barriers to women entering electrical trades. Furthermore, those women who did commence an apprenticeship in an electrical trade were found to be confronted by:

- masculine and sometimes hostile work environments
- discriminatory practices during training and in the workplace
- exposure to offensive or inappropriate materials (e.g., pornography), and
- an unwillingness on the part of some employers to adapt work conditions to accommodate female employees.

These findings suggest that the social context of work plays a very important role in the experience of apprentices. In relation to learning and skills development, apprentices sometimes experience restrictive learning opportunities at work (Fuller & Unwin, 2008). Apprentices' learning about working safely can be impacted, for example, by co-workers' use of unfamiliar jargon, inappropriate assumptions made about what is "common sense," and adverse work conditions (for example, damaged tools, poor work layout or unreasonable task requirements) (Laberge et al., 2014). Learning opportunities are also reduced when apprentices are not permitted sufficient time to practise and master work tasks and when work-based learning is narrowly focused on a single (usually boring, repetitive or unpleasant) task allocated to apprentices by more experienced workers (Laberge et al., 2014).

8.3 Young workers' safety experiences at work

8.3.1 Non-fatal injury incidence

International research and statistics consistently show that young workers (frequently defined as workers under the age of 25) experience disproportionately high rates of workplace incidents and injuries compared to older workers. This is particularly the case for young male workers (Salminen, 2004; Breslin & Smith, 2006). For example, Canadian research shows lost-time injury rates among adolescent workers (15–19 years) and young adult workers (20–24 years) to be markedly higher than among adult workers (> 25 years) (Breslin et al., 2003). When only considering male workers, young adult workers had the highest rate of workplace injury (43.2 per 1,000 workers), followed by adolescent males (39.3 per 1,000 workers). By comparison, the rate of injury among male workers over the age of 25 years was 34.6 per 1,000 workers (Breslin et al., 2003). Breslin et al. (2003) also report that, in the agriculture, manufacturing and construction industries, injury rates for young adult (47.2 per 1,000) and adolescent workers (41.8 per 1,000) were notably higher than for adult workers (35.3 per 1,000).

A similar pattern is noted in the European Union where the European Agency for Safety and Health at Work reports the incidence rate of workplace accidents (in which more than three days were lost) to be higher for young workers in all industry sectors. Notably, in Europe, young workers were reported to be at greater risk in construction, agriculture and manufacturing than in other industry sectors (European Agency for Safety and Health at Work, 2007).

In Australia, young workers constituted 17 per cent of the Australian workforce but accounted for 20 per cent of all workplace injuries (Safe Work Australia, 2013). Young Australian workers are reported to experience an injury rate of 66.1 work-related injuries per 1,000 workers, a figure that is 18 per cent higher than the rate for workers aged 25 years and over (Safe Work Australia, 2013). As in other countries, the risk of workplace injury for young workers is even higher in the construction industry. During 2009–2010, an injury rate of 67.3 was recorded for young construction workers, which was 1.2 higher than the injury rate for young workers across industries and 8.1 higher than the average rate for construction workers of all ages (Safe Work Australia, 2015).

Young workers are at greatest risk of injury when they first commence a job. Breslin and Smith (2006) report that the injury rate (adjusted for occupation, industry, and sex) of young workers in the first month of their job is three times higher than that of young workers who have been in their job for more than one year. However, other research suggests that the dangers associated with inexperience may last for much longer than one year. For example, Chau et al. (2010)

report that the injury rate among workers under the age of 25 increases for the first four years of work before beginning to decline.

8.3.2 Fatal injury incidence

International research shows that, in general, young workers have a lower probability of suffering a fatal workplace accident than older workers (Bande & López-Mourelo, 2015). However, the construction industry is a high-risk industry in which young workers are at greater risk of work-related fatality. From 2008 to 2011 the Australian construction industry recorded the highest number of young workers who died from a work-related traumatic injury (n=19, 26%), followed by the agriculture, forestry and fishing industry (n=18, 25%) and the manufacturing industry (n=13, 18%) (Safe Work Australia, 2013). The European Agency for Safety and Health at Work similarly reports that, although the rate of fatal workplace accidents is lower for young workers (compared to industry averages) in all sectors, the construction industry accounts for the highest number of occupational fatalities among people aged up to 24 years of all industries (European Agency for Safety and Health at Work, 2007). In the USA, Rauscher and Myers (2016) report that (after the agriculture sector) construction accounts for the second largest number of young worker fatalities.

8.4 Why young workers are a high-risk group for workplace safety incidents

Sometimes young workers' increased risk of workplace safety incidents has been attributed to physical or developmental factors (Okun et al., 2016). Others explain young workers' involvement in workplace incidents as arising from immaturity, risk-taking behaviour and a sense of invulnerability, suggesting these behaviours can be observed most frequently when young workers are in the presence of peer influence (Steinberg, 2004).

In these explanations, "youth" is seen as the principal risk factor, i.e., workers are more prone to injury or incident involvement simply because they are young (Nielsen, 2012). However, we suggest that attributing heightened risk to "being young" ignores factors in the work environment that are known to contribute to poor safety outcomes for young workers. Indeed, research evidence suggests that young workers' experiences of workplace safety are shaped by the job-related demands and conditions that they experience. Okun et al. (2016), for example, identify: (i) requirements to work too fast for their skill level; (ii) being provided with damaged or unsuitable work equipment; (iii) being provided with inadequate training and supervision; and/or (iv) having limited ability to control the way they work as job-related factors that contribute to the injury experience of young workers (many of whom are still engaged in on-the-job training). Breslin et al. (2007) similarly argue that young workers' high incidence of workplace injury is better explained by the type of work they are engaged in than by their biological age. Specifically, Breslin et al. (2007) report that young workers holding manual jobs were 2.6 times more likely to experience an injury compared to young workers engaging in non-manual jobs. Work hours and work schedules have also been linked to young workers' experience of injury (see also Chapter 4 on working time arrangements and health in construction). Breslin et al. (2007) found that, compared to working 0–60 hours in a month, the risk of experiencing an injury increases by 3.8 times for young workers who work 120–160 hours per month, and increases by 6.2 times for young workers who work more than 160 hours per month. Loudoun (2010) also reports that young male construction workers are at significantly increased risk of injury when they work a night shift compared to those who worked a day shift.

Research identifies particular hazard exposures and risk factors as being key factors in young workers' workplace safety experiences. For example, Hanvold et al. (2019) found that mechanical factors (e.g., heavy lifting), psychosocial factors (e.g., low control over work pace), and organisational factors (e.g., poor workplace safety culture) all increase the risk of young workers experiencing a safety incident/injury at work. Exposure to chemicals, heavy lifting, awkward postures, and high job demands were also related to occupational ill health among young workers (Hanvold et al., 2019).

Australian statistics suggest that young workers' exposure to workplace hazards is greater than that of older workers. Holding other factors constant (including working hours, employment type, industry, occupation and whether or not a job involves nightshift), Safe Work Australia (2015) reports that young Australian workers (aged between 15 and 24) are exposed to 30 per cent more workplace hazards than workers aged 55 or over. Young Australian workers are also more likely to be simultaneously exposed to noise and vibration, and chemical and airborne hazards than workers aged 55 or over (Safe Work Australia, 2015). Research in the Australian construction industry also suggests that young workers report being exposed to dangerous work conditions, including conducting work in environments with asbestos present, without being provided with suitable protective equipment (McCormack et al., 2013).

Young workers' risk-taking behaviour has also been explained by their employment conditions which are often precarious. Precarious employment is particularly likely to impact young workers who are unskilled or who have limited education. For example, Nielsen et al. (2017) describe how, when young workers feel "replaceable" at work they feel that they have to "earn" their unskilled job or trainee position by taking tasks that are potentially harmful to their health or safety. Precarious employment can also discourage young workers from reporting minor injuries or unsafe conditions which they come to accept as an inevitable part of the job (Breslin et al., 2007) and also increases young workers' experience of work stress (Nielsen et al., 2017).

Young workers' experiences of workplace safety also vary depending on their individual circumstances, particularly their reasons for working and their relationship with work. Nielsen et al. (2012) report differences between skilled workers, apprentices, sabbatical (or "gap year") workers, student workers, and a group they term "school dropouts." Apprentices, in particular, tended to take a long-term view of their employment and the investment they were making in their chosen job. Apprentices did not consider themselves to be risk-takers and viewed safety and maintaining their health and wellbeing as an important part of their development and mastery of their chosen job or trade. In contrast, student or gap year workers had a short-term view of their employment, perceived they could be easily replaced and were more likely to adapt to the "normal" conditions of work, which may include taking risks in some workplaces. Young workers who had dropped out of high school typically engaged in hard physical work or routine work. These workers often saw themselves as being at the bottom of the organisational hierarchy and accepted risk taking as an inevitable part of the work they performed. Breslin et al. (2011) similarly report that early school leavers have a higher rate of injury than other groups of young workers. These differences are partly attributable to the type of work performed by early school leavers (i.e., often unskilled, physically demanding manual work), but other factors, such as low levels of social support at work, are also likely to be contributing factors.

Breslin et al. (2011) observe that young workers who are no longer in formal education have already transitioned into "adult" roles and are not simply working for discretionary income. These workers may not be able to change jobs easily if they experience persistent unsafe, unhealthy or unpleasant conditions at work, increasing the likelihood that poor or unsafe conditions of work are accepted as "part of the job" (Breslin et al. 2011).

Turner et al. (2015) examined how young workers respond to workplace safety issues and requirements and found age-related differences. Three different types of response were considered in the study, i.e., safety voice, neglect and compliance behaviours (Turner et al., 2015). Safety compliance refers to fulfilling "core safety activities that need to be carried out" (p.40). Safety neglect refers to "taking short-cuts or work-arounds" (p.40) and safety voice refers to "speaking up about hazardous work" (p.40). Workers aged between 15 and 18 reported a significantly lower level of safety voice behaviour than workers aged between 19 and 22. Safety voice scores did not vary between workers aged 19–22 and 23–25. Workers aged between 15 and 18 also reported a lower level of safety compliance behaviour and more safety neglect than workers aged between 19 and 22. Workers aged between 19 and 22 reported a lower level of safety compliance and more safety neglect than workers aged between 23 and 25 (Turner et al., 2015). Gender differences in young workers' safety voice behaviour have also been found. Despite the fact that young male workers are statistically more likely to be injured at work even when factors linked to different risk exposures (e.g., types of occupations and industry sectors) are controlled for (Breslin & Smith, 2006), young women are reported to be more likely to raise work health and safety concerns with their supervisors than young men (Tucker & Turner, 2014).

Tucker and Turner (2013) examined young workers' responses to unsafe work in Canada, where the provincial government developed safety-related social marketing campaigns for youth, and many provincial governments also incorporated occupational safety education into the high school curriculum to address young worker injuries. It was expected that the social marketing campaign and high school curriculum would increase young workers' tendency to "speak out" against dangerous work. However, Tucker and Turner (2013) found that, instead of speaking up about harmful work-related hazards, many young workers used a "wait-and-see" approach when they had safety concerns. Young workers' reluctance to voice issues was related to the fear of losing their employment, their inexperience and "newcomer" status, and their sense of powerlessness. The finding is consistent with arguments that simply providing young workers with information about health, safety or wellbeing is insufficient because, as newcomers to a workplace, young workers may lack the self-confidence or ability to transfer information gained during training into practice in the workplace (Nyakänen et al., 2018). Breslin et al. (2007) express similar concerns about health, safety and wellbeing training programmes targeting young workers. Many such training programmes are predicated on the assumption that, once they are equipped to recognise workplace health or safety risks, young workers will assert their rights and act to reduce their personal exposure to danger (Breslin et al, 2007). In making this assumption, young workers are expected to take on an "internal responsibility" for their health, safety and wellbeing that may be unrealistic, given their "newcomer" status (Nyakänen et al., 2018). Although well-intentioned, Breslin et al. (2007) suggest this approach is limited by young workers' lack of self-confidence and practical ability to influence change in their workplaces.

The social environment of the workplace shapes the health and safety practices of young workers (Gherardi & Nicolini, 2002). It is partly through social interactions with others that young workers learn what health and safety-related behaviours are expected in a given context. For example, Nielsen (2012) argues that young workers "make sense" of the prevailing risk culture of their workplace, ultimately reproducing this and adapting to what is considered to be "the normal" or acceptable risk. Pek et al. (2017) similarly describe how young workers develop norms relating to workplace health and safety behaviour based on their social interactions with others, including their supervisors, co-workers and parents. Young workers who perceive that their supervisors, co-workers and parents expect them to work safely are less likely to take risks in the workplace (Pek et al., 2017).

Laberge et al. (2012) describe how workplace social frameworks (in providing formal and informal mentoring and support) contribute substantially to the work socialisation process, the development of work skills and the acquisition of "hands on" work experience.

Being able to talk about work health and safety with others in the workplace is part of learning a craft and it is therefore particularly important that young workers in training (e.g., apprentices) are able to ask questions and talk openly about workplace health and safety with their supervisors and co-workers. Supportive supervision of apprentices is critical, yet effective supervisory/mentoring relationships may not develop organically within workplaces, creating the potential for haphazard learning experiences (Laberge et al., 2012). Some research suggests that supervisors are not always receptive to conversations about workplace health and safety when these are initiated by young workers. For example, Breslin et al. (2007) found that, even when young workers raise questions or concerns about work health and safety, these may be silenced by supervisors whose focus is on getting the job done. Laberge et al. (2012) also observe that apprentices may be uncomfortable initiating conversations with their supervisors and be more likely to seek advice from others who do not occupy positions of formal authority, including more experienced co-workers. Similarly, Zierold (2017) reports that some young workers do not feel comfortable talking to their supervisors about workplace health and safety issues. The "approachability" of supervisors is an important factor shaping young workers' health and safety-related behaviour (Zierold, 2017). Importantly, Zierold (2017) found that young male workers are particularly susceptible to social pressure from supervisors and are more likely than young women workers to perform unsafe work if requested to do so.

Case example 8.1 highlights the importance of having a supervisor who is approachable and easy to talk to about workplace health and safety issues.

CASE EXAMPLE 8.1 THE IMPORTANCE OF SUPPORTIVE SUPERVISION FOR YOUNG WORKERS' SAFETY AT WORK

Interviews were conducted with 30 construction apprentices in New South Wales (Australia). The apprentices were asked how they deal with workplace safety issues when these arise. Specifically, they were asked what they do if they feel unsafe at work or are unsure how to perform a task safely. The apprentices' comments illustrate the importance of having a supervisor who is supportive of safety and also who is non-judgemental and approachable.

A woman apprentice explained: "*Our boss is very … safety is number one. If he sees tradies being unsafe on site, like not wearing their PPE [personal protective equipment], he tells them. He tells me that if I happen to see it, I bring it up to the tradie straightaway and let them know that they're not being safe, and then they have to adjust – like, if they're not wearing PPE, they've got to put their PPE on. But if they don't put it on at all after I've told them, then I ring my boss and let them know that the tradie is not being safe and I have warned them, and then he reprimands them.*" Another male apprentice similarly reflected: "*I was working with a bloke named [supervisor's name]. He was pretty good. He was hard to work with 'cause everything like … he's a real perfectionist. But one good thing about him, he was really safety conscious, he'd make you wear your safeties all the time, your gloves, like long longs on all the time. He'd just drill it into you really. Which was a bit annoying, but at the same time it's also good. Good because if something does happen at least, you know, you've got your safety and it could save your eye or who knows."*

However, apprentices also noted that supervisory messages about safety can sometimes be ambiguous when under time pressure. A woman apprentice described how: *"If someone asked me to run over and do something, like grind up some rod or any other material, I would say, I would have to quickly run to my tool bag over at the shed to get my safety glasses. And he said, 'Oh, it's only one cut. You'll be alright'."*

The apprentices explained how they are more comfortable speaking up or asking questions about safety when their supervisors are approachable and non-judgemental. For example, a woman apprentice commented: *"[My supervisor is] absolutely really good with it. There's no real judgement if I can't do this work. If it's something I just can't do because I'm not strong or I'm not as sure, there's no actual judgement towards me about it. You know he's very understanding and he usually gets on top of it very quickly."*

Another male apprentice said of his supervisor: *"We get along well. He's pretty easy to talk to and pretty approachable sort of a man ... a couple of times, when I got confused on safety or just general stuff, like learning and you know he just explains it again, nice and thoroughly. Before each task, he'll go through and explain, he'll ask questions, like, what's the main problems here? and we have to try and figure it out. If we figure it out, it's all good, but if not, he'll tell us what needs to be done. And – if I'm doing a task and don't understand, I'll go and ask him a question, how the proper way to do it is, or if I'm doing something wrong and I don't understand, I'll go ask him to help."*

These comments show how, for young construction workers who are still undergoing on-the-job training, having a supportive supervisor is important in ensuring their safety at work and enabling them to develop their trade-specific skills in the workplace.

However, not all of the apprentices had supervisors who were supportive and approachable. One male apprentice explained: *"the only person that yells is* [my supervisor]. *The only time that he will yell is when he's told one of the guys how to do something – like explained. They've done something, and they've done it wrong. They've screwed up, maybe they've screwed up a cut or something the wrong way, wasted a bit of material, whatever it is. Look, not straightaway got angry. Been like, 'You're doing it wrong. This is how you're meant to do it' and then later on, they've gone and done the same mistake. That's what really ticks off* [my supervisor], *when he has to explain himself twice.* [My supervisor] *feels that the only way that they're going to really learn is if he, I guess, you could say loses his shit at them. Yesterday, he's like, 'How are they going to learn?' And that definitely has come up from [the] way he was taught. Like he's said that, his builders used to scream at him so, you know, it gets passed down."*

> It is unlikely that apprentices will speak openly and honestly or ask questions about work health and safety issues when their supervisors are dismissive or even verbally aggressive with young workers who make mistakes in their on-the-job training.

8.5 Young construction workers' health-related behaviour

There is evidence to indicate that young construction workers engage in behaviours that have the potential to negatively affect their physical and mental health and wellbeing. These include gambling (Dowling et al. 2005); hazardous drinking (du Plessis & Corney, 2011; Pidd et al., 2017); and the use of illicit substances (du Plessis & Corney, 2011; Pidd et al., 2017).

Excessive or problem gambling has been linked to negative health impacts, reflected in morbidity and mortality, emotional or psychological distress, financial difficulties, diverted financial resources, bankruptcy, reduced performance, loss of role at employment or study, relationship conflict, criminal activity and neglect of responsibilities (Browne et al., 2016). Dowling et al. (2005) studied gambling behaviour among construction apprentices aged 18 to 24 years. In this study most of the apprentices (90 per cent) reported that they gambled and 37 per cent indicated they had gambled regularly in the 12 months leading up to the survey. Approximately one-third of the apprentices who indicated they gamble regularly identified as having a gambling problem. This was indicated by borrowing money to gamble, lying about how much was spent on gambling, and/or spending money allocated to food, clothing or bills on gambling. Help-seeking among these gamblers was very low (approximately 1.5 per cent).

Excessive alcohol consumption is a significant global health issue. International data indicates that more than 3 million deaths occur as a result of alcohol consumption each year, with 29 per cent of these deaths occurring due to injuries (WHO, 2018). In a work environment, alcohol consumption is particularly dangerous because it slows the body's motor and sensory systems, and impairs balance, co-ordination, perception and decision making (Roche et al., 2020). Drinking to intoxication outside work hours can also have a direct impact on workers' ability to work safely (Berry et al., 2007). While national and international data reveal a downward trend in drinking alcohol among young people, Australian research in the construction industry reveals that risky drinking behaviour is high among young workers (<25 years of age) (Roche et al., 2020).

Chapman et al. (2019) also report on the use of drugs in the construction industry, highlighting that young construction workers are a high-risk group (compared to other age groups) for cocaine and cannabis use. The prevalence of young construction workers' use of cannabis and meth/amphetamine is also reported to be substantially higher than that reported by young people who do not work in the construction industry (Australian Institute of Health and Welfare, 2017; cited in Pidd et al., 2017).

Many behaviours with the potential to affect the health and wellbeing of young workers occur outside the workplace, highlighting challenges and ethical considerations in relation to what organisations can and should do to address these behaviours. Further, behaviours including drug and alcohol consumption have been explained as arising from a complicated mix of individual, social and work-related factors (Frone, 2008). The workplace has been identified as a suitable place for interventions to address unhealthy behaviours, with some programmes specifically targeting young workers' alcohol consumption (Doumas & Hannah, 2008).

In Chapter 1 we flagged some important ethical considerations associated with implementing workplace health promotion programmes designed to exert social control over workers' behaviour outside the workplace. Such programmes typically focus on workers "behaving well" not just "feeling well" (Holmqvist, 2009) and frame the prevention of illness (and therefore the occurrence of sickness) as an individual or personal responsibility (Zoller, 2003). Zoller (2003) argues that this can contribute to stigma and potentially reduce workers' "voice" relating to occupational health and work–life balance, which can contribute to unhealthy behaviour (Laberge & Ledouix, 2011)

Interviews conducted with supervisors of apprentices in the construction industry in New South Wales, Australia also revealed that informal support can, in some cases, encourage young workers to seek help to address unhealthy lifestyle behaviours. For example, one supervisor explained: *"I've had a couple of guys that have had gambling and alcohol and drug issues. They've never opened up and I said, 'Well, look, I can help', you know? So you're not weak if you go and get help. You know, don't think you're a weak person because, to be honest, I think it's the total opposite. You're actually stronger. Well, one of the guys, he went to see someone about it and he turned his whole life around. He stopped drinking and got back with his partner. All I did was tell him, you know, 'This is what you should maybe do' and he went and did it himself, I didn't tell him which direction to go. I just said, 'Go and get some help, mate'. Which he did."*

8.6 Young workers' mental health experiences

Research suggests that young workers are at high risk of psychological and mental ill health when transitioning into work (Milner et al., 2019). Kessler et al. (2005) report that adolescence and early adulthood are risky life stages for mental health illness, with 75 per cent of lifetime mental disorder cases starting by age 24 years. Workforce entry can be challenging for young workers, who are still in the stage of ongoing psychological and physical development. Mental health risks can be elevated by stressful work conditions, with research finding young workers to be more susceptible to psychosocial stressors in the workplace than older workers (Pidd et al., 2017). Young workers' susceptibility to work-related stressors is confirmed in empirical studies.

In Australia, Milner et al. (2017) observed that young people's mental health can be impaired by poor psychosocial quality jobs characterised by the adversities of low control, high demands, low security and unfair pay. Specifically, young people who experience two or more of these adversities when entering the workforce experienced a statistically significant decline in their mental health compared to when they were not in the workforce (Milner et al., 2017). In contrast, young workers who entered jobs without these adversities experienced a modest improvement in their mental health (Milner et al., 2017). In Belgium, De Witte et al. (2007) similarly found that psychological job demands, such as the combination of high work pace and high time pressure coupled with low control (i.e., the opportunity of deciding how to meet job demands), produce strain outcomes in young workers starting their first jobs. In New Zealand, Melchior et al. (2007) also found that young workers who are exposed to high psychological job demands (excessive workload, extreme time pressures) have a twofold risk of major depression or generalised anxiety disorder compared to those with low job demands.

Some researchers have specifically focused their attention on the mental health experiences of young construction workers. Importantly, these studies identify construction as a particularly high-risk context for young workers' mental ill health. For example, Pidd et al. (2017) found that construction apprentices experience a substantially higher level of psychological distress than is observed in Australian young men in general. Rates of suicide among Australian construction apprentices are also alarmingly high, with construction apprentices reported as being more than two times more likely to die by suicide than other young men their age (Mates in Construction, 2022).

Of particular note, Pidd et al. (2017) observe that job stress and workplace bullying are significant predictors of psychological distress among construction apprentices. McCormack et al. (2013) similarly report that construction apprentices experience a variety of bullying behaviours in their workplaces, including banter leading to further behaviours that are unacceptable and personal harassment in the form of inappropriate and unacceptable teasing.

McCormack et al. (2013) also found that building and construction apprentices feel reluctant to confront bullies or report instances of workplace bullying. Reasons for this reluctance to report bullying behaviour are attributed to workplace power relations in which young apprentices feel powerless when faced with older, more experienced workers. When the perpetrator of bullying is a supervisor or a respected co-worker, reporting may feel risky to apprentices who worry about repercussions. As a result of this power imbalance, young construction workers often adopt avoidance behaviour, rather than seeking formal help to resolve the situation or asserting themselves (Djurkovic et al., 2005).

McCormack et al. (2013) also suggest that construction apprentices fear that, if they report bullying behaviour they may be branded a "trouble-maker," potentially lose their job and/or experience difficulty finding a new training employer, which is essential to their ability to complete their apprenticeship training. Apprentices also fear that reporting the bullying may make the situation even worse and lead to more intense bullying. In some cases, apprentices do not know who they should report bullying to or are concerned about appearing to be "weak." This fear is driven, in part, by the construction industry's culture.

A survey conducted in Queensland, Australia revealed that bullying and low levels of mental health and wellbeing are problematic issues experienced by construction apprentices (Ross et al., 2020). Among 1,483 construction apprentices who completed the survey, nearly a third (27.3 per cent) of respondents had experienced bullying, with 20 per cent reporting to be a victim of severe workplace bullying. About 13 per cent of respondents reported high levels of psychological distress, suggesting probable serious mental illness. Nearly 30 per cent of apprentices who participated in the survey reported a poor quality of life that may indicate depression. More than half (55.2 per cent) of respondents also indicated that they knew someone who had died by suicide and approximately 30 per cent of respondents reported that they had personally experienced suicidal thoughts in the 12 months prior to participating in the survey (Ross et al., 2020). While not all of the apprentices in the study were young workers, apprentices between the ages of 18 and 25 were significantly more likely to be the victims of bullying than older apprentices (Ross et al., 2020). Other risk factors for being the victim of bullying included: (i) being identified as LGBTI+; (ii) working for a large employer; (iii) not having an employer or working for a group training organisation; (iv) not currently being in an apprenticeship programme or having an "other" apprentice status (e.g., dismissal); (v) working in the engineering construction or the "workshop" industry sectors; and (vi) undertaking extensive overnight work (Ross et al., 2020). The findings also showed that the experience of being bullied was a significant predictor of psychological distress.

Humour is a deeply ingrained characteristic of construction work environments, with sarcasm, banter, mocking and irony prevalent in office-based environments and joke-telling (often using crude language, mimicry and innuendo) commonly used on site (Watts, 2007). When it is appropriately used, humour in the workplace can have psychological and social benefits. For example, workplace banter can enhance group cohesiveness, communication and reduce stress (Plester, 2009a). However, there is no universal understanding of what is funny and what is not, meaning that what is perceived to be funny to one person can be insulting, offensive or hurtful to others. In some instances, workplace cultures develop in which humour that exceeds typical workplace levels of acceptability (e.g., sexist and aggressive humour) is normalised (Plester, 2009b). Djurkovic et al. (2022) suggest there is a "fine line" between what constitutes acceptable joking behaviours and what should be identified as bullying in the workplace. Aggressive workplace humour (which includes teasing) can be harmful to mental health (Hogh et al., 2005) and is particularly harmful when targeted workers are low in power or social status, such as those relatively new to a role, inexperienced or still undergoing education or training (Mortensen & Baarts, 2018). Case example 8.2 below reflects the culture of banter on Australian construction sites and how this often involves teasing inexperienced young workers.

CASE EXAMPLE 8.2 THE NORMALISATION OF BANTER AND TEASING IN CONSTRUCTION WORKPLACES

In the previously mentioned study of 30 construction apprentices in New South Wales, Australia participants' experiences of workplace humour were explored. The apprentices discussed both the benefits and drawbacks of *"having a laugh."* Most insisted that humour is a vital part of getting through the working day. One male apprentice commented *"Everyone has a banter. Everyone loves having jokes. Like, you know, it's not fun unless you get in it."*

However, the apprentices also acknowledged that boundaries need to be maintained and not everyone likes the banter. A woman apprentice observed: *"I have seen guys who maybe aren't as much the 'bantery' type of boy. They might be more reserved and more quiet. I more see then they won't say much or won't contribute. But generally when it comes down to it, everyone on site can tell when they've taken a joke too far."*

Another apprentice observed how workplace humour often targets workers who have made a mistake: *"the banter's high. Yeah, there's some good banter. It just comes up, like if one of the apprentices does something dumb on the site and you just, you know, you give them a bit of banter or like if it's happened previously and you just give 'em shit for it, but you know, it's all a joke … Depends on how you give it. So … okay, if you go too far then they won't be happy about it, but if you go too far then you know you've gone too far, so you normally just apologise or something like that."*

The apprentices accepted being the subject of teasing on site. One apprentice explained: *"Obviously, you get ripped on [teased] too, but that's part of the fun, like, you wait your turn and when someone else stuffs up on the site, that's when you get him back, and, you know, that's the whole fun of it really … You know there's always banter going on, always shit talk, but at the end of the day we're all there to help each other, so no one's taking it like – no one's, obviously, trying to make anyone feel bad, we're all just having a bit of a laugh."*

The apprentices observed that banter can be particularly challenging for workers new to construction worksites. A male apprentice commented: *"I guess if you're working on a big site with a bunch of blokes, everyone has a high ego, everyone wants to be just throwing shots out there, but, you know, got to have a laugh. You know, you've just got to give people a heads up of how far some people can take it and some people can't … Yeah, you wouldn't want someone feeling like everyone's taking out of them just for being new, when, that's never the case, it's always just a bit of banter … but when you first start, you know, it's just typical for it to shock you."* Another male apprentice reflected: *"When I first started … my dad's a carpenter, so I've been around with him for a bit and I've been on the job site, so I knew what I was getting myself into with banter, but with a couple of other people I see, when they first start, they're not sure if someone's joking or not. Like if someone says, 'Oh mate, Christmas is coming before you finish digging this hole' some people think, 'Oh, he's making me feel bad because I can't dig fast' you know what I mean?"*

The interviews with apprentices also highlight the different ways in which men and women can interpret sexual humour in the workplace. Two carpentry apprentices working in the same company were interviewed. One man and one woman. The male apprentice described feeling concerned about offending the woman apprentice when she joined the company but was relieved when she joined in with the banter: *"I said to [training employer] 'Are you sure, 'cause you know, like stuff could go wrong?' … But when she did start, I was actually pretty impressed. Evidently, everyone – like everyone showed respect for her, and it, kind of just eased in, like what kind of banter they said with her, kind of like sussed her out first and – what her banter is like. And it turned out she liked it just as much as us, so by the end of it, no-one was really holding back. So, it was pretty good in the end and she was happy in the end."*

However, the woman apprentice reported a different experience: *"Well, it was kind of bad, but if you don't have a sense of humour with the boys in this industry you generally will not get along with them. Mainly it was about females, you know, like sexual jokes and all of that … Like they will somewhat hurt you, like rattle you in a way, but then at the same time you're like 'I'm going to hear this for the rest of my life from other people' … because I'm a female, they're going to call me different things. But, saying 'you stupid bitch' or the 'C' word – It's just swear words … nothing too bad, not to the point where it's racist or discriminative or anything like that."* The different experiences of the apprentices in this organisation illustrate how teasing (which in this case involved sexualised humour and offensive name calling) can be interpreted differently by perpetrators and the targets of this humour. Often what seems like innocent banter has the potential to be degrading, discriminatory and harmful.

8.7 Social support and mental health and wellbeing

The importance of social support in the workplace for psychological health and wellbeing is discussed in Chapter 10 in which a health-promoting sense of place is described. Support from within the workplace can help people to deal with stressful aspects of their work (Beehr, 1985; Johnson & Hall, 1988). Support from supervisors has been identified as being important for workers' health and wellbeing at work. For example, the absence of support in a supervisor-subordinate relationship has been linked to lower levels of workforce engagement and performance, reduced work satisfaction and increased burnout (Baruch-Feldman et al, 2002; Neves & Eisenberger, 2014).

The availability of social support in a work environment has been identified as a key factor shaping young workers' mental health and wellbeing, particularly when undertaking apprenticeship training (Buchanan et al., 2016). When social supports are available in a workplace, young workers are able to thrive, i.e., experience positive meaning and a sense of wellbeing at work; however, unsupportive environments are detrimental to mental health and wellbeing (Conway & Foskey, 2015).

Blewett et al. (2013) suggest that, for young workers, a supportive environment is one in which: (i) they feel safe, comfortable and respected at work; (ii) they are able to take a longer time to complete a task in a safe manner; (iii) they feel included in the workplace; (iv) they are engaged in health and safety processes; and (v) they feel able to speak up and be heard. Importantly, informal support that is embedded in daily interactions between apprentices, supervisors and experienced co-workers has been identified as being of greater benefit to the health, wellbeing and satisfaction of construction apprentices than formal support (for example, that provided through organisational mentoring programmes) (Buchanan et al., 2016).

Case example 8.3 highlights how having an understanding supervisor who demonstrates care and concern for their workers and tries to help them with personal difficulties is appreciated by young workers.

CASE EXAMPLE 8.3 SUPPORTIVE SUPERVISION OF APPRENTICES

Thirty construction apprentices engaged in a Group Training Programme in New South Wales, Australia were interviewed about their experiences of health, safety and wellbeing. In addition, ten frontline supervisors with responsibility for directing apprentices in their training workplaces were interviewed.

Comments made by many of the apprentices suggested that they experience high levels of social support from their supervisors and co-workers. Importantly, the apprentices identified trust and confidentiality as important elements of this support. One woman apprentice explained: *"At [training employer name] they're quite a tight-knit community, and like a family, so we all look out for each other … if we aren't feeling fantastic we can always go to our boss and have some discussion, or if we need advice, they're happy to give some which is really good. The [training employer name] really treats all their employees like a part of a family. We can be very confidential towards each other if one of us shares something publicly between multiple people, then we're happy to share it with the rest of the company but unless we get that specific permission, we don't go around sharing other people's business."*

A 21-year-old male apprentice described how his supervisor had initiated a conversation after noticing a behaviour change in the apprentice. The supervisor showed empathy and helped the apprentice navigate this difficult point in his life: *"[My supervisor is] actually a very good mate of mine. He's probably 40 something. He's helped me out a lot over the years or over the year I've known* him ... *the last job I wasn't turning up to work and every time he would be 'Come on, man, you've got to come into work' and that. Like 'we all want you to stay with* [company name]' ... *he's always there. It's just a lot of shit at home ... I've actually got two kids and one more on the way. It just sort of put too much on my plate."*

The supervisors we interviewed were mostly very understanding of apprentices' personal needs and were willing to provide practical adjustments and support when necessary: "*Most of the time they've* [the apprentices] *come to me with a personal issue, mum and dad got divorced or I've got issues with my girlfriend, all that sort of stuff. So usually, the best thing I can do for them is to give them time off, to be honest with you, to collect their thoughts and get some time away from the job."*

Some supervisors were aware of the boundary between work and personal life and did not want to "cross the boundary": "*If I can see there's something wrong and I think that something mightn't be right, I'll ask them 'Is everything okay? You know, you're not your usual self'. I won't push 'em but I'll definitely ask because at the end of the day I'd rather ask the question than not ask the question. Some say, 'Yeah, I'm fine' but some will open up."*

Supervisors who had received formal training in addressing workplace mental health issues felt more confident initiating conversations with young workers if they believed they were experiencing personal difficulties or emotional distress. This confidence was increased by the knowledge that they could ask whether someone is okay without taking on the role of a counsellor themselves. Understanding the limitations of their role and the importance of connecting young workers with appropriate professional services was a crucial component of supervisors' feeling prepared and able to initiate a conversation with a worker in relation to their mental health.

However, not all of the apprentices we interviewed experienced supportive supervision. Case example 8.4 describes a situation in which a young apprentice was told by co-workers that he was being given unpleasant work tasks to perform as "punishment" for asking for time off work following a family bereavement. Research shows that hostile treatment at work is significantly related to job satisfaction, affective commitment, turnover intention, general health, emotional exhaustion (burnout), depression and physical wellbeing, interpersonal deviance, organisational deviance and performance (Hershcovis & Barling, 2010).

The experience of abusive leadership has been linked to young workers' health and wellbeing (including the experience of anxiety inside and outside work) (Starratt & Grandy 2010). Abusive leadership was characterised as:

- playing favourites
- dealing dirty work as punishment

- threatening workers
- blurring the lines between professional and personal
- talking behind workers' backs
- putting workers down
- engaging in public criticism of workers
- setting unrealistic work expectations
- telling lies, and
- engaging in illegal practices.

CASE EXAMPLE 8.4 UNSUPPORTIVE SUPERVISION OF AN APPRENTICE

A 21-year-old plumbing apprentice described going through a period of personal difficulty. Despite a series of distressing events in this apprentice's personal life he did not speak to people at work about his situation: *"I had a pretty hard year last year. Oh, it was a terrible year really. My parents split up then both my dogs passed away. Then my Nan passed away and then we moved houses. That was a pretty full-on year. But I didn't really talk to any of my colleagues about it. I kept sort of quiet, I suppose."*

When asked if he thought he could speak to his supervisor about personal issues, he explained that he didn't think his supervisor would understand, and that project-related time pressure would cause his supervisor to insist that he should come to work, even if he needed to take leave: *"The problem is I feel like, oh some supervisors, they're not understanding, if that makes sense. Like, you say, 'Oh, I don't know, I've got a bit of shit going on', you're still under the pump or, you know. Like 'nah, you've got to do this, you've got to do that'. Say everything that was happening with me last year. If I said, 'Oh, can I have some time off without pay or something like, I'm not feeling right?' my boss'd be like, 'Nah, I need ya. Are you coming to work?'"*

The apprentice explained that it was difficult to talk to people at work: *"I think maybe just pulling them aside and saying, 'How you going?' 'Are you all right? Like, how do you honestly feel?' 'How's working going, are you learning?' If someone just pulls you aside and just have a one on one. I just think if there was something was going on, that person might probably open up a bit and tell them how they sort of feel a bit … if you've got a bunch of people listening, you're not going to open up as much because you've got everyone listening. If you say something with people around it's just, you know, it makes you sort of look stupid."*

The apprentice also described how he was told by co-workers that he was being given unpleasant work tasks as punishment for requesting to take time off when his grandmother died: *"Probably good to take a little bit of time off. When my Nan passed away – I had two days off. Because that was Dad's Mum and I was pretty close with her. And then as soon as I come back to work, I was sent to the Central Coast for a month. Just digging potholes. Because my boss got the shits with me for that. And I was just like, 'Really mate? I just lost my Nan'. That was a bit annoying. I found out why I was down there because one of the boys said, 'Oh, [supervisor's name] got the shits with you for having two days off'. And then I was just like, well come on, my Nan – I was pretty close to her and that. And Dad, you know, he was split up with Mum and – and his Mum's passed away. Wasn't real good."*

This case shows a number of features of abusive leadership as defined by Starratt and Grandy (2010). Not only was unpleasant work allocated to the apprentice as punishment for taking time off but it appears that the supervisor had also discussed this matter with other workers in the group behind the apprentice's back.

8.8   Protecting and promoting the health and wellbeing of young workers

There are numerous examples of work-based training programmes designed to equip young workers with the knowledge, skills and abilities that they need to ensure their health, safety and wellbeing as they enter the world of work. Increasingly, occupational health and safety training programmes targeting young workers go beyond providing information about workplace risks, policies and procedures, and address issues of self-advocacy and self-determination (Chin et al., 2010). For example, Chin et al. (2010) argue that "to reframe workers' expectations about injury on the job, youth need to be engaged in safety learning that questions their beliefs, rights and knowledge of self, and teaches them how to communicate with colleagues, employers, unions, and compensation agencies, as well as their family and friends" (p.572). Increasingly, programmes are designed to develop young workers' "soft skills" in order to appropriately respond to work environments or practices that concern them or are unsafe (Kincl et al., 2016).

One such programme, the Safety Voice for Ergonomics programme, provides masonry apprentices with training in ergonomic principles to counteract the high prevalence of musculoskeletal injury in masonry work. It incorporates elements of self-direction, self-control, accountability, responsibility, communication, and leadership to help apprentice workers to develop their "safety voice." The Safety Voice for Ergonomics programme is delivered using a blended learning approach and incorporates e-learning with interactive problem-solving and face-to-face delivery. Knowledge of safe and healthy work techniques is supplemented with "safety voice" activities in which apprentices practise dealing with situations in which they have to raise health or safety-related issues with "difficult" co-workers or supervisors (Kincl et al. 2016).

A similar programme has been implemented in Finland. The Attitude to Work programme focuses on the delivery of psychosocial resources for young workers and is designed to provide young workers with readiness and confidence to put their skills into practice and advocate for their health, safety and wellbeing in unfamiliar work environments. An important component of the programme is the development of "safety preparedness," defined as the "readiness to implement actions that support occupational safety, and their resilience to deal with barriers or problems related to occupational safety and safe working" (Nykänen et al., 2018, p. 46). The safety preparedness concept combines self-efficacy with "inoculation" against setbacks, or "skills that help an individual maintain active behaviour when facing barriers or setbacks" (Nykänen et al., 2018, p. 46). Potential barriers include unclear instructions, risky work behaviour of co-workers, unfamiliar work tasks or pressure to work faster than young workers' skills allow them to work safely. The content and delivery approach used in the Attitude to Work programme is presented in Table 8.1.

Nykänen et al. (2018) undertook a randomised controlled trial to evaluate the impact of the Attitude to Work programme. They report that participants in the programme showed a greater increase in safety preparedness and internal locus of control (i.e., the belief that they can individually influence their safety at work) at follow-up compared to a group of matched-paired participants who received some of the training content without the active learning delivery component.

Sámano-Ríos et al. (2019) conducted a systematic review of preventive health, safety and wellbeing programmes focused on young workers. Sámano-Ríos et al. (2019) observed that, of the 39 studies incorporated in the review, most of the programmes aimed to change young workers' health and safety beliefs, attitudes and behaviours through education and learning. However, very few programmes targeted environmental factors, such as workplace, organisational or legislative change. This is limiting because, as pointed out by Hanvold et al. (2019), to prevent workplace safety incidents and work-related illness among young workers, there is a need to focus on organisational risk factors, as addressing these factors will have a greater impact than focusing solely on the characteristics of being young. Most of the programmes also focused solely on young workers themselves, with a limited number of programmes involving others with the potential to influence young workers' health, safety and wellbeing, such as families, employers, supervisors and educators. Importantly, fewer than half of the programmes were rigorously evaluated, substantially weakening the evidence of their impact/effectiveness.

8.9 Conclusion

Young workers are a particularly vulnerable group in construction and are subject to worse health and wellbeing than their older counterparts. Rather than prepare

TABLE 8.1 Attitude to Work training content and delivery

Topic	Purpose	Method
Day 1		
Introduction to behaviours that support workplace safety	To share beliefs and experiences about safety at work	Group discussion with opinion line-up exercise
Identifying hazards at the workplace	To increase awareness of job-specific hazards and preventive actions	Small group exercise, hazard visualisation with flip charts
Analysing factors preceding accidents, relationship between unsafe behaviour and accidents, identifying behavioural strategies for preventing accidents	To strengthen positive attitudes towards accident prevention and safety	Group discussions about case stories, sharing previous experiences of accidents, near misses or safety-related events
Day 2		
Negative consequences of staying silent about safety issues and positive consequences of information seeking and speaking about safety at work	To identify how workers can communicate with co-workers, supervisors and safety representatives, ask questions and report problems. To practise social skills that support safe behaviour at work and to strengthen positive attitudes towards workplace safety	Group discussion, role-playing exercises
Safety inoculation training	To develop behavioural strategies to help overcome barriers to safe work and strengthen workers' self-confidence when faced with such barriers	Problem-solving exercises based on case stories
Personal safety goals	To foster personal commitment and motivation towards safe work and accident prevention	Group discussion with goal-setting activity

Source: Nyakänen et al. (2018).

young workers to cope with the challenging work factors they may experience as they navigate through the early stages of their career, the construction industry must take a different approach. That is, to create a workplace that enables young workers to learn, work, and flourish in a safe and supportive environment.

8.10 Discussion and review questions

1. Is it fair to assume that young workers are at greater risk of work-related injury because of their biological age? Why/why not? What other factors contribute to the higher incidence of injury among young workers?
2. Why is the health of young construction workers more precarious than that of other young people? What employment or job characteristics contribute to this? What role does the industry culture play in shaping health outcomes of young construction workers?
3. How do relationships with others in the workplace (e.g., supervisors and more experienced co-workers) shape young construction workers' experiences of health, safety and wellbeing at work? What are the characteristics of supportive workplaces for young workers?
4. Are training programmes that provide work health and safety information to young workers sufficient to protect their health, safety and wellbeing at work? Why/why not? What else could construction organisations do to ensure the health, safety and wellbeing of young workers?

8.11 Acknowledgements

Case examples 8.1, 8.2, 8.3 and 8.4 draw on work that was funded by icare New South Wales in Australia and supported by the Master Builders Association of New South Wales and the NSW Centre for Work Health and Safety.

References

Australian Government. (2021). *Australian Apprenticeships Incentives Programme Guidelines* (effective 9 March 2021). Accessed 29 June 2021 from: www.dese.gov.au/skills-sup portindividuals/resources/australian-apprenticeships-incentives-program-guidelines

Australian Industry Group. (2016). *Making Apprenticeships Work*. Accessed 12 September 2018 from: http://cdn.aigroup.com.au/Reports/2016/15160_apprenticeships_poli cy_full.pdf

Bakkevig Dagsland, Å. H., Mykletun, R. J., & Einarsen, S. (2015). "We're not slaves— we are actually the future!" A follow-up study of apprentices' experiences in the Norwegian hospitality industry. *Journal of Vocational Education & Training, 67*(4), 460–481.

Bande, R., & López-Mourelo, E. (2015). The impact of worker's age on the consequences of occupational accidents: Empirical evidence using Spanish data. *Journal of Labor Research, 36*(2), 129–174.

Baruch-Feldman, C., Brondolo, E., Ben-Dayan, D., & Schwartz, J. (2002). Sources of social support and burnout, job satisfaction, and productivity. *Journal of Occupational Health Psychology, 7*(1), 84–93.

Bednarz, A. (2014). *Understanding The Non-Completion of Apprentices*. National Centre for Vocational Education Research.

Beehr, T. A. (1985). The role of social support in coping with organisational stress. In: T.A Beehr and R.S Bhagat (Eds.), *Human Stress and Cognition in Organisations: An Integrated Perspective*, Wiley (pp. 375–398).

Berry, J. G., Pidd, K., Roche, A. M., & Harrison, J. E. (2007). Prevalence and patterns of alcohol use in the Australian workforce: Findings from the 2001 National Drug Strategy Household Survey. *Addiction*, 102(9), 1399–1410.

Blewett, V., Rainbird, S., Clarkson, L., Paterson, J., & Etherton, H. (2013). *Developing the Youth Health and Safety Strategy for South Australia*. Appleton Institute, Central Queensland University.

Breslin, C., Koehoorn, M., Smith, P., & Manno, M. (2003). Age related differences in work injuries and permanent impairment: a comparison of workers' compensation claims among adolescents, young adults, and adults. *Occupational and Environmental Medicine*, 60(9), e10–e10.

Breslin, F. C., & Smith, P. (2006). Trial by fire: A multivariate examination of the relation between job tenure and work injuries. *Occupational and Environmental Medicine*, 63(1), 27–32.

Breslin, F. C., Morassaei, S., Wood, M., & Mustard, C. A. (2011). Assessing occupational health and safety of young workers who use youth employment centers. *American Journal of Industrial Medicine*, 54(4), 325–337.

Breslin, F. C., Pole, J. D., Tompa, E., Amick III, B. C., Smith, P., & Johnson, S. H. (2007). Antecedents of work disability absence among young people: A prospective study. *Annals of Epidemiology*, 17(10), 814–820.

Breslin, F. C., Polzer, J., MacEachen, E., Morrongiello, B., & Shannon, H. (2007). Workplace injury or "part of the job"? Towards a gendered understanding of injuries and complaints among young workers. *Social Science & Medicine*, 64(4), 782–793.

Browne, M., Langham, E., Rawat, V., Greer, N., Li, E., Rose, J.,... & Bryden, G. (2016). *Assessing Gambling-Related Harm in Victoria: A Public Health Perspective*. Victorian Responsible Gambling Foundation.

Buchanan, J., Raffaele, C., Glozier, N., & Kanagaratnam, A. (2016). *Beyond Mentoring: Social Support Structures for Young Australian Carpentry Apprentices. Research Report*. National Centre for Vocational Education Research.

Burke, R. J. (2017), Work and well-being. In R. J. Burke & K. M. Page (Eds.), *Research Handbook on Work and Wellbeing*. Edward Elgar (pp. 3–36).

Chapman, J., Roche, A., Pidd, K., Ledner, B., & Finnane, J. (2019). Alcohol and drug use among construction workers: Which drugs and which workers? In *Public Health Association, Australia: Celebrating 50 Years, Poised to Meet the Challenges of the Next 50* (p. 55). Public Health Association of Australia.

Chau, N., Wild, P., Dehaene, D., Benamghar, L., Mur, J. M., & Touron, C. (2010). Roles of age, length of service and job in work-related injury: a prospective study of 446 120 person-years in railway workers. *Occupational and Environmental Medicine*, 67(3), 147–153.

Chin, P., DeLuca, C., Poth, C., Chadwick, I., Hutchinson, N., & Munby, H. (2010). Enabling youth to advocate for workplace safety. *Safety Science*, 48(5), 570–579.

Construction Skills Queensland (CSQ). (2018). *Women in Construction: An Opportunity Lost?* Accessed 29 August 2022 from: www.csq.org.au/wp-content/uploads/2018/11/CSQ2531-Women-in-Construction_2.pdf

Conway, M. L., & Foskey, R. (2015). Apprentices thriving at work: Looking through an appreciative lens. *Journal of Vocational Education & Training*, 67(3), 332–348.

Couldrey M. & Loveder P. (2016). *The Future of Australian Apprenticeships*. National Vocational Education and Training Research.

Dagsland, Å. H. B., Mykletun, R., & Einarsen, S. (2011). Apprentices' expectations and experiences in the socialisation process in their meeting with the hospitality industry. *Scandinavian Journal of Hospitality and Tourism*, 11(4), 395–415.

De Witte, H. D., Verhofstadt, E., & Omey, E. (2007). Testing Karasek's learning and strain hypotheses on young workers in their first job. *Work & Stress, 21*(2), 131–141.

Djurkovic, N., McCormack, D., & Casimir, G. (2005). The behavioral reactions of victims to different types of workplace bullying. *International Journal of Organization Theory & Behavior, 8*(4), 439–460.

Djurkovic, N., McCormack, D., Hoel, H., & Salin, D. (2022). Joking behaviours and bullying from the perspective of Australian human resource professionals. *Asia Pacific Journal of Human Resources, 60*(2), 381–404.

Doumas, D. M., & Hannah, E. (2008). Preventing high-risk drinking in youth in the workplace: A web-based normative feedback program. *Journal of Substance Abuse Treatment, 34*(3), 263–271.

Dowling, N., Clark, D., Memery, L., & Corney, T. (2005). Australian apprentices and gambling. *Youth Studies Australia, 24*(3), 17–23.

du Plessis, K., & Corney, T. (2011). Construction industry apprentices' substance use: A survey of prevalence rates, reasons for use, and regional and age differences. *Youth Studies Australia, 30*(4), 40–50.

Einboden, R., Choi, I., Ryan, R., Petrie, K., Johnston, D., Harvey, S. B., Glozier., N., Wray, A., & Deady, M. (2021). "Having a thick skin is essential": mental health challenges for young apprentices in Australia. *Journal of Youth Studies, 24*(3), 355–371.

European Agency for Safety and Health at Work. (2007). OSH in the figures: *Young Workers – Facts and Figures: Exposure to Risks and Health Effects.* Accessed 1 September 2022 from: https://osha.europa.eu/en/tools-and-publications/publications/repo rts/7606507

Fisher, C. D. (1986). Organisational socialisation: An integrative review. In K. M. Rowland & G. R. Ferris (Eds.), *Research in Personal and Human Resource Management.* JAI Press.

Frone, M. R. (2008). Employee alcohol and illicit drug use: Scope, causes, and organizational consequences. *Handbook of Organizational Behavior, 1,* 519–540.

Fuller, A., & Unwin, L. (2008). *Towards Expansive Apprenticeships: A Commentary by the Teaching and Learning Research Programme.* Institute of Education, London: Teaching and Learning Research Programme.

Gherardi, S., & Nicolini, D. (2002). Learning the trade: A culture of safety in practice. *Organisation, 9*(2), 191–223.

Gow, K., Hinschen, C., Anthony, D., & Warren, C. (2008). Work expectations and other factors influencing male apprentices' intentions to quit their trade. *Asia Pacific Journal of Human Resources, 46*(1), 99–121.

Hanvold, T. N., Kines, P., Nykänen, M., Thomée, S., Holte, K. A., Vuori, J.,... & Veiersted, K. B. (2019). Occupational safety and health among young workers in the Nordic countries: a systematic literature review. *Safety and Health at Work, 10*(1), 3–20.

Hershcovis, M. S., & Barling, J. (2010). Towards a multi-foci approach to workplace aggression: A meta-analytic review of outcomes from different perpetrators. *Journal of Organizational Behavior, 31*(1), 24–44.

Hogh, A., Henriksson, M.E. and Burr, H. (2005), A 5-year follow-up study of aggression at work and psychological health, *International Journal of Behavioral Medicine, 12*(4), 256–265.

Holmqvist, M. (2009). Corporate social responsibility as corporate social control: The case of work-site health promotion. *Scandinavian Journal of Management, 25*(1), 68–72.

Johnson, J. V., & Hall, E. M. (1988). Job strain, work place social support, and cardiovascular disease: a cross-sectional study of a random sample of the Swedish working population. *American Journal of Public Health, 78*(10), 1336–1342.

Jones, A., Clayton, B., Pfitzner, N., & Guthrie, H. (2017). *Perfect for a Woman: Increasing the Participation of Women in Electrical Trades*. Victoria University.

Kessler, R. C., Berglund, P., Demler, O., Jin, R., Merikangas, K. R., & Walters, E. E. (2005). Lifetime prevalence and age-of-onset distributions of DSM-IV disorders in the National Comorbidity Survey Replication. *Archives of General Psychiatry*, 62(6), 593–602.

Kincl, L. D., Anton, D., Hess, J. A., & Weeks, D. L. (2016). Safety voice for ergonomics (SAVE) project: Protocol for a workplace cluster-randomized controlled trial to reduce musculoskeletal disorders in masonry apprentices. *BMC Public Health*, 16(1), 362.

Laberge, M., & Ledoux, E. (2011). Occupational health and safety issues affecting young workers: A literature review. *Work*, 39(3), 215–232.

Laberge, M., MacEachen, E., & Calvet, B. (2014). Why are occupational health and safety training approaches not effective? Understanding young worker learning processes using an ergonomic lens. *Safety Science*, 68, 250–257.

Laberge, M., Vézina, N., Calvet, B., Lévesque, S., & Vézina-Nadon, L. (2012). Supervision of apprentices in semiskilled trades: program stipulations and workplace realities. *Relations industrielles/Industrial Relations*, 67(2), 199–221.

Lopata, J., Maclachlan, C., Dishke Hondzel, C., Mountenay, D., Halyk, J., Mayer, V., & Kaattari, T. (2015). *Barriers to Attracting Apprentices and Completing Their Apprenticeships*, Employment Ontario. Accessed 15 July 2022 from. www.voced.edu.au/content/ngv:72704

Loudoun, R. J. (2010). Injuries sustained by young males in construction during day and night work. *Construction Management and Economics*, 28(12), 1313–1320.

Marchand, T. H. (2008). Muscles, morals and mind: Craft apprenticeship and the formation of person. *British Journal of Educational Studies*, 56(3), 245–271.

Mates in Construction. (2022). *Why Mates Exists: The Problem*. Accessed 1 September 2022 from: https://mates.org.au/construction/the-problem

McCormack, D., Djurkovic, N., & Casimir, G. (2013). Workplace bullying: The experiences of building and construction apprentices. *Asia Pacific Journal of Human Resources*, 51(4), 406–420.

Melchior, M., Caspi, A., Milne, B. J., Danese, A., Poulton, R., & Moffitt, T. E. (2007). Work stress precipitates depression and anxiety in young, working women and men. *Psychological Medicine*, 37(8), 1119–1129.

Milner, A., Krnjacki, L., & LaMontagne, A. D. (2017). Psychosocial job quality and mental health among young workers: A fixed-effects regression analysis using 13 waves of annual data. *Scandinavian Journal of Work, Environment & Health*, 43(1), 50–58.

Milner, A., Law, P., & Reavley, N. (2019). *Young Workers and Mental Health: A Systematic Review of the Effect of Employment and Transition into Employment on Mental Health*. Victorian Health Promotion Foundation.

Mortensen, M., & Baarts, C. A. (2018). Killing ourselves with laughter … mapping the interplay of organizational teasing and workplace bullying in hospital work life. *Qualitative Research in Organizations and Management: An International Journal*, 13(1), 10–31.

National Centre for Vocational Education Research. (2018). *Completion and Attrition Rates for Apprentices and Trainees 2018 Data Tables*. Accessed 1 September 2022 from: www.voced.edu.au/content/ngv%3A8370

Neves, P., & Eisenberger, R. (2014). Perceived organisational support and risk taking. *Journal of Managerial Psychology*, 29(2), 187–205.

Nielsen, M. L. (2012). Adapting 'the normal'–examining relations between youth, risk and accidents at work. *Nordic Journal of Working Life Studies*, 2(2), 71–85.

Nielsen, M. L., Görlich, A., Grytnes, R., & Dyreborg, J. (2017). Without a safety net: Precarization among young Danish employees. *Nordic Journal of Working Life Studies*, 7(3), 3–22.

Nykänen, M., Sund, R., & Vuori, J. (2018). Enhancing safety competencies of young adults. A randomized field trial (RCT). *Journal of Safety Research*, 67, 45–56.

Okun, A. H., Guerin, R. J., & Schulte, P. A. (2016). Foundational workplace safety and health competencies for the emerging workforce. *Journal of Safety Research*, 59, 43–51.

Pek, S., Turner, N., Tucker, S., Kelloway, E. K., & Morrish, J. (2017). Injunctive safety norms, young worker risk-taking behaviors, and workplace injuries. *Accident Analysis & Prevention*, 106, 202–210.

Pidd, K., Duraisingam, V., Roche, A., & Trifonoff, A. (2017). Young construction workers: Substance use, mental health, and workplace psychosocial factors. *Advances in Dual Diagnosis*, 10(4), 155–168.

Plester, B. (2009a). Healthy humour: Using humour to cope at work. *Kōtuitui: New Zealand Journal of Social Sciences Online*, 4(1), 89–102.

Plester, B. (2009b), Crossing the line: boundaries of workplace humour and fun. *Employee Relations*, 31(6), 584–599.

Rauscher, K. J., & Myers, D. J. (2016). Occupational fatalities among young workers in the United States: 2001–2012. *American Journal of Industrial Medicine*, 59(6), 445–452.

Roche, A. M., Chapman, J., Duraisingam, V., Phillips, B., Finnane, J., & Pidd, K. (2020). Construction workers' alcohol use, knowledge, perceptions of risk and workplace norms. Drug and Alcohol *Review*, 39(7), 941–949.

Ross, V., Wardhani, R., & Kõlves, K. (2020). *The Impact of Workplace Bullying on Mental Health and Suicidality in Queensland Construction Industry Apprentices.* Australian Institute for Suicide Research and Prevention: Griffith University.

Safe Work Australia (2013). *Work-Related Injuries Experienced by Young Workers in Australia, 2009–10.* Safe Work Australia.

Safe Work Australia (2015). *Exposure to multiple hazards among Australian workers.* Safe Work Australia.

Salminen, S. (2004). Have young workers more injuries than older ones? An international literature review. *Journal of Safety Research*, 35(5), 513–521.

Sámano-Ríos, M. L., Ijaz, S., Ruotsalainen, J., Breslin, F. C., Gummesson, K., & Verbeek, J. (2019). Occupational safety and health interventions to protect young workers from hazardous work – A scoping review. *Safety Science*, 113, 389–403.

Starratt, A., & Grandy, G. (2010). Young workers' experiences of abusive leadership. *Leadership & Organisation Development Journal*, 31(2), 136–158.

Steinberg, L. (2004). Risk-taking in adolescence: What changes, and why? *Annals of the New York Academy of Sciences,* 1021, 51–58.

Tucker, S., & Turner, N. (2013). Waiting for safety: Responses by young Canadian workers to unsafe work. *Journal of Safety Research*, 45, 103–110.

Tucker, S., & Turner, N. (2014). Safety voice among young workers facing dangerous work: A policy-capturing approach. *Safety Science*, 62, 530–537.

Turner, N., Tucker, S., & Kelloway, E. K. (2015). Prevalence and demographic differences in microaccidents and safety behaviors among young workers in Canada. *Journal of Safety Research*, 53, 39–43.

Watts, J. (2007). IV. Can't Take a Joke? Humour as Resistance, Refuge and Exclusion in a Highly Gendered Workplace. *Feminism & Psychology,* 17(2), 259–266.

World Health Organization. (2018). *Global Status Report on Alcohol and Health 2018*. World Health Organization.

Zierold, K. M. (2017). Youth doing dangerous tasks: Supervision matters. *American Journal of Industrial Medicine, 60*(9), 789–797.

Zoller, H. M. (2003). Working out: Managerialism in workplace health promotion. *Management Communication Quarterly, 17*(2), 171–205.

9

HEALTHY AGEING AT WORK

Helen Lingard, Rita Peihua Zhang, Payam Pirzadeh and Michelle Turner

School of Property, Construction & Project Management, RMIT University, Melbourne, Australia

9.1 Introduction

Protecting and supporting the health and wellbeing of construction workers throughout their working lives is important. Yet the needs and experiences of workers in different age groups and life stages are likely to vary. In Chapter 8 we described the factors that shape health and wellbeing among young workers and considered ways that young workers might be better protected from adverse health outcomes associated with working in the construction industry. In this chapter we focus on the health and wellbeing of manual/non-managerial construction workers as they age and strategies that can support construction workers to stay healthy and well throughout their working lives.

9.2 The ageing population

According to the United Nations, population ageing is a global phenomenon occurring in nearly every country across the world due to declining birth rates and longer life expectancy. The proportion of the global population aged 65 years or over increased from 6 per cent in 1990 to 9 per cent in 2019 and is projected to climb to 16 per cent by 2050 (United Nations, 2019). This would mean one in six people in the world will be aged 65 years or over (United Nations, 2019). Population ageing is typically measured using the old-age dependency ratio (OADR), which reflects the number of old-age dependents (persons aged 65 years or over) per 100 persons of working age (aged 20 to 64 years). As the relative size of older age groups increases in many countries, concerns have been raised about how older persons will be supported financially and socially (Kenny et al., 2008). Increasing the retirement age is one measure that is often suggested to address this challenge. However, this may not always be possible or safe in physically demanding jobs.

DOI: 10.1201/9780367814236-9

Consistent with broader demographic trends, there is evidence that the construction industry workforce is also ageing in many countries. For example, in the UK the Chartered Institute of Building (CIOB) observes two important labour force trends: 1) the total number of construction workers over 60 has increased more than any other age group; and 2) the biggest reduction in construction worker numbers has occurred in those under 30 years of age (CIOB, 2021). In Australia, it is estimated that over 40 per cent of current workers in infrastructure construction are likely to retire over the next 15 years and more than 40 per cent of project management professionals and workers in the structures and civil trades are over the age of 45 (Infrastructure Australia, 2021). In the USA the average age of construction workers reached 42.6 in 2017 which was greater than the average age of all US workers (42.2 years) and was 3.5 years older than the average age of construction workers in 2003 and 6.4 years older than the average age of construction workers in the 1980s (Sokas et al., 2019).

O'Neill (2020) argues that construction employers should recognise the value of older workers whose skills and experience can contribute substantially to construction work. However, construction employers also need to understand the way that age affects workers' physical and cognitive capacity and provide appropriate organisational and workplace supports to enable older workers to work in safe, healthy and productive ways. O'Neill (2020) points out that catering for an age-diverse workforce is, in fact, legally required by equality and anti-discrimination legislation.

9.3 The ageing process

As they age, people naturally experience a decline in physical capacity resulting from molecular and cellular damage that accumulates over time. The ageing process produces a progressive deterioration of a range of components of fitness, such as aerobic/cardiovascular capacity, muscular mass strength and endurance, and flexibility (Kenny et al., 2008). Ageing is also accompanied by changes to body composition, bone mass and strength, degeneration of intervertebral discs, tendons and ligaments and increased risk of damage to articular cartilage (Boros & Freemont, 2017). Changes to the sensory system and muscle activation patterns associated with ageing can also contribute to impaired balance (Gomes et al., 2013). All of these physical changes can combine over time to reduce functional capacity and increase the likelihood of musculoskeletal injury (Boros & Freemont, 2017).

Ilmarinen (2002) reports that the average physical work capacity of a 65-year-old is approximately half that of an average 25-year-old worker (Ilmarinen, 2002). However, age-related health impacts can occur among much younger workers. For example, age-related physical health is reported to decline by about 20 per cent between the ages of 40 and 60 years (Ilmarinen, 2002) and, although declines in cardiovascular, respiratory, metabolic and muscular functions are

TABLE 9.1 Ability to conduct work tasks according to age group

Work ability indicator	20–29	30–39	40–49	50 and over
Ability to meet the physical demands of your work	8.76	8.30	7.92	8.29
Capability to perform the tasks and activities necessary for your work	8.65	8.33	7.92	8.57

Note: Rating is from 1 to 10 with higher scores indicating better capacity.

initially small, they build up to produce a substantial decrease in functional capacity between the ages of 40 and 50 (Kenny et al., 2008).

Age-related decline in physical work capacity exceeds and outpaces age-related declines in mental and social ability, with the result that the work ability of people in physically demanding job roles is impacted more acutely and at a younger age than that of workers whose jobs are less physically demanding. This has implications for the construction industry because site-based manual/non-managerial work is often physically demanding in nature.

Australian research by Turner and Lingard (2020) found that the proportion of manual/non-managerial construction workers who rate their ability to undertake physical tasks as being "very good" steadily declines with age, as does the capability to perform the tasks and activities necessary for their work. The exception to this is the 50 and over age group who report a higher ability than the 40–49 age group to conduct work tasks and may be due to a transition into less demanding physical roles and/or supervision roles. The decline in ability to conduct work tasks according to age group is shown in Table 9.1.

Research also suggests that, in addition to the natural ageing process, construction workers often experience bodily pain arising as a result of cumulative exposures to the physical demands of their work. Importantly, this can occur at a relatively young age. Of the workers who participated in the Turner and Lingard (2020) study, 17.6 per cent of those aged 20–29 years experienced lower back pain or joint pain in the fingers, shoulders, hips, knees, and/or ankles daily; 13.3 per cent of those aged 30–39 years experienced lower back pain daily; and 16.7 per cent of those aged 30–39 years experienced daily joint pain in the fingers, shoulders, hips, knees, and/or ankles.

Although the United Nations considers persons of working age to be between the ages of 20 and 64 years, Hoonakker and van Duivenbooden (2010) observe that construction workers differ from workers in other industries because they start working at a relatively young age (15 or 16). This means that, by the time they are 65 they will have worked for 50 years and cumulative exposure to adverse work conditions may have particularly significant effects on construction workers' health and wellbeing. Importantly, the cumulative exposure to physically and psychologically demanding work plays a significant role in shaping health and wellbeing over the working lives of construction workers, over and above the impacts of ageing. For example, Arndt et al. (2005) report the results of longitudinal research showing that, even though the incidence of work disability in construction workers increases with age, the dose–response relationship between work exposure to health risks and work disability persists even when age is controlled for (Arndt et al., 2005).

Case example 9.1 reveals that manual/non-managerial workers are resigned to experiencing increasing bodily pain and long-term debilitating deterioration in physical functioning as they age.

CASE EXAMPLE 9.1 MANUAL/NON-MANAGERIAL CONSTRUCTION WORKERS' EXPECTATION THAT WORK-RELATED BODILY PAIN WILL INCREASE WITH AGE

A study examined the link between bodily pain and mental health among manual/non-managerial construction workers in Victoria, Australia. A total of 67 workers participated in a survey and 18 of these workers participated in a follow-up interview.

All participants interviewed experienced physical pain arising from their job, irrespective of their age or occupation (trade). The frequency of pain ranged from occasional aches to ongoing shoulder, back, and joint pain. The interview participants all believed pain to be a normal part of manual/ non-managerial construction work. For example, one participant commented: "*Can't blame the [construction] industry. It's just the way it is*" (roof plumber, 45 years old). However, pain was also linked to age and years spent in the industry. Another participant commented: "*I think it wears you out over time unfortunately. Most blokes in the trade end up like that [in pain]*" (electrician, 48 years old). Participants observed that they expect their levels of pain to increase with the natural ageing process. One participant commented: "*I tend to get sore more often with age. But it's not just the back, it's the knees*" (electrician, 48 years old). Another participant explained: "[pain occurs] *not so much 'cause the work has changed or anything like that, but just age, and just always working the body*" (cable technician, 50 years old).

Participants believed an increase in debilitating pain is an inevitable part of working in the construction industry. For example, one participant reflected on the experience of his father who had worked as a roof plumber: "*My father actually did this for 47 years. And he's nearly 70 now and he can hardly walk. He can't use his hands anymore. What else can't he do? He gets gout bad and he's got arthritis in his fingers. So, that's what I've got to look forward to*" (roof plumber, 45 years old). Participants also commented that age increased their levels of pain when working in certain environmental conditions, e.g., cold weather: "*Getting to my age the cold hurts my knees and that. After so many*

> *years of going up and down roofs I get sore knees ... I feel like I'm getting a little bit of arthritis in my fingers and that's because I've been doing it for so long, but when it's colder they get sore"* (roof plumber, 45 years old).
>
> Many participants believed that they would be unable to stay in their role in the long term due to injury and associated pain. With this is mind, many were actively planning to move into a less physically demanding role. For example, this participant commented: *"I've sort of spent probably the last four or five years starting to work towards that, where I'm not going to be on the tools so much, because of the pain that my body is in, the pain that I come across some-times"* (carpenter, 29 years). Some participants were planning on moving off the "tools" into a supervisory role. For example, a participant explained: *"If I can get into a role where you're not on the tools anymore and it's sort of just managing the jobs or something like that, I think I could stay [working]. But, if it didn't turn out like that, I don't reckon the body would be able to handle it. You know, I don't want to retire when I'm 65 and can't stand up straight"* (bricklayer, 31 years old).
>
> The survey results also demonstrated a significant link between the experience of work-related bodily pain and workers' experience of higher levels of depression and anxiety, highlighting the interdependence between physical and mental health.
>
> *Turner & Lingard (2020)*

Ageing is also associated with cognitive decline and related to reduced processing speed, reasoning, memory and executive functions (Deary et al., 2009). It is argued that a decline in information processing speed can be explained by two underlying mechanisms:

1. the limited time mechanism – which refers to increased difficulty in completing cognitive tasks under time pressure, and
2. the simultaneity mechanism – which refers to increased difficulty in retrieving information from the early stages of a cognitive task performance for use in later stages of cognitive task performance (Ng & Feldman, 2013).

Ng and Feldman (2013) argue that the change in information processing speed could potentially make it harder for older workers to engage in multiple tasks simultaneously, especially when working under time pressure. However, despite this, no consistent negative relationship has been found between age and job performance suggesting that deterioration in certain types of cognitive function may be offset by performance improvements in other areas. For example, Ng and Feldman (2013) suggest that experience-based judgement can compensate for a potential decline in cognitive capacity and can be a positive predictor for workplace performance. It is argued that, with increasing age, people accumulate a variety of experiences and more nuanced understanding of their work environment, which enables older workers to make better decisions about appropriate actions for a given set of circumstances (Cornelius & Caspi, 1987; cited in Ng & Feldman 2013). Improved experience-based judgement may explain why older workers are reported to have a lower incidence of non-fatal injuries compared to young workers.

Truxillo et al. (2015) also categorised cognitive change in terms of the type of intelligence that is impacted. Fluid intelligence describes cognitive processing speed, reaction time, working memory and selective attention. These are believed to be negatively associated with age (Truxillo et al. 2015; Varianou-Mikellidou et al., 2019). However, crystallised intelligence describes accumulated knowledge, skills, and wisdom which typically increase with age (Truxillo et al. 2015).

The extent to which cognitive decline occurs as an inevitable part of the ageing process is also disputed, with some people arguing that cognitive decline is actually related to other unrecognised issues rather than attributable to ageing per se (Lindeboom & Weinstein, 2004). Others argue that cognitive decline can be influenced and reduced by healthy lifestyle choices, such as engaging in physical activity and having sufficient sleep (Yaffe et al., 2014). It is also important to note that the rate of ageing is dependent on a wide range of other non-age-related disease risk and protective factors (Adams & White, 2004). Also, exposure to these factors is believed to be more important with regard to ageing healthily than chronological age (Adams & White, 2004).

9.4   Age and work ability

Age is commonly understood in chronological terms. However, it can also be conceptualised using different dimensions, one of which is functional age (Sterns & Doverspike, 1989; cited in Varianou-Mikellidou, Boustras et al., 2019). This means, even with the same chronological age, individuals can vary widely in terms of their functional capabilities (Crawford et al., 2016). Therefore, work ability has been recommended as an alternative method of measuring age for the purposes of understanding performance and fitness at work (Tepas & Barnes-Farrell, 2002).

Work ability takes into account individuals' human resources and related associations with work demands and work conditions (Varianou-Mikellidou et al., 2019). Work ability has been defined as "a dynamic process that changes through its components throughout life, and it is the result of the interaction between individual resources (including health, functional capacity, education, know-out [sic], motivation), working conditions (environment, tools, human relations), and the surrounding society" (Costa and Sartori, 2007; p.1916).

Costa and Sartori (2007) examined the health conditions and work ability of 1,449 workers across different working sectors in Italy. A work ability index (WAI) was calculated for each worker by assessing the following perceptions or experiences:

- current work ability compared with lifetime best
- work ability in relation to job demands (mental, physical)
- number of current diseases diagnosed by a physician
- estimated work impairment due to diseases
- sick leave during the past 12 months
- own prognosis of work ability two years from now, and
- mental resources.

The results indicate that WAI scores declined progressively over the age groups, from an average WAI score of 41.2 for workers under 25 years old to an average score of 37.8 for workers over 55 years old. Specifically, the most notable decline in WAI over age was recorded for workers engaged in heavy manual work, primarily represented by construction workers (Costa & Sartori, 2007).

Healthy ageing at work is directly linked to work ability, which describes a situation in which someone has the health and basic competence required for managing work tasks, assuming that the work tasks are reasonable and the work environment is acceptable (Tengland, 2011). Work ability is a product of the interaction that occurs between:

(i) the physical and mental demands placed on people by their work;
(ii) workers' general health, including limitations to their ability to perform a job due to disease or ill health or declines in physical capacity; and
(iii) the resources available to workers to meet the demands of their work (Ilmarinen, 2009).

Poor work ability reflects a situation in which job demands exceed health resources and physical capacity (Sell, 2009). Poor work ability is a strong predictor of sickness absence and early retirement among construction workers, with particularly strong effects for workers over the age of 50 (Alavinia et al., 2009; Welch et al., 2010). This suggests that strategies to better retain construction workers in employment longer into their lives could focus on improving work ability through:

(i) helping older workers to maintain their physical and psychological health as they age (Jebens et al., 2015), and
(ii) designing jobs to ensure the demands of work better match workers' health resources (Peng & Chan, 2020).

9.5 Are health risk factors individual or environmental?

Construction workers' poor health and experience of work disability are often attributed to risk factors related to lifestyle behaviours and individual biomedical characteristics. For example, Claessen et al. (2009) describe a longitudinal cohort study of construction workers which revealed a body mass index indicating obesity was related, in a follow-up period of approximately 10 years, to occupational disability due to osteoarthritis and/or cardiovascular disease. Similarly, Alavinia et al. (2007) report health status determined by the physical health examination of 19,507 Dutch construction workers (including high body mass index, the presence of pulmonary problems, and a 10-year risk for cardiovascular disease) was a significant predictor of workers' longer-term ability to work. However, there is growing evidence to suggest that the interplay between occupational risk factors and individuals' health-related behaviours shape work disability outcomes (van den Berg et al. 2010). Older workers' experiences of health, safety and wellbeing have previously been attributed to both individual (e.g. biological and behavioural) and contextual factors (organisational and job-related characteristics) (Truxillo et al 2015). Arndt et al. (2005) identify musculoskeletal disorders (MSDs), cardiovascular disease, and mental disorders as causes of occupational disability among construction workers in Germany. They link these to occupational risk factors as well as individual lifestyle factors. Oude Hengel et al. (2012) similarly report a combination of occupational and individual factors that predict Dutch construction workers' ability and willingness to work until they reach the pension age (65 years). These findings are important because they highlight the need for a two-pronged approach by which organisations seek to reduce environmental risk factors through good job design while also supporting health promotion programmes focused on individual behaviours. Arguably, there has traditionally been a strong focus on individual behaviour-change programmes which fail to address or acknowledge the work-related causes of ill health and the need to address these as a component of an organisation's responsibilities under work health and safety legislation.

9.6 Older construction workers' physical work health experiences

There is no consensus at what age a worker should be considered to be an older worker. The Australian Bureau of Statistics refers to older workers as those who are 55 years old and above (Australian Bureau of Statistics, 2016). However, the term "older worker" is inconsistently defined in the literature. For example, the age at which workers are considered to be "older workers" ranges from 40 years and over (Ng & Feldman, 2013), 50 years and over (Black et al., 2017), 55 years and over (Costa & Sartori, 2007), to 65 and over (Bande & López-Mourelo, 2015). Ng and Feldman (2013) also refer to individuals who are 60–74 as the "young-old" and individuals who are age 75 or over as "old-old."

However, a growing body of research suggests that, irrespective of their age, manual/non-managerial construction workers are adversely affected by their exposure to occupational health hazards. For example, in the USA, manual/non-managerial construction workers are more susceptible to physical health complaints than other blue-collar workers (Petersen & Zwerling, 1998). In the UK, Stocks et al. (2010) analysed instances of medically reported work-related ill health among construction workers and found elevated rates of contact dermatitis, all types of skin neoplasma, nonmalignant pleural disease, mesothelioma, lung cancer, pneumoconiosis and musculoskeletal disorders.

The impacts of exposure to certain occupational health risks are also reported to increase with age. For example, analysis of hearing loss among 19,127 trade-based construction workers in the USA reveals that hearing loss among construction workers increases rapidly with age, with 86.4 per cent of trade-based workers older than 65 experiencing hearing loss. The duration of trade-based work was also a strong and significant risk factor for hearing loss which affected 19.1 per cent of workers who had worked in a construction trade for less than 15 years, but 67.8 per cent who had worked in a construction trade for more than 33 years (Dement et al., 2018). Importantly, hearing loss has been linked to increased risk of workplace accidents and injuries (Picard et al., 2008). Farrow and Reynolds (2012) suggest that older workers should participate in regular hearing assessments and be allocated tasks that do not involve working in noisy environments so as not to exacerbate hearing loss that may occur as part of the normal ageing process.

The prevalence of musculoskeletal disorders (MSDs) also increases with age. The incidence of MSDs among construction workers is disproportionately high in all age groups (Inyang et al., 2012) but US research found that 40 per cent of construction workers over the age of 50 experience chronic back pain (Dong et al., 2012a). In a study of Dutch construction workers between 1993 and 2003, Hoonakker and van Duivenbooden (2010) reported that musculoskeletal complaints in the back and neck increase steadily with age. However, older workers (55+ years) did not experience more complaints than workers aged 45–55, suggesting that the increased risk for back and neck injury begins at a younger age threshold than 55 years. In the Dutch study, complaints in the upper and lower extremities (arms and legs) also increased with age. The majority of upper extremity complaints related to the shoulder (20%), while the majority of lower extremity complaints related to the knee (18%). Interestingly, the older Dutch construction workers (aged 55+) had fewer complaints about the physical or psychological demands of their work compared to workers in other age groups, but had more complaints about working in awkward postures.

The increased prevalence of musculoskeletal disorders in older workers has been attributed to:

- biological changes related to ageing,
- elevated risk due to increasing years of exposure to harmful work demands, and
- chronic overload caused by an imbalance between physical workload and physical work capacity (DeZwart et al., 1997).

However, it is also important to note that MSDs, linked to poor lifting and manual handling practices, can begin early in the working life of construction workers (Merlino et al., 2003). The early experience of a musculoskeletal injury also predicts the occurrence of future injuries and the duration of work disability that occurs as a result (Dasinger et al., 2000). Thus, it is important that the health, safety and wellbeing of construction workers are protected from the beginning of their working lives, and that this includes the provision of pathways for healthy ageing (Schmitt & Unger, 2019).

Given the physically demanding nature of manual/non-managerial work, many construction workers suffer from permanent work incapacity and are forced to stop working due to health problems before they reach the statutory pension age (Brenner & Ahern, 2000; Welch, 2009; Oude Hengel et al., 2012). In Germany it is estimated that 63 per cent of construction workers retire early due to permanent disability (Siebert et al., 2001). Even compared to other blue-collar occupations, construction workers experience high levels of work incapacity at a relatively young age (Arndt et al., 2005). It is also important to note that construction workers' experience of physical and mental health symptoms is linked in complicated and causal ways (Abbe et al., 2011; Turner & Lingard, 2020). For example, Borsting Jacobsen et al. (2013) report that mental distress in construction workers is strongly and significantly associated with the experience of lower back pain, having two or more pain sites and the experience of injury. Research also suggests that physical and psychosocial risk factors interact with one another to produce occupational disability and early retirement among construction workers. For example, in a prospective study of 389,000 Swedish construction workers, Stattin and Jarvholm (2005) report that physical, ergonomic and psychosocial work demands all substantially increased the odds ratio of construction workers seeking a disability pension. Importantly, the effects of physical and ergonomic risk factors were exacerbated when workers reported the presence of psychosocial risk factors. Similarly, a Danish study revealed that both physical and psychosocial risk factors predicted the early retirement of workers in physically heavy occupations. Extreme bending of the back, low skill discretion and low decision authority were all associated with early retirement (Lund et al., 2001). All of this previous work points to the fact that the health, safety and wellbeing of older construction workers are impacted by a complex mix of organisational, job-related (physical and psychosocial) and individual (biomedical) risk factors.

9.7 The workplace safety of older construction workers

Australian data reveals that older construction workers are a high-risk group for workplace fatalities and severe injuries. Safe Work Australia reports that, between 2013 and 2016, of the 123 construction workers killed at work, workers aged 55–64 years accounted for 22 per cent and those aged 45–54 years accounted for 20 per cent of all deaths. Construction workers aged 55–64 also recorded the highest rate of serious injuries (9.9 serious claims per million hours worked) in the period from 2012–13 to 2015–16 (Safe Work Australia, 2018). In the

USA, although younger construction workers are reported to be more likely to experience a fall, older construction workers are more likely to be seriously injured in fall incidents, even when the fall is from a small distance or on the same level (Dong et al., 2012b). Dong et al. (2012b) analysed fatality data from the US Census of Fatal Occupational Injuries for 1992 to 2008 and found that older workers (aged 55+ years) had significantly higher rates of fatal falls than younger workers (16–54 years) for 11 of 14 construction trades. Roofers were at the highest risk of fatal falls and, among roofers, the rate of fatal falls among older workers was 60.5 per 100,000 FTEs[1] compared to 23.2 per 100,000 FTEs among younger roofers (Dong et al., 2012b). However, Dong et al. (2012b) also report that, compared to younger construction workers, fatal falls among older workers were less likely to be from roofs (25.4% compared to 34.3%) and more likely to be from ladders (22.7% compared to 15.4%).

9.8 Older workers' experience of psychosocial health risk factors

In addition to physical harm, research also suggests that older construction workers are vulnerable to psychosocial risk exposures that affect their mental health and wellbeing in various ways. For example, research shows that, compared to younger workers, older workers are more adversely affected by psychosocial job demands, including working under time pressure, a lack of employment security, and a concern about unfavourable changes in the work environment (De Zwart et al., 1999). These are all characteristics associated with working in project-based construction jobs. Similarly, a Dutch study of manual/non-managerial construction workers reports high levels of burnout among older workers leading to early retirement (Oude Hengel et al., 2012).

To understand the experiences of construction workers in different age groups an analysis was undertaken of data collected in the Household, Income and Labour Dynamics in Australia (HILDA) longitudinal panel study. In the HILDA study data is collected in annual waves from over 13,000 individuals within over 7,000 Australian households. The analysis of the HILDA data set is presented in case examples 9.2 and 9.3.

CASE EXAMPLE 9.2 EXAMINING THE MENTAL ILL HEALTH OF CONSTRUCTION WORKERS IN RELATION TO AGE AND JOB QUALITY

Data collected over a ten-year period (2010–2019) was analysed to explore the way in which mental health changes as workers in different age groups experience an increasing number of adverse job conditions. Comparisons were made between construction and non-construction workers. Only participants aged 18 and over who were employed and had non-missing job quality data were included in the analysis. Participants were divided into three groups based on their age in 2010:

(i) younger than 24,
(ii) between 24–45, and
(iii) older than 45.

These age categories have been referred to as the exploration, establishment and maintenance stages of a working lifespan (Schmitt & Unger, 2019).

Construction workers were distinguished from the rest of employed participants (based on classification codes in ANZSIC 2006 and ANZSCO 2006). The final sample included in the analysis comprised 63,636 observations from 11,491 non-construction employees and 4,229 observations from 924 construction workers. Five aspects of job quality were included in the analysis:

(i) job demands and complexity,
(ii) job control,
(iii) job security,
(iv) perceived fairness of efforts-rewards (pay), and
(v) time pressure.

Following an approach previously used by Butterworth et al. (2011), for each participant, a mean score was calculated for each aspect of job quality (by averaging the survey items for each component). Using the range of mean scores for each job quality category, the worst quartile score was calculated and was used to identify participants experiencing adverse job conditions with regard to the five job quality aspects (i.e., high job demand and complexity, low job control, etc.). For each individual, the total number of job adversities was calculated. This variable was then used to identify four job categories:

(i) jobs with no adverse conditions,
(ii) jobs with 1 adverse condition,
(iii) jobs with 2–3 adverse conditions, and
(iv) jobs with 4–5 adverse conditions.

Mental health is measured in HILDA using a subscale of the SF-36 general health survey, which has been previously validated (see Butterworth & Crosier, 2004). The mental health scale includes five items and measures how often in the past four weeks respondents experienced positive emotions (e.g., feeling happy or calm) and negative emotions (e.g., feeling nervous or down).

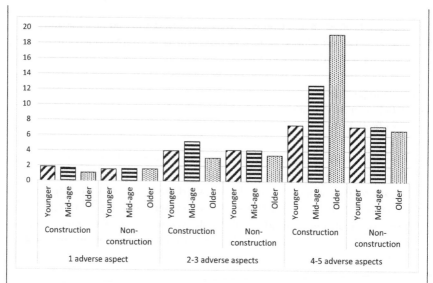

FIGURE 9.1 Decline in mental health scores of construction and non-construction participants by age groups and job quality

In the HILDA data set, the mental health scale is transformed, based on the procedure suggested by Ware et al. (2000), to reflect a 1–100 range. In this analysis the focus was on the decline in mental health. That is the extent to which mental health deteriorated over the ten waves of data. The higher the value the greater the decline in mental health.

Figure 9.1 compares the average decline in mental health scores for people in different age groups and job quality categories. The construction participants' results were also compared with non-construction industry (i.e., general population) data.

Construction and non-construction participants expressed similar levels of decline in mental health scores when experiencing jobs with one adverse condition. These scores did not vary substantially among the three age groups. When experiencing jobs with two or three adverse conditions, middle-aged construction workers indicated (on average) slightly poorer mental health compared to workers in other age groups and non-construction workers. However, when facing the worst jobs (jobs with four or five adverse conditions), two significant patterns were identified.

1. Construction workers indicated significantly poorer mental health compared to non-construction workers, and
2. Membership in different age groups had a significant effect on the decline in mental health experienced by construction workers, with the older

construction workers experiencing the highest level of decline followed by middle-aged construction workers.

This analysis suggests that poor quality jobs have a substantial negative impact on the mental health of construction workers and this impact increases with age. Strategies that directly address adverse conditions of work and improve job quality are recommended to protect the mental health of older construction workers.

Next, analysis was conducted to identify the extent to which construction workers in the HILDA data set are impacted by specific psychosocial risk factors and the extent to which this varies by age.

Case example 9.3 presents an analysis of the relationship between psychosocial risk factors experienced by manual/non-managerial construction workers and mental health experiences. This case example shows important differences in the psychosocial risk factors associated with mental health in different age groups. These differences have particular implications for ways to reduce the risk of psychological harm among older – compared to younger – construction workers.

CASE EXAMPLE 9.3 AGE DIFFERENCES IN THE EXPERIENCE OF JOB QUALITY COMPONENTS AND MENTAL HEALTH

The data included in this analysis was extracted from ten waves of HILDA data from 2009 to 2018. HILDA participants working in the construction industry (based on the ANZSIC 2006 industry classification code) were identified. Further, manual/non-managerial workers (technicians and trade workers, machinery operators and drivers, and labourers) were identified based on ANZSCO 2006 occupation classification codes. Participants aged 18 and over were included in the sample. Due to the longitudinal nature of the study, individuals who had only participated in one wave of the survey were excluded from the analysis. Cases with missing data were excluded on an analysis-by-analysis basis. The final data set included 4,850 responses from 1,221 individuals. There were 1,186 men and 35 women. Of the respondents, 430 were younger than 24 years old, 513 were aged between 25 and 45, and 278 were older than 45.

Job characteristics reflecting various aspects of job quality were also considered in the analysis (Butterworth et al., 2011). These were:

(i) job demands and complexity (four items, e.g., My job is complex and difficult; My job often requires me to learn new skills);

(ii) job control (three items, e.g., I have a lot of freedom to decide how I do my own work);

(iii) job security (three items, e.g., I have a secure future in my job), and

(iv) effort-reward fairness (one item: I get paid fairly for the things I do in my job).

To compare relationships between age groups, participants were divided into three age groups: younger than 24; between 25 and 45; and older than 45. A number of control variables were included in the analysis, including participants' age in the first wave of the survey which was included in this study (2009), household structure, education level, household income, gender, years worked in construction, having a disability or long-term health condition or providing care for another person due to a health condition, or because they are elderly or have a disability for which they require care.

Statistical methods (random intercept linear regression analysis) were used to examine the association between the four aspects of job quality and mental health of workers in different age groups. Results are shown in Table 9.2.

There was a positive and significant association between job security and mental health in all age groups, and the association was stronger among younger participants. Perceived fairness of effort and reward (pay) was positively and significantly associated with mental health in young (18–24) and middle-aged (25–45) workers. The associations between job control and job demands and complexity and mental health were statistically significant in middle-aged (25–45) and older (>45) workers. There was a positive association between job control and mental health and a negative association between job demands and complexity and mental health.

After controlling for potential confounders (Table 9.3), the positive association between job security and mental health remained significant for all age groups, but the positive association between job control and mental health was only statistically significant for older workers. Higher job demands

TABLE 9.2 Job quality correlates of mental health by age

Aspects of job quality	Age group 1 (<24)	Age group 2 (25–45)	Age group 3 (>45)
Job demands and complexity		-	-
Job control		+	+
Job security	+	+	+
Effort-reward fairness	+	+	

TABLE 9.3 Job quality correlates of mental health by age after controlling for demographic characteristics

Aspects of job quality	Age group 1 (<24)	Age group 2 (25–45)	Age group 3 (>45)
Job demands and complexity			-
Job control			+
Job security	+	+	+
Effort-reward fairness			

and complexity was associated with poorer mental health among the older workers, but not among workers below the age of 45. Having a disability or health condition was (statistically) significantly associated with poorer mental health in middle-aged and older workers but not among younger workers. In addition, being a single person was a statistically significant predictor of poor mental health for middle-aged and older workers, but not for younger workers. Satisfaction with work–life balance was also positively and significantly associated with mental health in workers older than 25, but not in those below the age of 25.

Case example 9.3 shows that the mental health of manual/non-managerial construction workers in Australia is influenced by various psychosocial job quality factors. In this respect, our findings are consistent with previous research that has focused on contextual/environmental determinants of health (Marmot, 2005).

Overall, the results indicate a positive association between job security and mental health in all age groups. After controlling for demographic and individual characteristics of workers, job control and job demands and complexity were significant predictors of mental health in the older age group (workers older than 45) but did not predict the mental health of younger or middle-aged workers.

As a project-based industry, job security is a particular concern as continued employment depends upon successfully winning work in a highly competitive commercial environment. Precarious employment (characterised by job insecurity) can increase workers' exposure to hazardous working conditions (including physical and psychosocial risks) while also contributing to material deprivation relating to income, wealth and savings, housing quality, superannuation, etc. (Benach et al., 2016). The links between job insecurity and mental health across all age groups found in the current study suggest that employment policies and practices should be carefully considered to reduce the adverse mental health outcomes that precarious employment practices can create.

After controlling for confounding variables in case example 9.3, job control and demands and complexity remained significant predictors of mental health for older workers. This is consistent with previous research that older workers are more adversely affected by working under time pressure (De Zwart et al., 1999). Previous research (Ng & Feldman, 2015) has also found age-related differences in the relationships between job autonomy (control) and work-related outcomes. However, they did not specifically focus on workers' health.

In case example 9.3, the direct effects of job demands and complexity, job control and effort-reward fairness on mental health were not significant after controlling for confounding variables. However, these job quality components were indirectly related to mental health through workers' satisfaction with their work–life balance among middle-aged survey participants. Workers in this age group (25–45) may have significant caring responsibilities for dependent children. Previous research has linked parental demands during mid-life to poor health (Evandrou et al., 2003). This may be one explanation for the way that satisfaction with work–life balance acts as the pathway through which job demands and complexity, job control and effort-reward fairness influence mental health among middle-aged workers.

Importantly, the results of the analysis outlined in case example 9.3 show that the impact of job quality on the mental health of construction workers is nuanced. Aspects of job quality that are predictive of mental health vary between workers in different age groups. This is important information when considering the strategies that can be implemented to protect the mental health of workers across the lifespan.

9.9 A lifespan perspective

The previous case example shows that health-related experiences and impacts change as workers progress through their working lives because the psychosocial risk factors that affect workers vary significantly according to their age group. These findings have important implications for the protection of mental health in the construction industry because, just as poor quality work has a negative impact on mental health, it is possible that improving the quality of work can have a positive impact on mental health among manual/non-managerial workers. However, the relationships between various components of psychosocial job quality and mental health are not "age neutral." The lifespan developmental theoretical perspective acknowledges that workers' experiences of job characteristics are shaped – at least to some extent – by their age.

Results presented in the case studies suggest that workers in all groups would likely benefit from policies designed to improve job security. However, interventions targeting middle-aged and older workers may need to focus on other job quality characteristics that predicted mental health in their age groups. For example, middle-aged workers may benefit from more flexible work practices that would help them to achieve a balance between their work and non-work lives. On the other hand, older workers may benefit from strategies designed to reduce job demands and complexity and/or increase their control over how their work is done.

Griffiths et al. (2009) similarly suggest that providing older workers with greater control over the pace at which they work, the level of their involvement in work, the length and timing of shifts worked and work-rest schedules is likely to be beneficial for their health, work ability and workforce participation. Griffiths et al. (2009) also recommend reducing job demands and complexity to ensure tasks are age-appropriate and reduce the need to work overtime, night shifts, etc., that are known to have a negative influence on the health of older manual/non-managerial workers (Costa & Sartori, 2007).

A lifespan developmental theoretical perspective can be helpful in understanding workers' work and health-related experiences as it seeks to explain the individual's life experiences by studying the sequence of interactions between individual (biological and psychological) and contextual (social and environmental) determinants of development (Zacher et al., 2019). According to Zacher et al. (2019), a lifespan developmental perspective does not comprise a single theory but, rather, is a broad way of thinking (meta-theory) about human development from childhood to maturity. A lifespan developmental perspective has informed numerous mid-range theories about how people can age successfully in ways that minimise their loss of functionality (both physical and cognitive) and maximise subjective (e.g., life and work satisfaction) and objective (e.g., mental health and physical functioning) life outcomes.

More recently, the concept of successful ageing has been refocused to consider the determinants of subjective and objective work-related outcomes that are valued and important to employees and their organisations (Olson & Schultz, 2019). Age is regarded as a key antecedent of these outcomes, but a variety of personal and contextual variables is also believed to influence workers' experiences. In the case of health outcomes, these variables may be more important than chronological age. Understanding the factors that interplay to shape important outcomes, including workers' health, is therefore a critical first step to developing strategies that enable successful ageing at work.

Changes to workers' physical, cognitive, emotional and motivational resources that occur with age may mean that the individual resources that workers bring to a job no longer fit well with their job demands (Schmitt & Unger, 2019). For example, Kanfer and Ackerman (2004) suggest that older workers experience stress in jobs that involve intensive short-term processing of information due to age-related changes in cognitive function, while Truxillo et al. (2012) suggest that deterioration of physical capacity, fitness and sensory capabilities can contribute to occupational injuries in workers whose jobs require these capabilities.

Kooij (2015) developed a theoretical position on successful ageing at work that focused on employees' proactive behaviours to maintain their person-job fit, for example, by maintaining their physical fitness and work ability. Baltes and Baltes (1990) also suggest that workers engage in adaptive behaviour to trade-off the impacts of resource depletion associated with ageing and maintain an effective fit with their job demands. Thus, older workers can: (i) actively choose the life and work goals that they will pursue to avoid stressful situations (selection); (ii) seek to attain, develop and use particular resources to help them achieve their goals (optimisation); and (iii) apply strategies to make up for resource losses or the limitations they may experience that are associated with ageing (compensation) (Schmitt & Unger, 2019).

9.10   The social context of work

Older workers' health and wellbeing can also be affected by the social context of ageing. Age stereotypes, age discrimination, and the organisational age climate are all believed to negatively affect older workers (Truxillo et al., 2015).

Age stereotypes are beliefs and expectations about workers that are related to the age of employees, irrespective of actual job performance (Posthuma & Campion, 2009). They are judgements made about workers based on their age rather than based on actual knowledge, skills, and capabilities. Age stereotypes can lead to unlawful age discrimination behaviour in the workplace. Posthuma and Campion (2009) identified a few common stereotypes concerning older workers, including that they:

- demonstrate poorer job performance
- are resistant to change
- have a lower ability to learn
- are likely to have shorter job tenure (when taking new employment), and
- are more costly.

However, in a meta-analysis, Ng and Feldman (2012) reported that these age stereotypes are not empirically supported. Notwithstanding the lack of evidence for them, age stereotypes are known to influence decisions about the allocation of resources and support to employees. For example, older workers may be given restricted or differential access to work health and safety (WHS) and other work-related training due to the erroneous belief that older workers are less ready to accept new technology, less adaptable to change, less able to learn new ideas, and less interested in training (Bohle et al., 2010). Johnson et al. (2011) reported that older workers (aged 55 and over) receive less formal training from their employers and obtain less intensive instruction than their younger counterparts because employers think older workers are slow to learn new skills and have the fear that the training cost will not be recouped via learning and improved performance (Johnson et al., 2011). These age-based decisions, driven by stereotypes, constitute age discrimination, i.e., decisions made about older workers are different from those made about younger workers (Truxillo et al., 2015).

The potential for discriminatory behaviour has an impact on the way that older workers interact with employers in relation to health and safety-related issues. For example, Drake et al. (2017) interviewed UK employers to understand concerns regarding the ageing workforce. One key theme that emerged from these interviews was the poor reporting culture and the consequent "hidden" health problems experienced by older workers. Specifically, older workers were reported to be less likely to disclose information about health-related problems due to fear of discrimination. In one case, Drake et al. (2017) report that a worker was overlooked for promotion after advising his manager about a degenerative knee condition. Older workers were also unwilling to self-report taking medication that could have safety-relevant side-effects (e.g., drowsiness, dizziness and inability to concentrate) – even when they were involved in operating machinery or vehicles – because they feared they would be discriminated against. Older workers reported:

- they have witnessed colleagues, who previously reported health issues, either being "sacked" or made redundant,
- they do not trust their managers and feared breach of confidentiality and potential ridicule from other workers, and
- they experience a lack of respect from younger managers and feel a "loss of dignity" in relation to the way others perceive their work capacity and performance (Drake et al., 2017).

Older workers also believed all workers, but particularly supervisors and managers, should receive age awareness training (Drake et al., 2017). Such training could provide information about the challenges that older workers face in the workplace and measures that organisations can take to better manage and support the older workforce.

Research has also found that older workers are more likely to be engaged in contingent (precarious) work and to experience job insecurity, which is closely associated with poor work health and safety outcomes (Bohle et al., 2010). Job insecurity has been found to be related to decreased safety motivation and unsafe behaviour, which is, in turn, linked to a higher incidence of workplace injuries and accidents (Probst & Brubaker, 2001).

9.11   Effective age management

Age management refers to the consideration of "age related factors … in daily management, including work arrangements and individual work tasks, so that everybody, regardless of age, feels empowered in reaching [their] own and corporate goals" (Ilmarinen, 2012, p.2). By recognising that age-related physiological and psychological changes have implications for workers' health, wellbeing and work ability, Varianou-Mikellidou et al. (2019) argue that an age-sensitive risk assessment, which considers workforce diversity and older workers' needs, should be included in organisational work health and safety management processes.

Varianou-Mikellidou et al. (2019) proposed a P-D-C-A approach to incorporating age management into existing work health and safety management systems. This would involve the following steps:

- Plan – policy should recognise ageing issues (recruitment, career development), structure of organisation and risk assessment should consider new risks due to ageing; plan knowledge transfer.
- Do – safety committees should include representatives from all age groups, training methods are adapted to older workers, develop a workplace culture without age discrimination; carry out knowledge transfer; use flexible working time practices.
- Check – health monitoring, measure performance; accident investigation (consider age in these); check whether age-related plans are also carried out.
- Act – review performance, lessons learned, adaptation measures (flexible working time, job rotation, adjustment of the workplace with, e.g., use of ergonomic tools); strive for continuous improvement.

Varianou-Mikellidou et al. (2019) suggest that the work ability index be used as a supporting tool to monitor performance in age management and ensure that factors that support the work ability of older workers are systematically identified and addressed. Regular work ability checks are also advocated by Griffiths et al. (2009).

9.12 Interventions designed to protect and promote the health and wellbeing of older workers

Truxillo et al. (2015) argue that workplace interventions or programmes should be put in place to support older workers and promote an age-diverse workforce. Interventions suggested as being useful vary in their focus. Some suggested strategies are shown in Table 9.4.

Some strategies focus on the provision of training to older workers to enable them to reduce the risks of work-related harm and continue to work productively and healthily. For example, Kenny et al. (2008) suggest that exercise and regular physical training can attenuate or slow down age-related declines in physical capacity, particularly between the ages of 45 and 65, improve functional ability and physical work capacity, and protect against lower back pain. Kenny et al. (2008) suggest that exercise programmes have generally led to improved fitness and decreased health risk amongst participants, as well as reducing sick leave, improving morale and reducing staff turnover. However, Kenny et al. (2008) note that workers are unlikely to take part in fitness training programmes unless time is allowed during the working day for them to engage in physical exercise activities. Similarly, when physical fitness facilities are not available at the workplace, and additional time is required to travel to and from exercise locations,

TABLE 9.4 Suggested interventions to support older workers

Intervention category	Examples
Selection, optimisation, and compensation (SOC) training programmes	• Training for older workers on how to best select skills and tasks that fit their abilities and interests • Organisational reflection as to the limits regarding what tasks might be offloaded by older workers
Work redesign	• Increased autonomy and skill variety • Decreased task variety • Support older workers in crafting their jobs to fit their needs with co-operation from supervisors and co-workers • Increase older workers' intrinsic motivation such as mentoring young workers
Increasing positive relations between groups	• Positive intergenerational exposure • Team interventions • Improved age diversity climate through training of supervisors and teams • Leadership training for supervisors to deal with age differences • Reduction of negative stereotypes (explicit and implicit)
Age-supportive human resources (HR) practices	• Interventions to allow flexible human resource (HR) practices for different age groups • Emphasis on different HR bundles for different age groups
Work–life supportive policies	• Flexible work arrangements • Part-time work • Eldercare support
Training practices for older workers	• Additional time • Smaller groups • Self-paced learning • Emphasis on learning goal orientation • Error management training (allow participants to make mistakes in training)

Source: Adapted from Truxillo et al., 2015.

workers are unlikely to participate in physical fitness training programmes. Consequently, for a physical fitness training programme to have the best chance of success, strong management support and resourcing is required so that time is made available within the workday and facilities are provided at, or at least very close to, the worksite. Another challenge associated with the provision of physical fitness training programmes for workers is that those who choose to participate may be those who are already active and in better health (Kenny et al., 2008). Older, less fit or less healthy workers may choose not to participate, citing their lack of physical fitness as a reason for this. Kenny et al. (2008) also highlight low participation rates in physical fitness programmes among men and people of lower education. To overcome some of these challenges, it is recommended that physical fitness programmes be well communicated and part of an integrated and comprehensive health and wellness intervention. Ideally, individual health and fitness assessments could be undertaken and form the basis of customised exercise programmes tailored to individual workers' fitness levels and needs. Others advocate the encouragement of physical exercise and relaxation among older workers (Griffiths et al. 2009) and/or the provision of counselling and training on the best coping strategies concerning sleep (Costa & Sartori, 2007).

Leisink and Knies (2011) recommend the implementation of programmes focused on creating a supportive and respectful workplace culture to protect the health and wellbeing of an age-diverse workforce. Such programmes seek to: promote an age-aware and age-tolerant organisational culture; communicate the unacceptability of direct and indirect age discrimination; provide training for managers and workers about ageing and its implications for work, health and wellbeing; and challenge age stereotypes in the workplace (Griffiths et al., 2009).

However, the most effective way to protect and promote the health and wellbeing of older workers is through ensuring that work is designed to remove or reduce sources of psychological or physical harm. For example, Costa and Sartori (2007) recommend that modified work time practices be implemented for older workers, including limiting or eliminating the expectation of night work after 45–50 years of age, transferring older workers to day work, allowing older workers to choose their preferred shifts and shortening working hours or providing more rest breaks. Importantly, if work hours are reduced this must be accompanied by a commensurate reduction in workload to prevent work intensification and stress. Given the finding that job control, demands and complexity affect older construction workers' mental health through their experience of work–life balance, it is important to recognise that older workers may have particular needs in relation to balancing their work and family lives and these should be taken into consideration (see also, Griffiths et al., 2009). Costa and Sartori (2007) also recommend organisations can tailor work to suit older workers if they provide periodic health/work ability assessments and use individuals' results to inform the design (and potentially redesign) of work.

Organisations can also help older workers maintain their health and wellbeing as they transition into retirement by helping older workers re-craft jobs to make them more compatible with their changing needs, desires, and capabilities. For example, Buyens et al. (2009) observe that employers can help older employees transition out of the workforce in psychologically healthier ways by allowing them to cut back on work hours, giving them more scheduling flexibility, and providing them with part-time bridge employment after age 65. Such findings are consistent with the earlier work of Herzog et al. (1991), who found that older workers whose patterns of workforce participation matched their personal preferences reported greater physical and psychological wellbeing.

Ergonomic work design interventions are also strongly recommended as a way to protect the health and wellbeing of older workers. For example, McMahan and Phillips (1999; cited in Kowalski-Trakofler et al., 2005) recommend work tasks be reviewed and where possible redesigned to:

- reduce extreme joint movement – for example, keep movements within acceptable range of motion, minimise twisting and reaching,
- reduce the need to use excessive force – for example, opt for mechanical assist devices, use padding to reduce pressures, keep cutting edges sharp, and
- reduce highly repetitive tasks – for example, use power tools, implement job rotation and ensure a variety of work.

Glimskär and Lundberg (2013) observe that, even when developed and offered to market, the take-up and use of ergonomically designed construction tools is low. Van der Molen et al. (2005) attribute this to the way that work is organised, in particular, the reliance on temporary employment and multilevel contracting. Notwithstanding this, the ergonomic assessment of work tasks is critical in the construction industry, in which the prevalence of work-related musculoskeletal disorders is extremely high. Research shows that careful selection of tools or redesign of work processes can substantially reduce the risk of injury in physically demanding construction tasks (Lingard et al., 2017). In particular, consideration should be paid to the design of work tasks so that they are age-appropriate (Griffiths et al., 2009).

9.13   Conclusion

Consistent with broader demographic trends across the globe, there is evidence that the construction industry workforce is ageing in many countries. Together with this, construction workers in manual roles can start to experience daily physical pain arising from work-related tasks very early in their working life. This means that older workers may have suffered from work-related pain and injury for decades which can seriously affect their work ability, health and wellbeing. Taking a lifespan perspective can help organisations to proactively allocate tasks which take into consideration changes to workers' physical, cognitive, emotional and motivational resources that occur with age. This is important as the social and economic hardship associated with poor mental or physical health and, in some cases, early withdrawal from the labour force is substantial. The construction industry therefore has a responsibility to protect the health, safety and wellbeing of older workers and to support them in providing pathways to healthy ageing at work.

9.14   Discussion and review questions

1. Why should construction organisations consider age when assessing health and safety risks in their workplaces?
2. Why do you think job characteristics (demands and complexity, work–life balance, job control, etc.) affect workers in different age groups differently?

What are the implications of these differences for managing workers' health and wellbeing?

3. What strategies can employers implement to support the employment and healthy ageing of older construction workers? What benefits could be achieved (for workers and organisations) through the implementation of such strategies?

9.15 Acknowledgements

This paper uses unit record data from Household, Income and Labour Dynamics in Australia Survey [HILDA] conducted by the Australian Government Department of Social Services (DSS). The findings and views reported in this paper, however, are those of the authors and should not be attributed to the Australian Government, DSS, or any of DSS' contractors or partners.

Note

1 Full-time equivalent.

References

Abbe, O. O., et al. (2011). Modeling the relationship between occupational stressors, psychosocial/physical symptoms and injuries in the construction industry. *International Journal of Industrial Ergonomics, 41*(2), 106–117.

Adams, J. M., & White, M. (2004). Biological ageing: A fundamental, biological link between socio-economic status and health? *The European Journal of Public Health, 14*(3), 331–334.

Ajslev, J. Z., Lund, H. L., Møller, J. L., Persson, R., & Andersen, L. L. (2013). Habituating pain: Questioning pain and physical strain as inextricable conditions in the construction industry. *Nordic Journal of Working Life Studies, 3*(3), 195–218.

Alavinia, S., van den Berg, T., van Duivenbooden, C., Elders, L., & Burdorf, A. (2009). Impact of work-related factors, lifestyle, and work ability on sickness absence among Dutch construction workers. *Scandinavian Journal of Work, Environment & Health, 35*(5), 325–333.

Alavinia, S. M., van Duivenbooden, C., & Burdorf, A. (2007). Influence of work-related factors and individual characteristics on work ability among Dutch construction workers. *Scandinavian Journal of Work, Environment & Health, 33*(5), 351–357.

Arndt, V., Rothenbacher, D., Daniel, U., Zschenderlein, B., Schuberth, S., & Brenner, H. (2005). Construction work and risk of occupational disability: A ten year follow up of 14 474 male workers. *Occupational and Environmental Medicine, 62*, 559–566.

Australian Bureau of Statistics. (2016). Older workers finding more acceptance. Retrieved from www.abs.gov.au/AUSSTATS/abs@.nsf/mediareleasesbyCatalogue/AF302 A921D62B018CA2581F000191700?OpenDocument

Baltes, P. B., & Baltes, M. M. (1990). Psychological perspectives on successful aging: The model of selective optimization with compensation. In P. B. Baltes and M. M. Baltes (Eds.), *Successful Aging: Perspectives from the Behavioral Sciences*. Cambridge University Press (pp.1–34).

Bande, R., & López-Mourelo, E. (2015). The impact of worker's age on the consequences of occupational accidents: Empirical evidence using Spanish data. *Journal of Labor Research*, 36(2), 129–174.

Benach, J., Vives, A., Tarafa, G., Delclos, C., & Muntaner, C. (2016). What should we know about precarious employment and health in 2025? Framing the agenda for the next decade of research. *International Journal of Epidemiology*, 45(1), 232–238.

Black, J. K., Balanos, G. M., & Whittaker, A. C. (2017). Resilience, work engagement and stress reactivity in a middle-aged manual worker population. *International Journal of Psychophysiology*, 116, 9–15.

Bohle, P., Pitts, C., & Quinlan, M. (2010). Time to call it quits? The safety and health of older workers. *International Journal of Health Services*, 40(1), 23–41.

Boros, K., & Freemont, T. (2017). Physiology of ageing of the musculoskeletal system. *Best Practice & Research Clinical Rheumatology*, 31(2), 203–217.

Borsting Jacobsen, H., et al. (2013). Construction workers struggle with a high prevalence of mental distress, and this is associated with their pain and injuries. *Journal of Occupational and Environmental Medicine*, 55 (10), 1197–1204.

Brenner, H., & Ahern, W. (2000). Sickness absence and early retirement on health grounds in the construction industry in Ireland. *Occupational and Environmental Medicine*, 57(9), 615–20.

Butterworth, P., & Crosier, T. (2004). The validity of the SF-36 in an Australian National Household Survey: Demonstrating the applicability of the Household Income and Labour Dynamics in Australia (HILDA) Survey to examination of health inequalities. *BMC Public Health*, 4(1), 44.

Butterworth, P., Leach, L. S., Rodgers, B., Broom, D. H., Olesen, S. C., & Strazdins, L. (2011). Psychosocial job adversity and health in Australia: Analysis of data from the HILDA Survey. *Australian and New Zealand Jjournal of Public Health*, 35(6), 564–571.

Buyens, D., Van Dijk, H., Dewilde, T., & De Vos, A. (2009). The aging workforce: Perceptions of career ending. *Journal of Managerial Psychology*, 24(2), 102–117

Chartered Institute of Building. (2021). The *Impact of the Ageing Population on the Construction Industry*. Accessed 1 September 2022 from: www.ciob.org/sites/default/files/CIOB%20research%20-%20The%20Impact%20of%20the%20Ageing%20Population%20on%20the%20Construction%20Industry_0.pdf,

Claessen, H., Arndt, V., Drath, C., & Brenner, H. (2009). Overweight, obesity and risk of work disability: A cohort study of construction workers in Germany. *Occupational and Environmental Medicine*, 66(6), 402–409.

Cornelius, S. W., & Caspi, A. (1987). Everyday problem solving in adulthood and old age. Psychology and Aging, 2(2), 144.

Costa, G., & Sartori, S. (2007). Ageing, working hours and work ability. *Ergonomics*, 50(11), 1914–1930.

Crawford, J. O., Davis, A., Cowie, H., Dixon, K., Mikkelsen, S. H., Bongers, P. M.,... Dupont, C. (2016). *The ageing workforce: Implications for occupational safety and health: A research review*. European Agency for Safety and Health at Work.

Dasinger, L. K., Krause, N., Deegan, L. J., Brand, R. J., & Rudolph, L. (2000). Physical Workplace Factors and Return to Work After Compensated Low Back Injury: A Disability Phase-Specific Analysis. *Journal of Occupational and Environmental Medicine*, 42(3), 323–333.

Deary, I. J., Corley, J., Gow, A. J., Harris, S. E., Houlihan, L. M., Marioni, R. E.,... Starr, J. M. (2009). Age-associated cognitive decline. *British Medical Bulletin*, 92(1), 135–152.

Dement, J., Welch, L. S., Ringen, K., Cranford, K., & Quinn, P. (2018). Hearing loss among older construction workers: Updated analyses. *American Journal of Industrial Medicine*, 61(4), 326–335.

De Zwart, B. C., Broersen, J. P., Frings-Dresen, M. H., & Van Dijk, F. J. (1997). Repeated survey on changes in musculoskeletal complaints relative to age and work demands. *Occupational and Environmental Medicine*, 54(11), 793–799.

De Zwart, B.C.H., Frings-Dresen, M.H. and van Duivenbooden, C. (1999). Senior workers in the Dutch construction industry: A search for age-related work and health issues. *Experimental Aging Research*, 25(4), 385–391.

Dong, X.S., et al. (2012a). Chronic back pain among older construction workers in the United States: A longitudinal study. *International Journal of Occupational and Environmental Health*, 18 (2), 99–109.

Dong, X. S., Wang, X., & Daw, C. (2012b). Fatal falls among older construction workers. *Human Factors*, 54(3), 303–315.

Drake, C., Haslam, R., & Haslam, C. (2017). Facilitators and barriers to the protection and promotion of the health and safety of older workers. *Policy and Practice in Health and Safety*, 15(1), 84–84.

Evandrou, M., & Glaser, K. (2003). Combining work and family life: The pension penalty of caring. *Ageing & Society*, 23(5), 583–601.

Farrow, A., & Reynolds, F. (2012). Health and safety of the older worker. *Occupational Medicine*, 62(1), 4–11.

Glimskär, B., & Lundberg, S., 2013. Barriers to adoption of ergonomic innovations in the construction industry. *Ergonomics in Design*, 21(4), 26–30.

Gomes, M. M., Reis, J. G., Neves, T. M., Petrella, M., & de Abreu, D. C. (2013). Impact of aging on balance and pattern of muscle activation in elderly women from different age groups. *International Journal of Gerontology*, 7(2), 106–111.

Griffiths, A., Knight, A., & Mahudin, D. N. M. (2009). *Ageing, Work-Related Stress and Health*. The Age and Employment Network.

Herzog, A., House, J. S., & Morgan, J. N. (1991). Relation of work and retirement to health and well-being in older age. *Psychology and Aging*, 6(2), 202–211.

Hoonakker, P., & van Duivenbooden, C. (2010). Monitoring working conditions and health of older workers in Dutch construction industry. *American Journal of Industrial Medicine*, 53(6), 641–653.

Ilmarinen, J. (2002). Physical requirements associated with the work of aging workers in the European Union. *Experimental Aging Research*, 28, 7–23.

Ilmarinen, J. (2009). Work ability – a comprehensive concept for occupational health research and prevention. *Scandinavian Journal of Work, Environment & Health*, 35(1), 1–5.

Ilmarinen, J. (2012). *Promoting Active Ageing in the Workplace*. European Agency for Safety and Health at Work.

Infrastructure Australia. (2021). *Infrastructure workforce and skills supply*. Australian Government.

Inyang, N., Al-Hussein, M., El-Rich, M., & Al-Jibouri, S. (2012). Ergonomic analysis and the need for its integration for planning and assessing construction tasks. *Journal of Construction Engineering and Management*, 138(12), 1370–1376.

Jebens, E., Mamen, A., Medbø, J. I., Knudsen, O., & Veiersted, K. B. (2015). Are elderly construction workers sufficiently fit for heavy manual labour? *Ergonomics*, 58(3), 450–462.

Johnson, R. W., Mermin, G. B., & Resseger, M. (2011). Job demands and work ability at older ages. *Journal of Aging & Social Policy*, 23(2), 101–118.

Kanfer, R., & Ackerman, P. L. (2004). Aging, adult development, and work motivation. *Academy of Management Review*, 29(3), 440–458.

Kenny, G. P., Yardley, J. E., Martineau, L., & Jay, O. (2008). Physical work capacity in older adults: implications for the aging worker. *American Journal of Industrial Medicine*, 51(8), 610–625.

Kooij, D. T. (2015). Successful aging at work: The active role of employees. *Work, Aging and Retirement,* 1(4), 309–319.

Kowalski-Trakofler, K. M., Steiner, L. J., & Schwerha, D. J. (2005). Safety considerations for the aging workforce. *Safety Science*, 43(10), 779–793.

Leisink, P. L., & Knies, E. (2011). Line managers' support for older workers. *International Journal of Human Resource Management*, 22(9), 1902–1917.

Lindeboom, J., & Weinstein, H. (2004). Neuropsychology of cognitive ageing, minimal cognitive impairment, Alzheimer's disease, and vascular cognitive impairment. *European Journal of Pharmacology*, 490(1–3), 83–86.

Lingard, H., Lythgo, N., Troynikov, O., Selva Raj, I., & Fitzgerald, C. (2017). *Musculoskeletal Injury Reduction in the Construction Industry.* Centre for Construction Work Health and Safety Research, RMIT University.

Lund, T., Iversen, L., & Poulsen, K.B. (2001). Work environment factors, health, lifestyle and marital status as predictors of job change and early retirement in physically heavy occupations. *American Journal of Industrial Medicine*, 40(2), 161–169.

Marmot, M. (2005). Social determinants of health inequalities. *The Lancet*, 365(9464), 1099–1104.

McMahan, S., & Phillips, K. (1999). America's Aging Workforce: Ergonomic Solutions for Reducing the Risk of CTDs. *American Journal of Health Studies*, 15(4), 199–202.

Merlino, L. A., Rosecrance, J. C., Anton, D., & Cook, T. M. (2003). Symptoms of musculoskeletal disorders among apprentice construction workers. *Applied Occupational and Environmental Hygiene*, 18(1), 57–64.

Ng, T. W., & Feldman, D. C. (2012). Evaluating six common stereotypes about older workers with meta-analytical data. *Personnel Psychology*, 65(4), 821–858.

Ng, T. W. H., & Feldman, D. C. (2013). How do within-person changes due to aging affect job performance? *Journal of Vocational Behavior*, 83(3), 500–513.

Ng, T. W., & Feldman, D. C. (2015). The moderating effects of age in the relationships of job autonomy to work outcomes. *Work, Aging and Retirement*, 1(1), 64–78.

Olson, D. A. & Shultz, K. S. (2019). Lifespan perspectives on successful aging at work. In B. Baltes, C.W. Rudolph and H. Zacher (Eds.), *Work Across the Lifespan*. Academic Press (pp. 215–234).

O'Neill, T. (2020). *Why older workers should be valued.* Accessed 1 September 2022 from: https://constructionmanagermagazine.com/why-older-construction-workers-should-be-valued/

Oude Hengel, K. M., Blatter, B. M., Joling, C. I., van der Beek, A. J., & Bongers, P. M. (2012). Effectiveness of an intervention at construction worksites on work engagement, social support, physical workload, and need for recovery: Results from a cluster randomized controlled trial. *BMC Public Health*, 12(1), 1008.

Peng, L., & Chan, A. H. (2020). Adjusting work conditions to meet the declined health and functional capacity of older construction workers in Hong Kong. *Safety Science*, 127, 104711.

Petersen, J. S., & Zwerling, C. (1998). Comparison of health outcomes among older construction and blue-collar employees in the United States. *American Journal of Industrial Medicine,* 34 (3), 280–287.

Picard, M., Girard, S.A., Simard, M. et al. (2008), Association of work-related accidents with noise exposure in the workplace and noise-induced hearing loss based on the experience of some 240,000 person-years of observation. *Accident Analysis and Prevention,* 40, 1644–1652.

Posthuma, R. A., & Campion, M. A. (2009). Age stereotypes in the workplace: Common stereotypes, moderators, and future research directions. *Journal of Management,* 35(1), 158–188.

Probst, T. M., & Brubaker, T. L. (2001). The effects of job insecurity on employee safety outcomes: Cross-sectional and longitudinal explorations. *Journal of Occupational Health Psychology,* 6(2), 139–159.

Safe Work Australia. (2018). Priority industry snapshot 2018 – Construction. www.safeworkaustralia.gov.au/system/files/documents/1807/construction-priority-industry-snapshot-2018.pdf, accessed 27 September 2022.

Schmitt, A., & Unger, D. (2019). Lifespan perspectives on occupational health. In B. Baltes, C.W. Rudolph and H. Zacher (Eds.), *Work Across the Lifespan.* Academic Press (pp. 369–393).

Sell, L. (2009). Predicting long-term sickness absence and early retirement pension from self-reported work ability. *International Archives of Occupational and Environmental Health,* 82, 1133–1138.

Siebert, U., Rothenbacher, D., Daniel, U., & Brenner, H. (2001). Demonstration of the healthy worker survivor effect in a cohort of workers in the construction industry. *Occupational and Environmental Medicine,* 58(9), 774–779.

Sokas, R. K., Dong, X. S., & Cain, C. T. (2019). Building a sustainable construction workforce. *International Journal of Environmental Research and Public Health,* 16(21), 4202.

Stattin, M., & Järvholm, B. (2005). Occupation, work environment, and disability pension: a prospective study of construction workers. *Scandinavian Journal of Public Health,* 33 (2), 84–90.

Sterns, H. L., & Doverspike, D. (1989). Aging and the retraining and learning process in organizations. In I. Goldstein, & R. Katzel (Eds.), *Training and Development in Work Organizations.* Jossey-Bass (pp. 229–332).

Stocks, S. J., McNamee, R., Carder, M., & Agius, R. M. (2010). The incidence of medically reported work-related ill health in the UK construction industry. *Occupational and Environmental Medicine,* 67(8), 574–576.

Tengland, P.A. (2011). The concept of work ability. *Journal of Occupational Rehabilitation,* 21(2), 275–285.

Tepas, D. I., & Barnes-Farrell, J. L. (2002). Is worker age a simple demographic variable? *Experimental Aging Research,* 28(1), 1–5.

Truxillo, D. M., Cadiz, D. M., & Hammer, L. B. (2015). Supporting the aging workforce: A review and recommendations for workplace intervention research. *Annual Review of Organizational Psychology and Organizational Behaviour,* 2(1), 351–381.

Truxillo, D. M., Cadiz, D. M., Rineer, J. R., Zaniboni, S., & Fraccaroli, F. (2012). A lifespan perspective on job design: Fitting the job and the worker to promote job satisfaction, engagement, and performance. *Organizational Psychology Review,* 2(4), 340–360.

Turner, M., & Lingard, H. (2020). Examining the interaction between bodily pain and mental health of construction workers. *Construction Management and Economics,* 38(11), 1009–1023.

United Nations, Department of Economic and Social Affairs, Population Division. (2019). *World Population Ageing 2019: Highlights* (ST/ESA/SER.A/430) van den Berg, T., Schuring, M., Avendano, M., Mackenbach, J., & Burdorf, A. (2010). The impact of ill health on exit from paid employment in Europe among older workers. *Occupational and Environmental Medicine*, 67(12), 845–852.

van der Molen, H.F., Koningsveld, E., Haslam, R., & Gibb, A., 2005. Editorial. Ergonomics in building and construction: time for implementation. *Applied Ergonomics*, 36(4), 387–389.

Varianou-Mikellidou, C., Boustras, G., Dimopoulos, C., Wybo, J.-L., Guldenmund, F. W., Nicolaidou, O., & Anyfantis, I. (2019). Occupational health and safety management in the context of an ageing workforce. *Safety Science*, 116, 231–244.

Welch, L., Haile, E., Boden, L. I., & Hunting, K. L. (2009). Musculoskeletal disorders among construction roofers – physical function and disability. *Scandinavian Journal of Work, Environment & Health*, 35(1), 56–63.

Welch, L., Haile, E., Boden, L. I., & Hunting, K. L. (2010). Impact of musculoskeletal and medical conditions on disability retirement – a longitudinal study among construction roofers. *American Journal of Industrial Medicine*, 53(6), 552–560.

Yaffe, K., Hoang, T. D., Byers, A. L., Barnes, D. E., & Friedl, K. E. (2014). Lifestyle and health-related risk factors and risk of cognitive aging among older veterans. *Alzheimer's & Dementia*, 10, S111–S121.

Zacher, H., Rudolph, C. W., & Baltes, B. B. (2019). An invitation to lifespan thinking, in B. Baltes, C. W. Rudolph and H. Zaher (Eds.), *Work Across the Lifespan*. Associated Press (pp.1–14).

10

BUILDING A SENSE OF PLACE

10.1 Introduction

In this chapter we focus on a positive approach to workers' health and well-being. We start by introducing the sense of place concept and how it has been framed within a work context. Taking a positive approach to mentally healthy workplaces is examined using a positive psychology lens. We then introduce a new sense of place model which comprises six elements: social support, community, life balance, engagement, respect, and employee resilience. We report on the results of a pilot study examining the reliability and validity of a bespoke, multidimensional measurement tool developed to measure sense of place. Finally, we describe how a sense of place at work is empirically linked to mental health.

10.2 What is sense of place (SoP)?

Sense of place (SoP) is used to describe the perception of place in connection with the qualities and attributes that distinguish a place from others, give it a sense of authenticity, and induce feelings of attachment and belonging (Foote & Azaryahu, 2009). SoP has been criticised due to the lack of conceptual clarity with which it has been used; however, Kudryavtsev et al. (2012) argue that SoP may be understood to combine two complementary concepts: place attachment and place meaning. Place attachment describes "the bond between people and places, or the degree to which a place is important to people" (Kudryavtsev et al., 2012, p. 231). Place meaning refers to "the symbolic meanings that people ascribe to settings" (Kudryavtsev et al., 2012, p. 232). Consistent with broader ecological understandings of health, SoP is often associated with a person's living environment and has been linked to quality of life, health and wellbeing (Gattino et al., 2013; DeMiglio & Williams, 2016).

DOI: 10.1201/9780367814236-10

SoP has been explored across many disciplines to describe the various aspects of human relationships with the natural environment (Hausmann et al., 2015). In the environmental psychology and sociology disciplines, SoP is focused on community, belonging and identity and is associated with: "exploring the dimensions of the people-place relationship; reduction of, and recovery from stress; psychological integrity and preventing mental illnesses" (Hausmann et al., 2015, p.121). SoP in the workplace has received minimal attention in the extant literature, and research has often focused on the physical components of the workplace associated with wellbeing. Furthermore, much of the research on SoP in the workplace has focused on the experiences of office-based and knowledge workers (Foley, 2007; Miller et al., 2001). For example, Miller et al. (2001) focused on the interior setting of a workplace and operationalised SoP of knowledge workers to include comfort, control, noise, privacy, and personalisation.

Much of the extant literature on SoP in the workplace has limited relevance to work in construction. Construction work is often project-based, and teams can consist of a wide variety of occupations dispersed across multiple locations (Langford et al., 1995). Therefore defining "place" in the construction workplace in a physical sense is somewhat challenging. Construction projects are temporary coalitions of permanent and temporary organisations working interdependently to achieve project outcomes, while also managing their own business interests (Berggren et al., 2001). There is a heavy reliance on subcontracting to undertake manual/non-managerial construction work and the workforce is heavily transient. Relationships between contributors to projects are arms-length, transactional and sometimes conflict-ridden. In this context, a health-promoting SoP may be difficult to realise.

10.3   Developing a sense of place in a dynamic workplace

In relation to SoP in the workplace, Foley (2007) considers the definition of work and this has relevance to construction as a "place" of work. Foley (2007, p.864) contends that the workplace should not be conceived "as zones or territories but as modes of workplace interaction and proximity – entered into or withdrawn for discrete purposes, and which incorporate a range of tasks, activities and social encounters." Foley's (2007) definition of the workplace challenges us to look beyond the physical and geographical place of work when considering SoP in construction and focus on the interactions and tasks of construction work. This is important because:

- The physical "place" of a construction project is constantly evolving throughout the construction process.
- Typically, work contributing to a construction project can occur simultaneously across multiple, geographically dispersed worksites. For example, work tasks contributing to one project may take place virtually (such as working from home), from a corporate office, offsite in a manufacturing facility, on site in the site office, and on site in direct construction activity.

Arguably, the development of a sense of attachment and meaning in relation to one's place of work is likely to be more difficult in project work than in more stable, routinised work situations. Projects are inherently temporary and involve people from different organisations and functions who may not have worked together before and who may only work with each other for a limited period of time (Borg & Söderlund, 2014). Consequently, it may take time for project workers to learn to work together effectively, build trust and establish a sense of belonging to a team. Moreover, project workers are typically employed in different organisations or departments whilst simultaneously performing their project roles. The requirement to work together to deliver a project outside normal organisational boundaries or functional groups creates "ambiguous belongings" that project workers experience as stressful (Borg & Söderlund, 2014). The lack of stability in project work, in terms of assignments, relationships and evaluations of performance has also been identified by Cicmil et al. (2016) as contributing to work stress and exhaustion. In juggling multiple project goals in the context of project complexity and finite resources, project workers reportedly experience a "work-life in which nothing is stable, nothing and no one is reliable, in which professional reputations, performances and senses of personal worthiness are repeatedly challenged and may be lost" (Cicmil et al., 2016, p. 59).

10.4 Positive approach to mentally healthy workplaces

10.4.1 Prevention and promotion

As explored in previous chapters, mental ill health in construction has emerged as a serious issue. Mental ill health is known to "cluster within" particular industries and occupations, with workers in male-dominated industries being at increased risk (Roche et al., 2016, p. 280). Construction is a male-dominated industry and its workers are a high-risk group for mental ill health (Roche et al., 2016). A recent report undertaken on behalf of the Chartered Institute of Building revealed that construction industry workers are worse off than workers in other industries in terms of experiencing poor work–life balance, high workload, excessive travel time, technology overload, and unrealistic deadlines (Cattell et al., 2017). In a systematic review of mental ill health risk factors in the construction industry, Chan et al. (2020) identified key risk factors for mental ill health as a lack of job control, welfare concerns, workplace hazards, job demands, workplace injustice, interference with family time, and lack of support.

There is an increasing emphasis on the workplace as a point of intervention for targeting the prevention of mental illness and the promotion of wellbeing (Harvey et al., 2014). The workplace is considered an effective site of intervention for mental health promotion programmes, particularly among men who are reported to have lower levels of mental health literacy and be less likely than women to seek help for personal difficulties (Roche et al., 2016). Roche et al. (2016) argue that:

- large numbers of people can be accessed through workplace interventions,
- workplaces already contain existing infrastructure and frameworks to support the implementation of mental health and wellbeing programmes, and
- addressing mental health as part of workplace occupational health and safety management activities reduces stigma and encourages help-seeking behaviour in relation to mental health.

While changing attitudes and behaviour in relation to mental ill health is important, long-term prevention measures also need to target the construction industry's culture and entrenched practices that contribute to the emergence of mental ill health. Dextras-Gauthier et al. (2012) argue that the behaviours, structures and processes that produce adverse conditions of work are shaped by the values, assumptions and beliefs inherent in an industry or organisational culture. They argue that "when dealing with mental health issues, including burnout, depression, and psychological distress, managers need to tread further upstream to identify those elements of organizational culture that are ultimately causing ill health" (Dextras-Gauthier et al., 2012, p.97).

Many occupational health initiatives focus on reducing sickness, presenteeism or sickness absence, which are all known to present a high cost to organisations. However, it is increasingly recognised that workers who are mentally and physically healthy are also more productive, shifting the emphasis from prevention of ill health to the promotion of good health in workplaces (Christensen, 2017). Hakanen and Schaufeli (2012) argue that workers' general wellbeing should be understood as being more than the absence of depressive symptoms. Rather, a state of general wellbeing also constitutes the presence of a positive state of life satisfaction, happiness, and a sense of belonging (Böhnke, 2005). Böhnke (2005) contends that lack of belonging can result in feeling alienated which is associated with self-reported pessimism, detachment from social order, social exclusion and anxiety (Böhnke, 2005).

There is an increasing call for research that investigates whether factors, other than those that cause ill health, predict positive health measures (Torp et al., 2013). Understanding the determinants of positive wellbeing will enable the design and implementation of interventions that can create a psychologically healthy workplace.

10.4.2   *Positive psychology in the workplace*

Understanding the "conditions and processes that contribute to the flourishing or optimal functioning of people, groups, and institutions" is the overarching goal of the positive psychology movement (Gable & Haidt, 2005, p.104). Positive psychology is based on the premise that there is a need to focus scientific research and interest "on understanding the entire breadth of human experience, from loss, suffering, illness, and distress through connection, fulfilment, health, and well-being" (Linley et al., 2006, p.6).

According to Seligman and Csikszentmihalyi (2000), positive psychology is comprised of three pillars:

(i) Positive institutions (families, schools, businesses, communities, societies).
(ii) Positive individual traits (character strengths, such as resilience, purpose, values, interests).
(iii) Positive subjective experiences (wellbeing and positive emotions).

The role of the institution is critical in facilitating the development and presence of positive traits, which in turn facilitate subjective experiences (Peterson, 2006). Within a work context, this places the organisation in a central role of enabling positive subjective experiences (Peterson, 2006). In considering the role of the "organisation" in construction, it is important to consider how work is structured and organised more broadly. Multiple organisations typically come together to deliver a construction project (Shirazi et al., 1996) which can span clients (e.g., tenants and financiers), consultants (e.g., architects, engineers and surveyors) and constructors (e.g., main contractor, subcontractors and suppliers) (Langford et al., 1995). The construction industry has been recognised as a "projectized industry" (Project Management Institute, 2021). It therefore may be more fitting to substitute "organisation" with "project" when considering the key components of positive psychology in the construction workplace environment, as projects are known to develop their own unique workplace cultures.

10.4.3 Positive psychology interventions

In relation to workplace interventions, the positive psychology movement has contributed to a relatively recent managerial focus on the creation of mentally healthy workplaces, defined as workplaces in which:

• "risk factors are acknowledged and appropriate action [is] taken to minimise their potential negative impact" and
• "protective or resilience factors are fostered and maximized" (Harvey et al., 2014, p.12).

Thus, in a mentally healthy workplace steps are taken to eliminate risk factors for loss, suffering, illness, and distress, as well as to create a context within which workers can flourish.

Meyers et al. (2013) draw on Seligman and Csikszentmihalyi's (2000) seminal description of positive psychology to develop their definition of a positive psychology intervention:

> Any intentional activity or method (training, coaching, etc.) based on (a) the cultivation of valued subjective experiences, (b) the building of positive individual traits, or (c) the building of civic virtue and positive institutions.
> p.620

Positive psychology interventions as defined by Meyers et al. (2013) seek to build or broaden any aspects of the three pillars (positive institutions, positive traits, positive subjective experience) at the individual, team, or organisational level (Donaldson et al., 2019).

Meyers et al. (2013) elaborate on their definition of a positive psychology intervention, stating that:

- Under part (a) of the definition falls any intervention that understands positive subjective experiences as part of the intervention method (e.g., remembering sacred moments) and not just as a by-product that happens to appear in consequence of the intervention.
- Part (b) of the definition encompasses interventions that aim at identifying, developing, broadening, and/or using valued individual traits or trait-like constructs (e.g. character strengths).
- Part (c) encompasses any intervention that aims at identifying, developing, broadening, and/or putting to practice valued characteristics of organizations or organizational subgroups.

p.620

Seligman (2011) proposed a theory of wellbeing intended to shape positive psychology interventions. The theory is known as PERMA (i.e., positive emotions, engagement, relationships, meaning, and accomplishment) and has been used to guide the development and implementation of workplace interventions. Henry (2005) draws on a positive psychology perspective (Seligman & Csikszentmihalyi, 2000) to consider the characteristics of a "healthy organisation." Henry (2005) contends that interventions can occur at four levels: the individual, the group, the organisation, and the inter-organisational.

At the individual level, interventions focus on improving the psychological health of workers and seek to build strengths, enhance positive individual resources such as emotional intelligence and resilience, and promote wellbeing (Di Fabio, 2017; Green et al., 2017). At the group level, interventions focus on team building (belonging and social support), group training (promotes identifying, accepting, and working with diversity), creative thinking (healthy groups are open to creative challenges from members), and workplace relational civility in terms of relational decency, relational culture, and relational readiness for positive interactions with other workers, which can reduce conflict in organisations (Di Fabio, 2017). At the organisation level, the focus is on making the organisation a more efficient and happy place to work in, creating an open culture characterised by sustained creativity and innovation, and promoting an organisational climate that supports positive relationships and leadership styles for the empowerment of employees through autonomy and self-organisation (Di Fabio, 2017). At the inter-organisation level, the focus is on making the boundaries of organisations more fluid and improving the relations between organisations. Partnerships, networking, and community involvement are emphasised at the inter-organisation level (Di Fabio, 2017).

10.5   Sense of place conceptual model

A comprehensive review of the peer-reviewed positive psychology literature was undertaken to identify the workplace conditions in construction that contribute to a SoP and enable high levels of mental health and wellbeing. The purpose of this review was to develop a multifaceted model that could be used as the basis of a performance measurement and benchmarking tool for use in construction project environments. The review applied a positive psychology approach to identify and define protective factors supportive of healthy functioning for workers. A critical review of the literature was undertaken to: 1) identify and define protective factors; 2) ensure factors are mutually exclusive; and 3) identify a set of metrics for each of the protective factors identified and defined.

From the literature, six elements were identified that were strongly empirically linked to positive mental health outcomes (see Figure 10.1). These are: social support, community, life balance, engagement, respect, and employee resilience.

10.5.1   Social support

Social support refers to situations in which one person or group needs help to achieve an objective and another person or group offers resources to provide help (Dovidio et al., 2006). According to Brough and Pears (2004, p.472), workplace social support focuses on "collaborative problem solving and sharing information, reappraising situations and obtaining advice from a variety of personnel

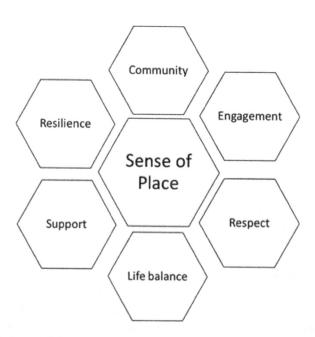

FIGURE 10.1 Sense of place conceptual model

such as colleagues, supervisors and managers (i.e. sources of social support)." In the workplace, social support is defined as the degree to which individuals perceive that their wellbeing is valued by workplace sources, such as supervisors and the broader organisation in which they are embedded, and the perception that these sources provide help to support this wellbeing (Eisenberger et al., 2002; Kossek et al., 2011). Kossek et al. (2011, p.292) conceptualise workplace social support as "(a) emanating from multiple sources, such as supervisors, co-workers, and employing organisations; and (b) distinguished by different types or foci of support that are either 'content general' or 'content specific'." General work support refers to the degree to which workers perceive that supervisors or employers care about their global wellbeing on the job through providing positive social interaction or resources. Content-specific support refers to perceptions of care and the provision of resources to reinforce a particular type of role demand (Kossek et al., 2011).

There is strong evidence of the association between social support and health, including mental health (Kawachi & Berkman, 2001). Perceived organisational support is positively linked to worker engagement and wellbeing (Caesens et al., 2016) and negatively related to burnout (Walters & Raybould, 2007). The absence of support in a supervisor-employee relationship has also been observed to have an impact on the performance of employees, their satisfaction at work and on the engagement and burnout of the affected employees (Baruch-Feldman et al., 2002; Neves & Eisenberger, 2014). Johnson and Hall (1988) incorporated social support into the Job Demand-Control model of occupational stress (Karasek, 1979) and demonstrated that, in environments characterised by high demands and low control, workers experienced reduced levels of strain when social support was high.

10.5.2   Community

Sense of community (SOC), also referred to as psychological sense of community, refers to the fundamental human phenomenon of collective experience (Peterson et al., 2008). McMillan (1976, p.9) describes SOC as "a feeling that members have of belonging, a feeling that members matter to one another and to the group, and a shared faith that members' needs will be met through their commitment to be together." A workplace community is identifiable as a set of formal and informal networks of individuals who share a common association (Burroughs & Eby, 1998). In a work setting, Lambert and Hopkins (1995, p.152) define a sense of community as "mutual commitment between workers and their employing organization." Lambert and Hopkins (1995) draw on Mowday et al. (1982, p.153) to clarify that mutual commitment can be understood within the context of organisational commitment, described as "the relative strength of an individual's identification with and involvement in a particular organization, which is characterized by belief and acceptance of organizational goals, and values, willingness to exert effort on behalf of the organization, and a desire to maintain a membership in that organization."

SOC is commonly described as a multidimensional construct in which reference is often made to McMillan and Chavis' (1986, p.9) four elements of: membership; influence; integration and fulfilment of needs; and shared emotional connection. A sense of community is positively related to experiencing higher levels of mental wellbeing (Boyd & Nowell, 2017; Peterson et al., 2008).

10.5.3   Life balance

Life balance describes a situation in which workers experience "satisfaction and perceptions of success in meeting work and nonwork role demands, low levels of conflict among roles, and opportunity for inter-role enrichment, meaning that experiences in one role can improve performance and satisfaction in other roles as well" (Kossek et al., 2014, p.301). Life balance is strongly and consistently positively related to job and life satisfaction and negatively related to anxiety and depression across samples from seven different countries/cultures (Haar et al., 2014).

Positive interaction between work and family has been linked to psychological wellbeing. For example, Allis and O'Driscoll (2008) report that nonwork-to-work facilitation is associated with higher levels of employee wellbeing, while Haar and Bardoel (2008) report that positive spillover between work and family life was negatively associated with psychological distress and turnover intention in a sample of Australian workers. Van Steenbergen et al. (2007) also found work-to-family facilitation contributed to the prediction of previously reported work–family outcomes, including work satisfaction, organisational commitment, job performance, home performance, home commitment, home satisfaction and general life satisfaction, over and above variance explained by traditional measures of work–family conflict. In a two-staged longitudinal study, Innstrand et al. (2008) similarly found that work-to-family facilitation at "time one" was associated with lower levels of employee burnout at "time two."

10.5.4   Engagement

Work engagement has been described as "a positive, fulfilling, affective-motivational state of work-related well-being" (Bakker et al., 2008, pp.187–188). Work engagement is often regarded as the opposite of job burnout. For example, Maslach and Leiter (1997) suggested engagement comprises energy, involvement and effectiveness, which are the direct opposites of the three burnout dimensions of exhaustion, cynicism and diminished personal efficacy.

Other researchers have defined and operationalised work engagement as a distinct construct from burnout. For example, Schaufeli et al. (2002) define work engagement as "a positive, fulfilling, work-related state of mind that is characterized by vigour, dedication and absorption" (p.74). The components of work engagement are further defined as follows:

- vigour is characterised by "high levels of mental resilience while working, the willingness to invest effort in one's work and persistence even in the face of difficulties";
- dedication describes "being strongly involved in one's work and experiencing a sense of significance, enthusiasm, inspiration, pride and challenge"; and
- absorption is characterised by "being fully concentrated and happily engrossed in one's work, whereby time passes quickly, and one has difficulties with detaching oneself from work" (Bakker et al., 2008, p.188).

Innstrand et al. (2012) directly tested for a relationship between work engagement and symptoms of anxiety or depression, using a two-wave longitudinal data set (with a two-year time interval). They report the statistical model that positioned work engagement as predicting low levels of anxiety or depression was stronger than an alternative model in which work engagement was positioned as an outcome of positive mental health. Thus, the direction of causality is likely to be from engagement to the absence of mental ill health. In particular, the lagged negative effect of vigour on symptoms of depression and anxiety over the two-year data collection period provides evidence that work engagement has a positive protective effect on mental health. Innstrand et al. (2012) argue that this suggests that, in addition to eliminating organisational risk factors for mental ill health, workplaces should also focus on creating the conditions in which workers can flourish. Hakanen and Schaufeli (2012) similarly report that a positive state of work engagement negatively predicted depressive symptoms over a seven-year longitudinal study.

10.5.5 Respect/civility

Respect has been defined and operationalised in various ways within the organisational literature. For example, Bies and Moag (1986) define respect as being treated politely, while disrespect includes inconsiderate actions, use of abusive language, and coercion (Grover, 2013). De Cremer and Tyler (2005) refer to respect as how worthy and recognised one feels, while van Quaquebeke and Eckloff (2010) define respectful leadership as "maintaining an appreciative attitude toward the other person and acting on the basis of this attitude even if one does not personally like or agree with the object of respect" (p. 344). Andersson and Pearson (1999) consider respect from a workplace incivility lens, defining incivility as "low intensity deviant behaviour with an ambiguous intent to harm the target, in violation of workplace norms for mutual respect" (p.457).

A respectful workplace is one in which people feel worthy and recognised and incivility is not tolerated. In contrast, workplace civility reflects "behavior that helps to preserve the norms for mutual respect at work; it comprises behaviors that are fundamental to positively connecting with another, building relationships, and empathizing" (Pearson et al., 2000, p.125). In the workplace, civility "demands that one speaks in ways that are respectful, responsible, restrained, and principled and avoid that which is offensive, rude, demeaning, and threatening"

(Gill & Sypher, 2009, p.55). Workplace incivility is associated with psychological distress, and strategies to improve respect and civility in the workplace can significantly reduce burnout (Leiter et al., 2011).

In the workplace, respect has been studied in the context of the organisational justice literature. Organisational justice refers to "employees' perception of fairness in the organizational work systems and workplace relationships" (Pattnaik & Tripathy, 2019, p.58). Organisational justice has also been described as a personal evaluation about the ethical and moral standing of managerial conduct (Cropanzano et al., 2007). Cropanzano et al. (2007) contend that while justice contributes to workers' relationships with their employer, injustice is reported to dissolve bonds within the work community. There is evidence that low organisational justice is a risk to the health of employees (Elovainio et al., 2002).

10.5.6 Employee resilience

Resilience is increasingly understood not as a stable set of personal characteristics but as a process arising from the interplay of the individual with their work environment (World Health Organization, 2017). In the workplace, resilience describes the ability of an individual worker or work group to respond to everyday problems and challenges associated with work and being able to "bounce back" when setbacks are encountered and remain effective in challenging situations. Beyond this, resilience in the workplace also incorporates the lasting benefit and learning that occurs through successfully coping with adverse situations (Cooper et al., 2013). Resilience in the workplace is positively linked to mental health (Kinman & Grant, 2011). Importantly, workers' resilience can be facilitated by the work environment, including leadership and the prevailing workplace culture (Näswall et al., 2015).

Central to models of resilience are the inclusion of protective factors which are critical for managing stressful events effectively to either mitigate or eliminate risk. According to Windle (2011), protective factors are the defining attributes of resilience. Some studies distinguish the individual level protective factors as assets, while resources are regarded as external to the individual (Fergus & Zimmerman, 2005; Sacker & Schoon, 2007):

- internal protective factors are individual qualities or characteristics/capabilities that are responsible for fostering resilience and are specific to the individual, and
- external protective factors are positive environmental support structures from the environment in which the individual is situated.

10.6 Sense of place tool

A review of scales was undertaken for each of the identified SoP components. The scales were selected according to the following criteria: satisfactory psychometric properties, alignment with component definitions, publicly available and

TABLE 10.1 Sense of place (SoP) scales

SoP component	Scale name	No. of items and factors	Citation
Community	Brief Sense of Community Scale	8(4)	Peterson et al. (2008)
Engagement	Oldenburg Burnout Inventory	8(2)	Demerouti et al. (2010)
Respect	Civility Norms Questionnaire-Brief	4(1)	Walsh et al. (2012)
Life balance	Work life balance	3(1)	Haar (2013)
Support (supervisor)	Social Support from Supervisor Index	4(1)	Caplan (1975)
Support (co-workers)	Social Support from Coworkers Index	4(1)	Caplan (1975)
Resilience	Employee Resilience Scale	9(1)	Näswall et al. (2015)

no charge for use, and length and number of items. Table 10.1 summarises a set of scales selected based on the described criteria.

A pilot project was conducted with members of a construction project to test the SoP conceptual model using the scales outlined in Table 10.1. All scales demonstrated good internal consistency reliability. Pearson product-moment correlations were conducted to ascertain the relationship between the SoP variables, and also the relationship between each of the SoP variables and employee wellbeing. The seven-item Warwick-Edinburgh Mental Wellbeing Short-Form was used in the survey to measure positive mental health (Stewart-Brown et al., 2009; Ng et al., 2017). The SoP components were found to be all statistically significantly correlated with employees' wellbeing. The correlations between the SoP components and wellbeing were all positive, i.e., as employees' perceptions of SoP increases so too does their wellbeing. The correlations with wellbeing ranged from $r=.355$ ($p=.003$) for the relationship between co-worker social support and wellbeing to $r=.680$ ($p=.000$) for the relationship between employee resilience and wellbeing. Thus, the statistical associations between the SoP components and employee wellbeing were all of medium or high strength. These findings further support the validity of the SoP survey items for use in the construction industry because they are all significantly related to wellbeing in a way that makes theoretical sense.

10.7 Link between sense of place and mental wellbeing

A clear and significant link has been established between SoP and mental wellbeing. In a pilot study (outlined above), significant and positive bivariate correlations were found between each of the SoP model components and mental wellbeing. This indicates that the SoP components, as operationalised in the

TABLE 10.2 Allocation of participants to high, medium and low wellbeing groupings

Grouping	No. of participants	Percentage
Low wellbeing	7	10
Medium wellbeing	49	70
High wellbeing	14	20
Total	70	100

survey tool, are linked in a significant way to mental wellbeing in a project work environment.

Participants of the pilot study were divided into three groups reflecting whether they reported low, medium or high wellbeing scores. The allocation of participants to groups was based upon the application of population norm scores for the short version of the Warwick-Edinburgh Mental Wellbeing Scale (SWEMWBS) used in the study. The SWEMWBS has a mean of 23.5 and a standard deviation of 3.9 in the United Kingdom general population samples (Ng et al., 2017). This means that 15 per cent of the population can be expected to have a score of >27.4, so we set the threshold for high wellbeing at 27.5. Conversely, 15 per cent of the population can be expected to have a score of <19.6, so we established a threshold point of 19.5, below which participants were deemed to have low wellbeing. Table 10.2 shows the distribution of participants into these groupings based on the threshold values applied. Our results are close to Ng's findings that the top 15 per cent of scores range from 27.5 to 35.0 (high) and the bottom 15 per cent from 7.0 to 19.5 (low).

Figure 10.2 shows the mean SoP component scores for participants reporting low, medium and high wellbeing scores. For all components the lowest mean scores were observed in participants reporting low wellbeing according to the SWEMWBS and highest mean scores were observed in participants reporting high wellbeing scores.

The statistical significance of the differences in mean SoP component scores between wellbeing groupings was tested using a one-way analysis of variance (ANOVA). Statistically significant differences were found between the mean scores of participants reporting low, medium and high levels of wellbeing for all of the SoP components, with the exception of co-worker support. To investigate these findings, post-hoc tests were undertaken to systematically compare each of the pairs of groups to indicate whether there was a significant difference between each pair. This was only carried out for ANOVAs that produced significant main effects for differences between groups. The results of the post-hoc tests are presented in Table 10.3.

Case example 10.1 demonstrates how a construction project in New Zealand focused on creating a Community of People which prioritised the welfare, and health and safety of workers.

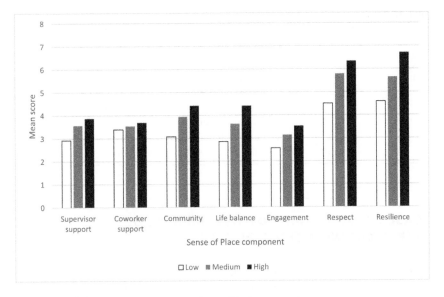

FIGURE 10.2 Mean component scores by wellbeing grouping

TABLE 10.3 Results of post-hoc tests showing pairwise differences in sense of place component scores

Sense of place component	*Significant pairwise differences*
Supervisor support	• People with low wellbeing had significantly lower supervisor support scores than people with medium wellbeing • People with low wellbeing had significantly lower supervisor support scores than people with high wellbeing
Community	• People with low wellbeing had significantly lower community scores than people with medium wellbeing • People with low wellbeing had significantly lower community scores than people with high wellbeing
Life balance	• People with low wellbeing had significantly lower life balance than people with high wellbeing
Engagement	• People with low wellbeing had significantly lower engagement scores than people with medium wellbeing • People with low wellbeing had significantly lower engagement scores than people with high wellbeing • People with medium wellbeing had significantly lower engagement scores than people with high wellbeing
Respect	• People with low wellbeing had significantly lower respect scores than people with medium wellbeing • People with low wellbeing scores had significantly lower respect scores than people with high wellbeing

(*continued*)

TABLE 10.3 Cont.

Sense of place component	Significant pairwise differences
Resilience	• People with low wellbeing had significantly lower resilience scores than people with medium wellbeing • People with low wellbeing had significantly lower resilience scores than people with high wellbeing • People with medium wellbeing scores had significantly lower resilience scores than people with high wellbeing

CASE EXAMPLE 10.1 POSITIVE IMPACTS OF EXPERIENCING A SENSE OF PLACE

Workers at the construction project experienced a strong SoP, and described feeling part of a team, enjoying the collaborative nature of the project, having positive relationships with others at the project and feeling a sense of pride and satisfaction associated with participation in the project. Workers' comments reflect the fact that the SoP concept is relevant to project workers. Several comments also reflect that working at the project positively affected workers' health and wellbeing. Emergent themes and illustrative comments made by workers at the project are summarised as follows:

Teamwork and collaboration

• *Being involved with a "one team ethos." Knowing there is support on all levels available. [Project name] willingness to engage and assist the contractor's needs and suggestions.*
• *It has been personally rewarding to be part of a team who have collectively worked through an extremely challenging project with multiple hurdles and big challenges, a team who have had open and honest conversations and have cared for one another, right to the end.*

Enjoyable and safe work environment

• *Now I come to work here because I enjoy working again and enjoy the environment I work in and the team I now work for.*
• *Thank you to the entire [company name] management team for creating a fun safe work environment. Being here has turned my life around!*
• *I enjoy my work life here. Excellent attempt to create a safer and more collaborative, safe and productive workplace. Impressed by management and their safety initiatives. Benefited greatly from the Workplace support counselling initiative.*

Sense of belonging and respect

- *The Contractor Compound is a unique space to be involved with. It has grown a workplace culture that gives me and my team a sense of belonging and self worth to the [project name].*
- *There was a real feeling of care and respect for all members engaged in the project. This is in contrast to many projects I have worked on in my early career.*
- *Loved being a part of the [project name]. The attitude and good manners of the team I've worked with has been the highlight.*

Relationships

- *[project name] is such a family-orientated project, every single person I have met on this project has made me feel welcome and appreciated, and all people involved here have got each others' backs 100%.*
- *The [project name] is a big whānau [extended family] where you get the respect from everyone.*
- *Well what can I say: it's been great, meeting a lot of people, awesome environment to have the opportunity to work at.*

10.8   Conclusion

Mentally healthy workplaces are described as those which foster and maximise protective factors. The SoP conceptual model is positioned within a positive psychology paradigm and offers an evidence-based framework through which organisations can create a context for workers to flourish. Mentally healthy workplaces are also described as those which seek to acknowledge risk factors and take appropriate action to minimise their potential negative impact. Construction is known as a high-demands industry in which work-based hazards can create adverse and hostile environments that are harmful to workers' mental health. In order to have a positive impact on mental health, implementation of a SoP in construction must be accompanied with the removal of harmful work conditions which lead to mental ill health. It is anticipated that initiatives designed specifically to create a sense of place in the construction project environment will yield benefits for workers' psychological wellbeing.

10.9   Discussion and review questions

1. How can the three pillars of positive psychology be applied on a construction project? Why is this potentially helpful to ensuring workers are mentally healthy and well?

2. Why are construction projects challenging environments in which to foster a sense of place? What are the potential benefits associated with effectively promoting a sense of place in a construction project?
3. What strategies can be implemented in a project to develop a sense of place? How can a project sense of place be measured or evaluated?

10.10 Acknowledgements

This work was supported by the Cross Yarra Partnership with funding by WorkSafe Victoria (Australia) under the WorkWell Mental Health Improvement Fund; RMIT University DSC ERA 2023 Proposal Scheme; Fonterra Co-operative Group Ltd.

References

Allis, P., & O'Driscoll, M. (2008). Positive effects of nonwork-to-work facilitation on well-being in work, family and personal domains. *Journal of Managerial Psychology,* 23(3), 273–291.

Andersson, L. M., & Pearson, C. M. (1999). Tit for tat? The spiraling effect of incivility in the workplace. *Academy of Management Review,* 24(3), 452–471.

Bakker, A. B., Schaufeli, W. B., Leiter, M. P., & Taris, T. W. (2008). Work engagement: An emerging concept in occupational health psychology. *Work & Stress,* 22(3), 187–200.

Baruch-Feldman, C., Brondolo, E., Ben-Dayan, D., & Schwartz, J. (2002). Sources of social support and burnout, job satisfaction, and productivity. *Journal of Occupational Health Psychology,* 7(1), 84–93.

Berggren, C., Söderlund, J., & Anderson, C. (2001). Clients, Contractors, and Consultants: The Consequences of Organizational Fragmentation in Contemporary Project Environments. *Project Management Journal,* 32(3), 39–48.

Bies, R. J., & Moag, J. F. (1986). Interactional justice: Communication criteria of fairness. In R. J. Lewicki, B. H. Sheppard, and M. H. Bazerman (Eds.), *Research on Negotiations in Organizations* (Vol. 1). JAI Press (pp. 43–55).

Böhnke, P. (2005). *First European Quality of Life Survey: Life Satisfaction, Happiness and Sense of Belonging.* European Foundation for the Improvement of Living and Working Conditions.

Borg, E., & Söderlund, J. (2014). Moving in, moving on: Liminality practices in project-based work. *Employee Relations,* 36(2), 182–197.

Boyd, N. M., & Nowell, B. (2017). Testing a theory of sense of community and community responsibility in organizations: An empirical assessment of predictive capacity on employee well-being and organizational citizenship. *Journal of Community Psychology,* 45(2), 210–229.

Brough, P. & Pears, J. (2004). Evaluating the influence of the type of social support on job satisfaction and work related psychological well-being. *International Journal of Organisational Behaviour,* 8, 472–485.

Burroughs, S. M., & Eby, L. T. (1998). Psychological sense of community at work: A measurement system and explanatory framework. *Journal of Community Psychology,* 26(6), 509–53.

Caesens, G., Stinglhamber, F., & Ohana, M. (2016). Perceived organizational support and well-being: A weekly study. *Journal of Managerial Psychology*, 31(7), 1214–1230.

Caplan, R. D., Cobb, S., French, J. R. P., Harrison, R.V., & Pinneau, S. R. (1975). *Job Demands and Worker Health*. National Institute for Occupational Safety and Health.

Cattell, K. S., Bowen, P. A., Cooper, C. L., & Edwards, P. J. (2017). The State of Well-Being in *the Construction Industry*. Chartered Institute of Building.

Chan, A., P. C., Nwaogu, J., M., & Naslund, J., A. (2020). Mental ill-health risk factors in the construction industry: Systematic review. *Journal of Construction Engineering and Management*, 146(3), 04020004.

Christensen, M. (2017). Healthy individuals in healthy organizations: The happy productive worker hypotheses. In M. Christensen, O. Saksvik and M. Kaanika-Murray (Eds.), *The Positive Side of Occupational Health Psychology*. Springer (pp. 155–169).

Cicmil, S., Lindgren, M., & Packendorff, J. (2016). The project (management) discourse and its consequences: on vulnerability and unsustainability in project-based work. *New Technology, Work and Employment*, 31(1), 58–76.

Cooper, C., Flint-Taylor, J., & Pearn, M. (2013). *Building Resilience for Success: A Resource for Managers and Organizations*. Palgrave Macmillan.

Cropanzano, R., Bowen, D. E., & Gilliland, S. W. (2007). The management of organizational justice. *Academy of Management Perspectives*, 21(4), 34–48.

De Cremer, D., & Tyler, T. R. (2005). Am I respected or not?: Inclusion and reputation as issues in group membership. *Social Justice Research*, 18(2), 121–153.

Demerouti, E., Mostert, K., & Bakker, A. B. (2010). Burnout and work engagement: A thorough investigation of the independency of both constructs. *Journal of Occupational Health Psychology*, 15(3), 209–222.

DeMiglio, L., & Williams, A. (2016). A sense of place, a sense of well-being. In *Sense of Place, Health and Quality of Life*. Routledge (pp. 35–50).

Dextras-Gauthier, J., Marchand, A., & Haines III, V. (2012). Organizational culture, work organization conditions, and mental health: A proposed integration. *International Journal of Stress Management*, 19(2), 81–104.

Di Fabio, A. (2017). Positive healthy organizations: Promoting well-being, meaningfulness, and sustainability in organizations. *Frontiers in Psychology*, 8(1938), 1–6.

Donaldson, S. I., Lee, J. Y., & Donaldson, S. I. (2019). Evaluating positive psychology interventions at work: A systematic review and meta-analysis. *International Journal of Applied Positive Psychology*, 4(3), 113–134.

Dovidio, J. F., Piliavin, J. A. Schroeder, D. A., & Penner, L. A. (2006). *The Social Psychology of Prosocial Behavior*. Lawrence Erlbaum Associates.

Eisenberger, R., Stinglhamber, F., Vandenberghe, C., Sucharski, I. L., & Rhoades, L. (2002). Perceived supervisor support: Contributions to perceived organizational support and employee retention. *Journal of Applied Psychology*, 87(3), 565–573.

Elovainio, M., Kivimäki, M., & Vahtera, J. (2002). Organizational justice: Evidence of a new psychosocial predictor of health. *American Journal of Public Health*, 92(1), 105–108.

Fergus, S., & Zimmerman, M. A. (2005). Adolescent resilience: A framework for understanding healthy development in the face of risk. *Annual Review of Public Health*, 26, 399–419.

Foley, S. (2007). Understanding a sense of place in collaborative environments. In M. J. Smith and G. Salvendy (Eds.), *Human Interface and the Management of Information. Interacting in Information Environments*. Springer (pp. 863–872).

Foote, K. E., & Azaryahu, M. (2009). Sense of Place. In R. Kitchin and N. Thrift (Eds.), *International Encyclopaedia of Human Geography*. Elsevier (pp. 96–100).

Gable S. L., & Haidt, J. (2005). What (and why) is positive psychology. *Review of General Psychology*, 9, 103–110.

Gattino, S., De Piccoli, N., Fassio, O., & Rollero, C. (2013). Quality of life and sense of community. A study on health and place of residence. *Journal of Community Psychology*, 41(7), 811–826.

Gill, M. J., & Sypher, B. D. (2009). Workplace incivility and organizational trust. In P. Lutgen-Sandvik and B. D. Sypher (Eds.), *Destructive Organizational Communication: Processes, Consequences, and Constructive Ways of Organizing*. Routledge (pp. 53–73).

Green, S., Evans, O., & Williams, B. (2017). Positive psychology at work: Research and practice. In C. Proctor (ed.), *Positive Psychology Interventions in Practice*. Springer (pp. 185–206).

Grover, S. L. (2013). Unraveling respect in organization studies. *Human Relations*, 67(1), 27–51.

Haar, J. M. (2013). Testing a new measure of work–life balance: A study of parent and non-parent employees from New Zealand. *International Journal of Human Resource Management*, 24(17), 3305–3324.

Haar, J. M., & Bardoel, E. A. (2008). Positive spillover from the work - family interface: A study of Australian employees. *Asia Pacific Journal of Human Resources*, 46(3), 275–287.

Haar, J. M., Russo, M., Suñe, A., & Ollier-Malaterre, A. (2014). Outcomes of work–life balance on job satisfaction, life satisfaction and mental health: A study across seven cultures. *Journal of Vocational Behavior*, 85(3), 361–373.

Hakanen, J. J., & Schaufeli, W. B. (2012). Do burnout and work engagement predict depressive symptoms and life satisfaction? A three-wave seven-year prospective study. *Journal of Affective Disorders*, 141(2–3), 415–424.

Harvey, S. B., Joyce, S., Tan, L., Johnson, A., Nguyen, H., Modini, M., & Growth, M. (2014). Developing a mentally healthy workplace: A review of the literature. *A Report for the National Mental Health Commission and Mentally Healthy Workplace Alliance*. University of New South Wales.

Hausmann, A., Slotow, R. O. B., Burns, J. K., & Di Minin, E. (2015). The ecosystem service of sense of place: Benefits for human well-being and biodiversity conservation. *Environmental Conservation*, 43(2), 117–127.

Henry, J. (2005). The healthy organization. In A. Antoniou and C. Cooper (Eds.), *Research Companion to Organizational Health Psychology*. Edward Elgar (pp. 382–391).

Innstrand, S. T., Langballe, E. M., & Falkum, E. (2012). A longitudinal study of the relationship between work engagement and symptoms of anxiety and depression. *Stress Health*, 28(1), 1–10.

Innstrand, S. T., Langballe, E. M., Espnes, G. A., Falkum, E., & Aasland, O. G. (2008). Positive and negative work-family interaction and burnout: A longitudinal study of reciprocal relations. *Work & Stress*, 22(1), 1–15.

Johnson, J. V., & Hall, E. M. (1988). Job strain, work place social support, and cardiovascular disease: a cross-sectional study of a random sample of the Swedish working population. *American Journal of Public Health*, 78(10), 1336–1342.

Karasek, R. A. (1979). Job demands, job decision latitude, and mental strain: implications for job redesign. *Administrative Science Quarterly*, 24(2), 285–308.

Kawachi, I., & Berkman, L. F. (2000). Social cohesion, social capital, and health. In L. F. Berkman and I. Kawachi (Eds.), *Social Epidemiology*. Oxford University Press (pp. 174–190).

Kawachi, I., & Berkman, L. F. (2001). Social ties and mental health. Journal of Urban Health, 78(3), 458–467.

Kinman, G., & Grant, L. (2011). Exploring stress resilience in trainee social workers: The role of emotional and social competencies. *British Journal of Social Work*, 41(2), 261–275.

Kossek, E. E., Pichler, S., Bodner, T., & Hammer, L. B. (2011). Workplace social support and work-family conflict: A meta-analysis clarifying the influence of general and work-family-specific supervisor and organizational support. *Personnel Psychology*, 64(2), 289–313.

Kossek, E. E., Valcour, M., & Lirio, P. (2014). The sustainable workforce: Organizational strategies for promoting work–life balance and wellbeing. In P.Y. Chen & C. L. Cooper (Eds.), *Work and Wellbeing: A Complete Reference Guide, Volume III*. John Wiley & Sons (pp. 295–319).

Kudryavtsev, A., Stedman, R. C., & Krasny, M. E. (2012). Sense of place in environmental education. *Environmental Education Research*, 18(2), 229–250.

Lambert, S. J., & Hopkins, K. (1995). Occupational conditions and workers' sense of community: Variations by gender and race. *American Journal of Community Psychology*, 23(2), 151–179.

Langford, D., Hancock, M. R., Fellows, R., & Gale, A. W. (1995). *Human Resources Management in Construction*. Longman.

Leiter, M. P., Laschinger, H. K. S., Day, A., & Oore, D. G. (2011). The impact of civility interventions on employee social behavior, distress, and attitudes. *Journal of Applied Psychology*, 96(6), 1258–1274.

Linley, P. A., Joseph, S., Harrington, S., & Wood, A. M. (2006). Positive psychology: Past, present, and (possible) future. *Journal of Positive Psychology*, 1(1), 3–16.

Maslach, C., & Leiter, M. P. (1997). *The Truth About Burnout: How Organizations Cause Personal Stress and What To Do About It*. Jossey-Bass.

McMillan, D. W. (1976). *Sense of Community: An Attempt at Definition*. Unpublished manuscript: George Peabody College.

McMillan, D. W., & Chavis, D. M. (1986). Sense of community: A definition and theory. *Journal of Community Psychology*, 14(1), 6–23.

Meyers, M. C., van Woerkom, M., & Bakker, A. B. (2013). The added value of the positive: A literature review of positive psychology interventions in organizations. *European Journal of Work and Organizational Psychology*, 22(5), 618–632.

Miller, N. G., Erickson, A., & Yust, B. L. (2001). Sense of place in the workplace: The relationship between personal objects and job satisfaction and motivation. *Journal of Interior Design*, 27(1), 35–44.

Mowday, R. T., Porter, L. W., & Steers, R. M. (1982) *Employee–Organization Linkages*. Academic Press.

Näswall, K., Kuntz, J., & Malinen, S. (2015). Employee Resilience Scale (EmpRes): *Technical Report. Resilient Organisations Research Report 2015/04*. ISSN 1178-7279.

Neves, P., & Eisenberger, R. (2014). Perceived organizational support and risk taking. *Journal of Managerial Psychology*, 29(2), 187–205.

Ng F., L., Scholes, S., Boniface, S., Mindell, J., & Stewart-Brown, S. (2017). Evaluating and establishing national norms for mental wellbeing using the short Warwick–Edinburgh Mental Well-being Scale (SWEMWBS): findings from the Health Survey for England. *Quality of Life Research*, 26(5), 1129–1144.

Pattnaik, S., & Tripathy, S. K. (2019). The journey of justice: Recounting milestones over the past six decades. *Management and Labour Studies*, 44(1), 58–85.

Pearson, C., Andersson, L., & Porath, C. (2000). Assessing and attacking workplace incivility. *Organizational Dynamics, 29*, 123–137.

Peterson, C. (2006). *A Primer in Positive Psychology.* Oxford University Press.

Peterson, N. A., Speer, P. W., & McMillan, D. W. (2008). Validation of A brief sense of community scale: Confirmation of the principal theory of sense of community. *Journal of Community Psychology, 36*(1), 61–73.

Project Management Institute. (2021). *Talent Gap: Ten-Year Employment Trends, Costs, and Global Implications.* Project Management Institute.

Roche, A. M., Pidd, K., Fischer, J. A., Lee, N., Scarfe, A., & Kostadinov, V. (2016). Men, work, and mental health: A systematic review of depression in male-dominated industries and occupations. *Safety and Health at Work, 7*(4), 268–283.

Sacker, A., & Schoon, I. (2007). Educational resilience in later life: Resources and assets in adolescence and return to education after leaving school at age 16. *Social Science Research, 36*(3), 873–896.

Schaufeli, W. B., Salanova, M., González-Romá, V., & Bakker, A. B. (2002). The measurement of engagement and burnout: A two sample confirmatory factor analytic approach. *Journal of Happiness Studies, 3*(1), 71–92.

Seligman, M. (2011). *Flourish: A New Understanding of Happiness, Well-being – and How to Achieve Them.* Nicholas Brealey Publishing.

Seligman, M., & Csikszentmihalyi, M. (2000). Positive psychology: An introduction. *American Psychologist, 55*(1), 5–14.

Shirazi, B., Langford, D. A., & Rowlinson, S. M. (1996). Organizational structures in the construction industry. *Construction Management and Economics, 14*(3), 199–212.

Stewart-Brown, S., Tennant, A., Tennant, R., Platt, S., Parkinson, J., & Weich, S. (2009). Internal construct validity of the Warwick-Edinburgh Mental Well-being Scale (WEMWBS): a Rasch analysis using data from the Scottish Health Education Population Survey. *Health and Quality of Life Outcomes, 7*(1), 1–8.

Torp, S., Grimsmo, A., Hagen, S., Duran, A., & Gudbergsson, S. B. (2013). Work engagement: A practical measure for workplace health promotion? *Health Promotion International, 28*(3), 387–396.

van Quaquebeke, N., & Eckloff, T. (2010). Defining respectful leadership: What it is, how it can be measured, and another glimpse at what it is related to. *Journal of Business Ethics, 91*(3), 343–358.

van Steenbergen, E. F., Ellemers, N., & Mooijaart, A. (2007). How work and family can facilitate each other: Distinct types of work-family facilitation and outcomes for women and men. *Journal of Occupational Health Psychology, 12*(3), 279–300.

Walsh, B. M., Magley, V. J., Reeves, D. W., Davies-Schrils, K. A., Marmet, M. D., & Gallus, J. A. (2012). Assessing workgroup norms for civility: The development of the civility norms questionnaire-brief. *Journal of Business and Psychology, 27*(4), 407–420.

Walters, G., & Raybould, M. (2007). Burnout and perceived organisational support among front-line hospitality employees. *Journal of Hospitality and Tourism Management, 14*(2), 144–156.

Windle, G. (2011). What is resilience? A review and concept analysis. *Reviews in Clinical Gerontology, 21*(02), 152–169

World Health Organization. (2017). *Building Resilience: A Key Pillar of Health 2020 and the Sustainable Development Goals.* World Health Organization.

11

THINKING ABOUT THE FUTURE

11.1   An unexpected turn

We started writing this book before the COVID-19 viral disease spread across the world, causing unprecedented disruption to people's work and personal lives. The pandemic had a direct effect on the health of construction workers. For example, by early April 2020, COVID-19 transmission was rampant among migrant construction workers living in purpose-built dormitories in Singapore and, by 6 May 2020, migrant workers accounted for 88 per cent of the total confirmed COVID cases recorded in Singapore (Koh, 2020). Although the transmission of COVID-19 infections among this group was swiftly addressed by a comprehensive programme of measures, the initial situation in Singapore highlights the vulnerability of migrant workers and the importance of providing adequate housing and healthcare to prevent such occurrences in the future. The transmission of COVID-19 among construction workers in Singapore was attributed to a lack of physical distancing in dormitories, in which workers shared cooking, eating, recreation and sanitary facilities.

The response to the COVID-19 pandemic varied from country to country. While some countries implemented strict lockdowns, travel bans, quarantine periods, mandatory mask wearing and other measures, others adopted much less stringent containment policies. The need to consider the trade-off between public health and business continuity was a key feature of decision making for governments during this time. Indeed, it was the construction industry's implementation of transmission control measures that ensured construction sites were permitted to continue operating (albeit in a limited capacity) during the peak of the pandemic in Australia. These measures included vaccine mandates, capping attendance at worksites, improving ventilation and ensuring density limits (one

DOI: 10.1201/9780367814236-11

person per four square metres) in site facilities and establishing worker shift "bubbles" where practical.

Despite the implementation of containment measures, evidence suggests construction workers were relatively hard hit by COVID-19 and decisions taken to keep construction sites operating during the pandemic may have cost lives (particularly those of low skilled workers). In the US State of Texas, the continuation of construction work during a "lockdown" period is estimated to have produced a fivefold increase in hospitalisation of construction workers compared to non-construction workers (Pasco et al., 2020). Similarly, in the UK, site-based construction workers experienced higher mortality rates from COVID-19 than office-based construction professionals (who could work remotely during the pandemic). Between 9 March 2020 and 28 December 2020 in England and Wales, 70 low skilled construction workers died from COVID-19, a rate of 82.1/100,000 workers; 224 workers in construction building trades died from COVID-19, a rate of 37.3/100,000 workers; and 75 building finishing trade workers died from COVID-19, a rate of 42.6/100,000 workers. This compares with 34 engineering professionals (10.8/100,000 workers) and 20 architects, town planners and surveyors (12.1/100,000 workers) (Office For National Statistics, 2021). The continuation of construction work during the pandemic also potentially undermined the effectiveness of containment measures put in place to protect the broader community because locally integrated construction workers would then transmit the virus to family members and other people they interacted with outside the workplace (Pasco et al., 2020).

During the pandemic all workers faced a dual threat of economic stress and exposure to the virus (Sinclair et al., 2021). In some cases one threat may have been traded off against another, as workers in low income jobs or low security jobs may have been more likely to risk their physical health to maintain their employment. The willingness to work on site irrespective of perceived risk was observed among self-employed construction workers in the UK construction industry (Jones et al., 2021). Workers with limited financial resources at the start of the pandemic would also be less able to grapple with the disruption and demands created by lockdown conditions, such as the requirement to school children at home, the need to purchase protective equipment, and shortages of food and basic provisions. It is highly likely that, through the interaction of the dual threats identified by Sinclair et al. (2021), the pandemic has increased both health and economic inequalities within the construction workforce.

The COVID-19 pandemic also shone a bright light on the importance of managing workers' health and safety which became a fundamental organisational priority during this time (Sinclair et al., 2020). The continued operation, and in some cases survival, of businesses depended upon their ability to manage workers' health and safety. Never before has the health and safety of workers been elevated to such strategic importance within construction organisations.

During this time there has also been a blurring of occupational health and public health, as workplaces could become super-spreading environments and the effective management of workers' health was therefore critical to containing the virus in the broader community (Gross et al., 2021). The broadening of "occupational health" to "worker health" reflects a more public health-oriented approach in which the focus is on managing a population of workers more holistically, with consideration of exposures that occur at work, as well as exposures and effects that occur in workers' families and communities (see also Peckham et al., 2017).

A more holistic approach to understanding the exposures and effects of the COVID-19 pandemic includes a consideration of both physical and psychological health. There is considerable evidence that the pandemic has taken a substantial toll on psychological health in the general population. For example, a survey of 5,070 Australian adults during the pandemic found that 78 per cent of respondents experienced deteriorated mental health compared with the beginning of the pandemic. More than 50 per cent of participants reportedly experienced elevated psychological distress, depression, stress, and anxiety, which was attributed to feelings of uncertainty about the future, loneliness, and financial concerns (Newby et al., 2020).

Similar effects have been reported in the construction workforce. In the USA, data collected from construction workers in 2019 and 2020 revealed that 42.9 per cent of workers felt more anxious or depressed in 2020 than they did in 2019 (Brown et al., 2022). Particularly high increases were observed in younger workers, female workers, part-time workers and workers whose family income is below the poverty level. The more pronounced deterioration among part-time construction workers and those with low family incomes suggests that economic stressors may have exacerbated the damaging effects of the pandemic on the psychological health of construction workers.

Caponecchia and Mayland (2020) observe that the pandemic raised the profile of mental health, with more organisations now recognising the need to manage work-related risks to workers' mental health. They suggest that transitioning out of the pandemic[1] presents a golden opportunity to "maintain the rage" in relation to protecting workers' mental health and to radically redesign work tasks and structures in ways that eliminate psychosocial risk factors associated with poor mental health. This is an extremely important observation and it is critical that organisations do not lapse quickly back into "business as usual" without taking stock of the lessons learned during the pandemic. Unfortunately, in Australia, the construction industry is already experiencing "after-effects" of the pandemic. As case numbers decline and restrictions have gradually eased, Australian construction workers have been left facing significant project delays caused by labour shortages, supply chain disruptions and rising costs of materials. In the context of huge demand created by governments ostensibly to support the construction industry during lockdown, the pressures faced by construction workers are arguably greater than they were at the height of the pandemic (and stress-levels are reportedly worse than pre-COVID levels). The opportunities to significantly change the industry in ways that reduce the risk of psychological harm in the post-pandemic era may be lost if significant action does not occur quickly.

As economies emerge from the pandemic and COVID-19 containment measures come to an end, occupational health professionals are also focusing on return-to-work processes and the provision of social support to workers whose health may have been affected by the pandemic. It is important to recognise that the risk of serious health effects associated with COVID-19 has not magically disappeared. For example, people who suffer from chronic obstructive pulmonary disease (COPD) are particularly susceptible to severe COVID-19 (Johansen et al., 2022). The prevalence of COPD among construction workers is high (see Chapter 2), making workers with this particular condition a high-risk group whose health needs to be considered as workplaces return to full capacity and infection control measures are relaxed. Some workers may also be experiencing longer-term effects of COVID-19. So-called "long COVID" is reported to cause fatigue, shortness of breath, cardiac abnormalities, cognitive impairment, sleep disturbances, symptoms of post-traumatic stress disorder, muscle pain, concentration problems and headaches (Crook et al., 2021). Godeau et al. (2021) recommend that specific strategies be implemented to promote the safe return to work of workers experiencing these symptoms, some of which could have significant implications for workers in the high-risk construction work context.

In addition to managing the physical and mental health "fallout" from the pandemic, global economic impacts threaten to bring a second wave of health consequences that will also need to be managed (Burdorf et al., 2020). Economic recessions create hardship, including unemployment, income decline and unmanageable debt, all of which are significantly associated with poor psychological health, increased rates of common mental disorders, substance-related disorders and suicidal behaviours (Frasquilho et al., 2015; Karanikolos et al., 2016) As with the COVID-19 pandemic itself, the negative health effects of economic recession are likely to have a disproportionately more damaging effect on workers with particular vulnerabilities, including migrant workers and those in precarious forms of employment (Godderis & Luyten, 2020). It is likely that the pandemic will have a long tail with respect to the effects on sections of the construction industry's workforce.

Notwithstanding these ongoing challenges, the radically disruptive nature of the COVID-19 pandemic has been identified as an opportunity for policymakers, employers, unions and academics to rethink the construction industry's production systems with a particular focus on how to make the industry work better for its people (Sherratt & Dainty, 2022). Case study data collected during the height of the pandemic suggests that dramatically changing systems of work in construction projects, with a priority focus on workers' health and safety, can also improve productivity and workers' effectiveness (Jones et al., 2021). The question as to whether organisational and site-wide changes made during the pandemic can (and should) be sustained post-pandemic is an important one to consider.

11.2 Lessons learned about working from home during the COVID-19 pandemic

Working from home for white-collar construction workers is one practice that may be sustained in some organisations. However, the circumstances in which working from home is healthy and the extent to which new forms of risk are introduced by working remotely need to be understood.

During the COVID-19 pandemic, working from home was an effective COVID-19 containment approach. Teams could still operate as video-conferencing was introduced as a substitute for face-to-face interaction. Working from home in ordinary circumstances is regarded as having positive effects on health and wellbeing because it is purported to increase control over work hours, reduce feelings of being rushed, increase job satisfaction, lower stress, eliminate time spent commuting, and reduce work–life conflict (Gajendran & Harrison, 2007; Montreuil & Lippel, 2003). However, during the COVID-19 pandemic, the dramatic shift to working from home occurred under conditions that were far from normal. Work from home requirements were mandated swiftly, leaving workers and organisations little time to adjust (Bouziri et al., 2020). These involuntary work from home measures were also in place for an extended period of time (Caligiuri et al., 2020).

The health benefits associated with working from home are ambiguous and questions arise as to who benefits most, workers or their employing organisations (Wheatley, 2012). Despite the potential health benefits, working at home can reduce social support and contribute to social isolation and psychological strain (Cooper & Kurland, 2002; Bentley et al., 2016). Work hours are also longer amongst people who work from home frequently, with many reporting working in excess of their contracted work hours (Felstead & Henseke, 2017). Work–family boundaries can be blurred and negative spillover can arise whereby work interferes with family and personal time (Hallin, 2020). During the pandemic, evidence is also emerging to show that people working from home experienced a significant increase in sedentary behaviour, worsened sleep quality, increased mood disturbance, a reduction in quality of life and a decrease in work-related health (Barrone Gibbs et al., 2021).

Moreover, the health effects of working from home have a gendered aspect. Women who work from home can find themselves working a "double shift" in which hours spent in domestic and caring work added to those spent in paid work amount to a very long working day (Wheatley, 2012). This gendered effect was arguably exacerbated during the pandemic as the closure of schools and childcare facilities increased the demand for care work at home (Yavorsky et al., 2020). While childcare responsibilities increased for both men and women during the COVID-19 pandemic, some studies suggest that women were more severely affected than men in terms of their workload, health and wellbeing (Croda & Grossbard, 2021). A study undertaken in the UK found that parents of young children needed to provide the equivalent of a full-time working week of additional care during lockdown. Women provided approximately 10 hours more of this care each week than men, irrespective of their involvement in paid work (Sevilla & Smith, 2020). This is likely to have taken a toll on the psychological health of women working from home during the pandemic (Zamarro & Prados, 2021). (See also Chapter 4 for a discussion of work hours, caring responsibilities and women's health.)

Case example 11.1 highlights the ambiguous link between working from home and workers' health. It is important that, in the post-pandemic era, work from home arrangements are carefully designed and implemented to deliver positive health benefits and reduce the risks of overwork, social isolation and work–family conflict.

CASE EXAMPLE 11.1 WORKING TIME AND MENTAL HEALTH DURING THE COVID-19 PANDEMIC

During the COVID-19 pandemic, the construction industry was classified as an essential sector in Australia. This meant that, despite the social distancing requirements, construction activities were expected to continue, even when other non-essential industries were forced to close. In order to achieve this, flexible work arrangements, such as working from home or weekly alterations between working on site and working from home were implemented.

Data was collected from project-based workers who worked from home on alternate weeks in an effort to reduce the number of people in project offices. Data was collected weekly and subsequently fortnightly from 3 different project sites during this period and a total of 548 responses were received. Some participants also provided comments about their experiences. Participants in the study included construction workers, foremen, site managers, engineers, design managers, project leaders and employees in specialty support roles.

Mental health was observed to decline steadily and significantly during the data collection period. However, both positive and negative experiences of working from home during the pandemic were identified. Some employees preferred working from home because: (i) it saved time getting ready for work and commuting; (ii) they enjoyed being able to work flexibly and have more time available for family and other non-work activities; and (iii) they were able to eat more healthily and do more exercise than when working in the office. However, the study also highlighted some negative impacts on mental wellbeing including: (i) feeling time pressure; (ii) experiencing work interference with non-work activities; and (iii) working long hours.

Importantly the negative relationships between long work hours, feeling time pressured and work interfering with non-work life were all fully mediated by employees' satisfaction with their work–life balance. That is, the dissatisfaction with work–life balance created by long hours, perceived time pressure and work–life conflict was the pathway through which these experiences affected employees' mental health. Comments made by some of the employees suggest that working at home served to blur the boundaries between work and non-work life, reducing their satisfaction with work–life balance. For example, one employee commented: *"As our work is at home now, it becomes difficult to shut off work. Emails and correspondence are sent at all hours of the day and night and one never is able to get on top of it all."* Another explained: *"Separating work from life has become difficult, I have noticed that the smallest aspect of taking the train into the city allows me time to get into work mode and be ready to work for the day."* Employees with caring responsibilities experienced working from home as particularly challenging: *"The biggest issue I have is balancing care of a child, work and downtime. I feel downtime is getting less and less."*

Pirzadeh & Lingard (2021)

11.3   Future issues in work and health

Even before the COVID-19 pandemic, it was observed that rapid and substantial changes were occurring to the nature of work, workplaces and the workforce (Schulte et al., 2020). Some of these changes have been amplified by the COVID-19 pandemic – for example, organisations are more accepting of workers engaging in work remotely rather than from a dedicated location, the traditional workplace. These changes alter the way that "old" occupational hazards – i.e., those that have been known to exist for a long time – are experienced by workers. Irrespective of where work is undertaken, workers need access to ergonomically designed workstations and equipment. During COVID-19, workers frequently worked at dining tables and kitchen benchtops. The extent to which organisations intervened to ensure remote work was conducted in a safe and healthy work environment is unclear but it is likely that the risk of injury was increased for many workers as a result of a lack of attention to office ergonomics (Tamers et al., 2020).

It is worth noting here that the construction industry still has some way to go in improving the management of ergonomic hazards that are less "visible" than other occupational safety hazards. Many site-based work activities are performed today in the same way, using the same tools and equipment, as they have been performed for many decades. Researchers in the field of ergonomics have noted the construction industry's resistance to adopting new ways of working that reduce risks associated with poor design of work processes and equipment (Boatman et al., 2015; Sneller et al., 2018). Steel fixing is a case in point. Steel fixing involves positioning steel rods (sometimes referred to as rebar) and fixing them together using wire ties in preparation for concreting work.

Steel fixing is a high-risk activity for musculoskeletal injury as a result of awkward trunk postures, repetitive bending of the back, and twisting and flexion of the wrist when using traditional pincer-cutters to twist and cut steel wire ties. Ergonomically designed tools are available that significantly reduce the risk of back and wrist injury, yet Australian research showed that these tools are not in widespread use in the construction industry (Lingard et al., 2019). This is but one example of the construction industry's ambivalence in relation to preventing harm to workers. Although musculoskeletal injury is frequently experienced as debilitating (and sometimes career-ending) by construction workers, known ergonomic solutions to reduce the risk of harm to the musculoskeletal system are often not implemented. While ergonomic hazards in construction work are certainly not new, the prevalence of musculoskeletal injury in the industry highlights the need for ergonomics to be central to conversations about future issues in work and health in the sector.

Having noted that some "old" occupational health hazards faced by construction workers warrant greater management attention, it is also true that the profile and mix of hazards experienced by workers will change in the future as it is shaped by broader societal and environmental trends.

11.4 Climate change and workers' health

In 2009 the National Institute for Occupational Safety and Health (USA) developed a preliminary framework describing how workers' health and safety could be affected by climate change (Schulte & Chun, 2009). Seven categories of climate-related hazards were identified in this framework, as follows: (1) increased ambient temperature; (2) air pollution; (3) exposure to ultraviolet light radiation; (4) extreme weather; (5) vector-borne diseases and expanded habitats; (6) industrial transitions and emerging technologies; and (7) changes in the built environment (Schulte et al., 2016).

Heat stress causes serious acute and chronic health effects, including heat stroke, death and fatal chronic kidney disease, as well as increased accidental injury risk due to the effects of extreme heat on human performance (Kjellstrom et al., 2016). The normal core temperature of the human body is 37°C. Physical activity increases body heat through metabolic processes. This heat can be lost through sweating and convection (contact with cooler air). However, hot and humid conditions reduce the ability for heat to be lost and the core body temperature can increase in these conditions. Diminished work capacity occurs if the core temperature increases above 38°C and acute heat disorders (heatstroke) can occur if the core temperature reaches 39°C (Kjellstrom et al., 2009).

There is already evidence to suggest construction workers are a high-risk occupational group for work-related heat stress, due to the nature of their work, i.e., physically demanding work often undertaken in outdoor environments (Acharya et al., 2018). For example, in the USA between 1992 and 2016, construction workers made up 6 per cent of the workforce, but accounted for 19 per cent of all work-related deaths and 36 per cent of all work-related heat-related deaths (Dong et al, 2019). Moreover, while construction worker fatalities declined steadily between 1992 and 2016, heat-related work-related deaths increased significantly. The increase in heat-related work-related deaths among construction workers was significantly correlated with rising temperatures in the USA during this period (Dong et al., 2019).

It is also evident that particular groups of construction workers may be particularly at risk of heat-related health effects. For example, migrant workers, whose employment is often precarious, may be at greater risk. In the US construction industry, a statistically higher risk of heat-related deaths was found among Hispanic workers born in Mexico than among other worker groups (Dong et al., 2019). It is also reported that migrant construction workers in Qatar were required to work in temperatures of up to 45°C for up to 10 hours a day during the construction of infrastructure related to the FIFA World Cup (The Guardian, 2019). Pradhan et al. (2019) report an average annual death rate of 150/100,000 workers among Nepali construction workers in Qatar during the FIFA World Cup construction programme. These workers were aged between 25 and 35 years.

Many of these Nepali migrant worker deaths were attributed to cardiovascular disease and a strong correlation was found between average monthly afternoon heat levels and cardiovascular deaths.

Heat stress is preventable through measures such as stopping work during periods of high ambient temperature, taking rest breaks commensurate with work rate and temperature, staying hydrated, and wearing appropriate clothing (light-coloured, loose clothing made of natural fibres wherever possible) and wearing sunscreen, sunglasses and broad brimmed hats. It is noteworthy that Pradhan et al. (2019) estimate that up to 200 of the 571 Nepali migrant worker deaths recorded in Qatar between 2009 and 2017 could have been prevented if effective heat protection had been implemented. Importantly, Qatar introduced new laws in 2021 prohibiting work outside between 10:00 and 15:30 from 1 June to 15 September and requiring that all work must stop (irrespective of time) if the wet-bulb globe temperature[2] (WBGT) rises above 32.1°C in a workplace. Requirements for annual worker health checks and mandatory risk assessments by employers were also introduced in Qatar (ILO, 2021).

Technical guidelines identify maximum heat exposures for work undertaken at different levels of intensity. For example, the ISO 7243 (ISO, 1989) recommends the duration of rest breaks as a percentage of working time that should be taken based on the WBGT and work intensity in order to prevent workers' body core temperature rising above 38°C. For very heavy work, the international standard recommends a 25 per cent rest/hour ratio at a WBGT of 26.5°C, increasing to a 50 per cent rest/hour ratio at a WBGT of 28°C, 75 per cent rest/hour ratio at a WBGT of 31°C. US (NIOSH) guidance also specifies that no very heavy work should be performed at all at a WBGT of 34°C (Kjellstrom et al., 2009). Importantly, however, these guidelines do not have legal force (Xiang et al., 2016) and the extent to which they are followed is questionable.

Even when clear thresholds are included in binding industrial agreements, employers may resist requests to stop work. For example, enterprise agreements between construction industry unions and employers routinely specify that (unless in an air-conditioned environment) work is to stop when the ambient temperature reaches 35°C or where the temperature is 28°C and the humidity is 75 per cent. However, workers report pressure to continue working when temperatures reach these thresholds and it is unlikely that stop work measures will be implemented in workplaces without union representation (Newman & Humphrys, 2020). It is also reported that construction workers in precarious employment are less inclined to take rest and hydration breaks during hot weather due to concerns about the effect of this on their pay and/or employment security (Schulte et al., 2016). Migrant construction workers whose work is characterised by poor and dangerous working conditions, low and sometimes stolen wages and limited benefits are likely to be particularly susceptible to these concerns (Torres et al., 2013).

Rising temperatures in many parts of the world associated with climate change are increasing the risk of heat-related illness (Ansah et al., 2021) and climate change has been described as "a threat to safe, comfortable and productive thermal working environments for a significant part of the global population" (Kjellstrom et al., 2009 p.5). The challenge for construction is that, while it may be economically feasible to cool indoor working environments, working outdoors is much more challenging. Kjellstrom et al. (2016) estimate that climate change will reduce available work hours in all regions between 1975 and 2050, with the highest reductions in Southeast Asia (18.2%), Central America (18.6%), West Africa (15.8%), Central Africa (15.4%), Oceania (15.2%), the Caribbean (11.7%) and South Asia (11.5%). While not the most affected area, countries like Australia are not exempt from these effects. It is estimated that dangerous days for outdoor workers in Australia will increase from the present 1 day per year, to 15–27 days per year by 2070 (Xiang et al., 2016).

Increasing temperature linked to climate change has implications for the scheduling and management of construction projects. If more days are likely to be lost due to hot weather and workers require more frequent rest breaks during the workday (in order to work safely), this will affect the amount of work that can be done in a given day, week or month. Unless these factors are considered when estimating the realistic duration of a project, the likely result will be increased time pressures borne by workers – whose health is affected by already tight project timelines (see also Chapter 4). Moreover, in geographic areas where outside work can only be performed during cooler times of the day, more work may need to be undertaken outside daylight hours. This has the potential to increase conflict between work and non-work life and, in the case of nightwork, could also disrupt circadian rhythms and adversely affect workers' health (Costa, 1996).

It is not only rising temperatures linked to climate change that affect workers' health. Global warming is also reported to reduce air quality and increase air pollution which can affect outdoor workers. The effects of exposure to air pollution during outdoor work are amplified when work is physically demanding as respiratory rates are increased (Schulte et al., 2016). The interaction of greenhouse gases, climate change and ozone depletion also produce higher levels of ultraviolet radiation, increasing the risk to outdoor workers (Schulte et al., 2016). There is evidence that construction workers are a high-risk group for skin cancer. However, compared to other occupational groups, construction workers are less likely to adopt prevention measures for skin cancer, highlighting the need for interventions to better protect construction workers from exposure to ultraviolet radiation (Ragan et al., 2019). Climate change (through rising temperatures) also increases the risk to outdoor workers posed by vector-borne diseases and other biological hazards (e.g., moulds, pollens and fungal spores) (Schulte et al., 2016).

Climate change is linked to an increased frequency of extreme weather events, such as floods, landslides, droughts, and wildfires (Schulte et al., 2016). The safety of outdoor workers can be directly threatened by these events, but construction workers may also experience increased risks to health and safety during the clean-up and rebuilding activity that often follows these events (Uddin et al., 2021). For example, workers can be exposed to raw sewage, mould, asbestos, lead, dust and carbon monoxide, as well as traditional construction-related safety hazards (electrocution, slips, trips and falls, etc.) (Rosen et al. 2015).

Climate change can also adversely affect the psychological health of people who experience extreme heat or weather. This experience may be compounded by resource loss caused by drought, rising sea levels, etc. and social strain or anxiety associated with knowledge and awareness of the effects of climate change on the planet (Hayes & Poland, 2018).

Construction workers will inevitably be heavily involved in measures to decarbonise the built environment, including retrofitting buildings to conserve energy and the construction of new infrastructure to support the production of renewable energy. "Green" buildings are widely purported to improve the health and wellbeing of their occupants; however, the occupational health of those that construct green buildings has received far less attention. It is important that, as these changes occur, the occupational health (and safety) implications for construction workers are understood and managed. For example, the International Labour Organization (2019) identifies some new and significant health risks associated with "green" technologies. Wind turbine construction, for example, exposes workers to the risk of falls from heights, musculoskeletal disorders, awkward postures, physical load, electrocution, and injuries from working with rotating machinery and falling objects.

Construction workers' health is also starting to be recognised as an important component of a sustainable built environment. For example, in Australia, a rating system designed to improve the energy and environmental performance of buildings recognises and awards credit for evidence of Responsible Construction Practices. Criteria for the Responsible Construction Practices credit include a requirement that constructors of a building "promote positive mental and physical health outcomes of site activities and culture of site workers, through programs and solutions on site" (Green Building Council of Australia, 2022). The inclusion of construction workers' health in such schemes is welcome and acknowledges that buildings and other structures cannot in all fairness be considered to be sustainable if people are harmed during their construction.

11.5 New models of work and health

The previous discussion of climate change highlights the complex interrelationship that exists between the health of the planet and workers' health because industries and jobs of the future will inevitably be shaped by climate change in some way or other. Moreover, without serious and committed action to reduce emissions of carbon dioxide and other greenhouse gases, both work and health will become increasingly precarious for many people.

Given their global significance and far-reaching consequences, human-made disasters, including the COVID-19 pandemic and climate change, place increased focus on health (inside and outside the workplace). However, these occurrences also exposed weaknesses in the way that occupational health has historically been understood, i.e., with a narrow focus on the prevention of harm occurring within the confines of the workplace.

New models are proposed which expand the remit of work health and safety, by shifting from a narrow "labour approach" to a more strategic "public health approach" (Harrison & Dawson, 2016). Such a shift involves extending the remit of occupational health and safety both horizontally and vertically (Felknor et al., 2021). Horizontal expansion extends traditional models of occupational health and safety to include consideration of personal, social, and economic risk factors that affect workers' health and safety outside the workplace. This expansion recognises that workers' health and safety is shaped by interactions between experiences that occur in work as well as other life domains. Non-traditional hazards, such as low wages and imbalance between work and personal life, are recognised in this broader concept of work health and safety (Felknor et al., 2021).

The International Labour Organization (2019) similarly points out that occupational health and safety is not confined to the workplace because people's occupational health and safety experiences clearly affect people's general health and wellbeing, as well as social health in the communities in which workers live. The ILO calls for closer connections to be drawn between occupational and public health and suggests that occupational health can play a greater role in community health promotion as well as the prevention and management of psychosocial risks, mental health disorders and non-communicable diseases (such as hypertension, cardiovascular disease, gastrointestinal disorders, diabetes and other causes of mortality) (ILO, 2019).

There is also growing recognition that workers' needs and health outcomes are shaped not only by their own employment experiences, but by all the jobs held by people within their households (Tamers et al., 2020). Chapter 4 discussed the health implications of working long hours in construction jobs. It is no doubt true that construction workers' health is adversely affected by working long hours. However, we argue that, to appreciate the health effects of work hours in totality, long hours must be understood in relation to the combined work hours of all people within the same household (Jacobs & Gersen, 2001). Rather than one member of a household (usually a man) working up to 80 hours a week, it is worth considering what it would look like if both partners worked 35 hours a week and more equally shared domestic and caring work. Would this contribute to improved health and wellbeing of construction workers, their domestic partners and family members?

Vertical expansion of the occupational health concept also involves extending the traditional narrow focus of occupational health professionals on preventing work-related ill health to include an additional focus on the promotion of workers' positive wellbeing. Wellbeing is a broader concept than health which includes physically safe and healthy conditions of work but also "includes environmental factors affecting mental health and features social support, autonomy and self-determination in a more aspirational concept of holistic health" (Peckham et al., 2017, p. 9). Therefore, to adequately address wellbeing, organisations need to consider the design and provision of decent work, good quality jobs and opportunities for workers to have some control over the ways they work to ensure a good person-job "fit."

Vertical expansion of the traditional occupational health and safety concept includes consideration of the cumulative health effects that workers experience over their working life continuum, including those that occur pre- and post-employment. Rather than focusing solely on managing hazards and risks in a single workplace, this approach considers the way that periods of under- and over-employment shape health outcomes as workers transition through different ages, jobs and life stages (Felknor et al., 2021). The ILO (2019) points out that the norm for most workers is now to work for many employers and even work in several different jobs and careers over their working lives. Jobs and employment in construction are also more transient and temporary than in many other sectors. Over the life course, workers' health is shaped by occupational, personal, social and economic risk factors which interact in complex ways. Consequently, health (and safety) are best understood as cumulative products of a broad range of experiences across the entire work life continuum. Promoting positive health therefore involves supporting workers and investing in their capabilities and skills development to ensure that they are able to effectively manage the transitions that take place over their entire life course (ILO, 2019).

Adopting a public health (as opposed to a labour approach) to workers' health is not necessarily easy. There is an inherent danger that employers will opt to implement individual approaches such as vitality/fitness programmes and support for coping behaviours, instead of primary prevention programmes that focus on removing psychosocial hazards from workplaces and processes and improving the quality of work through job design (Schulte et al., 2019). It is therefore important that employers' responsibility for organising work in such a way as to protect and promote workers' health and wellbeing take precedence over strategies that attribute blame for poor health on individual workers (Schulte et al., 2019). For example, previous research in the construction industry highlights that well-intentioned strategies to promote healthy lifestyle behaviours in blue-collar workers (the provision of fruit and yoga classes) had little beneficial effect on health or health-related behaviour of workers who were overworked and concerned about their job security (Lingard & Turner, 2015). Adopting a higher level of conceptualisation of wellbeing requires that construction employers address organisational cultural and job-related factors that cause harm and prevent workers from achieving happy and fulfilled work and non-work lives. Dextras-Gauthier et al. (2012, p.97) similarly argue that "when dealing with mental health issues, including burnout, depression, and psychological distress, managers need to tread further upstream to identify those elements of organisational culture that are ultimately causing ill health."

Case example 11.2 provides an example of a collaborative industry-government initiative to address the cultural challenge of long work hours and wellbeing in the Australian construction industry.

CASE STUDY 11.2 SUPPORTING WELLBEING THROUGH A COLLABORATIVE CULTURE CHANGE INITIATIVE

In recognition that employment and labour patterns inherent in the Australian construction industry are harmful for workers, the Australian Constructors Association (representing construction employers) has partnered with two state governments (New South Wales and Victoria) to develop a Culture Standard that is expected to ultimately form part of government procurement requirements.

The aim of the Culture Standard is to drive cultural change and create a construction industry in which all workers feel valued, wellbeing is prioritised across all job roles, work hours are capped and everyone has access to flexible work options so they have time for life.

The Culture Standard focuses on three key challenges facing the industry that can be addressed through improved collaboration between clients and contractors: (i) time for life outside of work; (ii) gender diversity; and (iii) mental wellbeing. To meet the aims of the Culture Standard, contractors will programme their project to:

- target that all workers work 50 hours or less per week, and
- ensure that no workers work over 55 hours per week, and
- operate the site from Monday to Friday or, where this is not viable (such as projects requiring occupancy or continuous plant activity), demonstrate why and ensure all workers are working a five day per week programme.

The involvement of government (as a major client of the construction industry) and private construction organisations is critical to the success of the initiative. This case study highlights that an industry-wide approach is needed to introduce cultural change which supports and protects workers' health.

In this chapter we have highlighted the growing integration between public health and occupational health. Throughout this book we have also highlighted that health must be considered as the product of broader systems of organisation and work. In doing so, Chapter 1 referred to the social determinants of health and the need to address these in order to overcome health inequality. Some of the factors that have come to be recognised as having a direct impact on health at the individual level include education, employment, social environments, physical environments, and gender. Along with the individually based determinants, there are more broad-based determinants of health that act at the community, population, and national levels (Knibb-Lamouche, 2012). Culture, spiritual wellbeing and connectedness to nature and the environment have been identified as determinants of health for Indigenous populations (Hayes & Poland, 2018), yet this has received little attention in the context of workers' health and wellbeing. Arguably, there is a need to incorporate ecological, spiritual, historical and cultural factors into our understanding of the determinants of health, along with the more commonly cited social and economic factors. In case example 11.3, we describe a health and wellbeing programme which was implemented at a large construction organisation in New Zealand that is aligned with the country's Indigenous understanding of health.

There is growing recognition of the need for culturally safe care and support to improve the health outcomes of minority populations which may include first nations and Indigenous peoples (Knibb-Lamouche, 2012). Arguably, organisations employing workers from minority populations have an important role to play in creating culturally safe workplaces which are sensitive to and respect cultural values and beliefs and enable health and wellbeing. Importantly, health can have specific meanings amongst cultures (e.g., Durie, 1985) which can shape beliefs, values and associated behaviours.

CASE EXAMPLE 11.3 INCORPORATING THE CULTURAL DIMENSIONS OF HEALTH INTO A HEALTH AND WELLBEING PROGRAMME

The Māori are the Indigenous people of New Zealand, and Māori health is underpinned by four dimensions representing the basic beliefs of life – te taha hinengaro (mental health); te taha tinana (physical health); te taha whānau (family health); and te taha wairua (spiritual health) (Ministry of Health, 2017). Spiritual health is not necessarily aligned with a religion but can be understood as having a sense of meaning and value. The four dimensions of health are represented by the four walls of a house.

A health and wellbeing programme incorporating the four dimensions of Māori health was developed by Dr David Beaumont, who practised as a traditional physician prior to exploring a new way of thinking about health using a positive approach that is firmly embedded within New Zealand's cultural beliefs (Beaumont, 2021). The programme takes a whole-of-person approach and seeks to enable participants to live life to their full potential by taking control and flourishing: *"What the program does is actually to get people to map out what the next six months of their lives are going to look like in all four of those domains. Physical, psychological, family, and spiritual."*

In response to the mental health challenges arising from the COVID-19 pandemic, workers from a large construction organisation in New Zealand participated in the programme. At the commencement of the programme, participants were challenged to consider whether they took a passive role in their life: *"that is generally where we believe that life happens to you and that we're passive players in the world that happens around us. But it's not true. And actually, here is the opportunity for you to become the hero of your own journey and even more than that, the ability to shape your own destiny."* One of the ways in which this programme differs from other programmes is that it *"provides people with a framework of understanding and gives them some tools ... as health and wellbeing cannot be separated from our lives."*

One of the construction participants provided some feedback on the programme to Dr Beaumont: *"A big Māori guy came up to me at morning tea and he said: 'I've realized what you're doing, you know, if you told us what to do and we didn't do it or it didn't work, we'd blame you but because we're developing the plan ourselves if we don't make it happen, or if it doesn't work, we only have ourselves to blame.'."* This reflection highlights that individuals find a sense of meaning and value in different ways and that imposing solutions on people may not be beneficial for their health and wellbeing. Furthermore, it is critical for organisations that health is considered more broadly than just in the workplace, as health can have a cultural context and meaning which is illustrated in this case example.

As outlined in Chapter 1, the World Health Organization defines health broadly as "a state of complete physical, mental and social well-being, and not merely the absence of disease" (WHO, 2010, p. 15). This definition of health is widely cited, but has been criticised as being too narrow (e.g., Card, 2017; Charlier et al., 2017; Leonardi, 2018; Oleribe et al., 2018). A common criticism is the definition's requirement for "complete [...] well-being." A multitude of alternative health definitions have been proposed, yet there are still debates and disagreements on the precise meaning of health. Arguably, such debates are useful in challenging us to consider what health is and how it should be supported within a workforce. Leonardi (2018) cautions us to critically reflect on definitions of health and how they might be applied within different segments of the population: "if we construct health on the basis of Western society's upper-middle class ethic, people belonging to a different class or different ethnic group will be assessed by a cultural bias, and their own health will be underestimated" (p.740).

In response to the limitations of current health definitions, Leonardi (2018, pp.740–741) proposes nine features which should be incorporated into future health definitions:

1. Move beyond the absence of diseases or infirmities and the biophysical parameters to avoid the old well-established reductionism of medicine.
2. Be conceptualized as a capability, because health as a concept becomes coherent when it is conceived as a capability, or more precisely, a cluster of capabilities.
3. Be considered as an ongoing, iterative, and dynamic process, not as a state to reach to catch the complexity of this phenomenon, avoiding neglect of some dynamic and iterative aspects of healthy conditions.
4. Be potentially achievable for everyone in real life, in all circumstances, at every age, regardless of cultural or socioeconomic status, race, or religion, to avoid becoming a utopia.
5. Include both malaise and wellbeing, because most people cope daily with negative events and therefore feel unease, sorrow, and unpleasant emotions without reporting a loss of health. The inclusion of malaise in a definition of health is strategic for contrasting medicalization of society and reducing cultural bias to consider health as an ideal condition: it allows one to have realistic expectations about it and to be healthy even when one is coping with negative events. For older people or those affected by chronic illness, health can be understood only as the ability to live with restrictions, to accept physical deficits, and to find an arrangement with these.
6. Overcome individualistic approaches, because it can no longer be considered a property of an abstract individual independent from living context, but, at the same time, health cannot be solely reduced to an outcome of social determinants.
7. Be independent of moral and ethical discourse, even if it is unavoidable that each definition of health is an implicit expression of particular social-cultural norms. This aspect is very important because it allows one to avoid the problem of conflating morals with scientific assessments, but its concrete application might not be easy because value-laden statements are involved in several facets of health.
8. Be based on a person's priorities, values, needs, aspirations, and goals to integrate the patient's personal experience into medical practice and to take

account of those subjective factors which have an important role in a person's health (it may entail a loss in terms of measurability and standardisation, but it increases the construct validity). This implies the adoption of an idiographic perspective, based on the specific individual and his or her unique point of view, rejecting a nomothetic perspective aimed at finding general laws which explain health phenomena for all individuals.

9. Be operational and measurable by clear, concrete, and definite processes to become a useful concept in real situations. Of course, as with all abstract concepts, health cannot be measured directly but only by indicators, which must be constructed on the base of the definition of health.

Inclusion of these features "allow(s) one to construct many definitions of health, among which one can choose the most useful for achieving the knowledge and operational goals pursued in the different scopes of application" (Leonardi, 2018, p.741).

11.6 Technology

A key feature of construction now and into the future is the increasing use of technology. The effects of rapid technological change (for example, digitisation, automation and artificial intelligence) are frequently anticipated by researchers envisioning hazards in work of the future (Schulte et al., 2020). The adoption of new technology has the potential to improve work conditions and health for construction workers. For example, automated processes can remove people from hazardous environments and the use of robots can reduce the need for workers to carry out dangerous work activities (ILO, 2019). However, new health (and safety) hazards can also be introduced when implementing new technologies. Technological job displacement describes a situation in which human workers are replaced with technology which has the potential to cause psychological and financial hardship for workers (Tamers et al., 2020). Other hazards associated with new technology include increased ergonomic risk presented by new forms of human–machine interaction, increased likelihood of accidents due to loss of understanding, control and knowledge of work processes and/ or over-confidence in technology infallibility (ILO, 2019). While potentially useful to assist in the management and monitoring of occupational health risks, sensor technology, cloud-based human resource systems and machine-learning enabled data analytics also raise concerns about privacy and data security (Tamers et al., 2020).

The use of technology to realise productivity gains is the cornerstone of the Fourth Industrial Revolution (4IR), which is expected to change "the very essence of our human experience" (Barton, 2020, p.302). In construction, digitisation has been conceptualised as "the use of digital technologies and processes in the delivery of tangible and intangible services within a construction organisation with a view to gaining a competitive advantage over other competitors while providing better service delivery in the process" (Aghimien et al., 2019, p.85). Some of the expected benefits of digitisation in the construction industry are time and cost savings, efficiency in procurement systems, smart construction through the use of interconnected machinery, and effective project monitoring and planning (Aghimien et al., 2019). As a result of the 4IR and the implementation of technology to improve the efficiency of the construction industry, we have seen the emergence of a new concept in construction referred to as "Construction 4.0" (Kozlovska et al., 2021).

Despite the promise of productivity gains, of concern is that 4IR has emerged as disadvantaging particular segments of the working population, such as women, people of colour, and workers from developing countries. Barton (2020, p.303) contends that the "4IR threatens to promote anti-public interest technologies that are increasingly oppressive, exclusionary, and exploitative." While the use of technology may have productivity benefits for organisations, its positive impact on workers is more in doubt and this can be seen in Construction 4.0 where technology is expected to lead to job loss and unemployment, and negative changes in the quality of work (Sherratt et al., 2020; Aghimien et al., 2021).

Ideally, the use of technology will protect and improve construction workers' health and wellbeing. Yet, Barton (2021) argues that the 4IR is predicated on the "discredited logic of technological determinism: the idea that technologies contain futures and that the use of a particular technology implies the inevitability of the future dictated by that technology" (p.32). While reflecting on the impact of the COVID-19 pandemic on worker health, safety and wellbeing, Sherratt and Dainty (2022) suggest that the emerging Fifth Industrial Revolution may prioritise people over economic efficiency. The Fifth Industrial Revolution (5IR) encompasses the notion of harmonious human–machine collaborations, with a specific focus on the wellbeing of the multiple stakeholders (i.e., society, companies, employees, customers). According to Noble et al. (2022, p.199) the 5IR "paves the way for a (r)evolution in thinking about and leveraging human–machine collaborations for greater societal well-being."

Noble et al. (2022) identify that, as technological boundaries continue to be pushed in the 5IR, the ethical and humane use of technology will become even more important, and indeed, emerging technologies may require carefully designed restrictions. As new and unanticipated ethical issues continue to arise as the boundaries of technology are pushed, how can we protect the health and wellbeing of workers in construction? Noble et al. (2022, p.207) pose a number of questions which have direct relevance for the promotion and protection of construction workers' health:

- As technological capabilities reach new heights constantly, how can we define ethical and humane uses of technology?
- Do organisations need chief ethical and humane officers?
- Should organisations establish their own set of rules relating to the use of technology, or will industry guidelines emerge?

11.7 Conclusion

The future of work is uncertain. Climate change and technologically driven change will present new and undetermined challenges to the construction industry in what is already a challenging and complex work environment. How we plan and respond to these challenges will be integral in promoting and protecting the health of construction workers. As we continue to put workers' health at the forefront, it's imperative that health is understood within the broader environment, is contextual, and that a primary focus is prioritised. This will only be achieved through an industry-wide collaborative approach.

11.8 Discussion and review questions

1. What do you understand by the terms "health" and "wellbeing"? Is it possible that these things mean different things to different people? Why/ why not?
2. What societal trends are likely to shape the way that construction workers experience health and wellbeing in the future? How can construction organisations position themselves to manage new or emerging risks?
3. Should the remit of occupational health programmes be extended beyond the workplace to include consideration of social, economic and cultural determinants of wellbeing? What is the relationship between occupational health and public health? Should they be more closely aligned?

Notes

1 On 15 September 2022, the Director-General of the World Health Organization, Tedros Adhanom Ghebreyesus, stated the end of the pandemic "is in sight."
2 The WBGT index was developed by the US Army and is the most frequently used measure of thermal conditions in occupational health. It takes into account air temperature, radiant temperature, humidity and air movement.

References

Acharya, P., Boggess, B., & Zhang, K. (2018). Assessing heat stress and health among construction workers in a changing climate: a review. *International Journal of Environmental Research and Public Health*, 15(2), 247.

Aghimien, D., Aigbavboa, C., Meno, T., & Ikuabe, M. (2021). Unravelling the risks of construction digitalisation in developing countries. *Construction Innovation*, 21(3), 456–475.

Aghimien, D. O., Aigbavboa, C. O. and Oke, A. E. (2019). Viewing digitalisation in construction through the lens of past studies, advances in ICT in Design, Construction and Management in Architecture, Engineering, Construction and Operations (AECO), *Proceedings of the 36th CIB W78 2019 Conference*, Northumbria University at Newcastle, 18–20 September, pp. 84–93.

Ansah, E. W., Ankomah-Appiah, E., Amoadu, M., & Sarfo, J. O. (2021). Climate change, health and safety of workers in developing economies: A scoping review. *The Journal of Climate Change and Health*, 3, 100034.

Barone Gibbs, B., Kline, C. E., Huber, K. A., Paley, J. L., & Perera, S. J. O. M. (2021). COVID-19 shelter-at-home and work, lifestyle and well-being in desk workers. *Occupational Medicine*, 71(2), 86–94.

Barton, C. J. (2020). The Fourth Industrial Revolution: Promise or Peril? 2020 *IEEE International Symposium on Technology and Society* (ISTAS), 302–309.

Barton, C. J. (2021). The fourth industrial revolution will not bring the future we want. *IEEE Technology and Society Magazine,* 40(3), 31–33.

Beaumont, D. (2021). *Positive Medicine: Disrupting the Future of Medical Practice.* Oxford University Press: Oxford.

Bentley, T. A., Teo, S. T., McLeod, L., Tan, F., Bosua, R., & Gloet, M. (2016). The role of organisational support in teleworker wellbeing: A socio-technical systems approach. *Applied Ergonomics*, 52, 207–215.

Boatman, L., Chaplan, D., Teran, S., & Welch, L. S. (2015). Creating a climate for ergonomic changes in the construction industry. *American Journal of Industrial Medicine*, 58(8), 858–869.

Bouziri, H., Smith, D. R., Descatha, A., Dab, W., & Jean, K. (2020). Working from home in the time of COVID-19: How to best preserve occupational health? *Occupational and Environmental Medicine,* 77(7), 509–510.

Brown, S., Trueblood, A. B., Harris, W., & Dong, X. S. (2022). *Construction Worker Mental Health During the Covid-19 Pandemic.* Center for the Protection of Workers Rights.

Burdorf, A., Porru, F., & Rugulies, R. (2020). The COVID-19 (Coronavirus) pandemic: Consequences for occupational health. *Scandinavian Journal of Work, Environment & Health*, 46(3), 229–230.

Caligiuri, P., De Cieri, H., Minbaeva, D., Verbeke, A., & Zimmermann, A. (2020). International HRM insights for navigating the COVID-19 pandemic: Implications for future research and practice. *Journal of International Business Studies*, 51, 697–713.

Caponecchia, C., & Mayland, E. C. (2020). Transitioning to job redesign: Improving workplace health and safety in the COVID-19 era. *Occupational and Environmental Medicine*, 77(12), 868–868.

Card, A. J. (2017). Moving beyond the WHO definition of health: A new perspective for an aging world and the emerging era of value-based care. *World Medical & Health Policy,* 9(1), 127–137.

Charlier, P., Coppens, Y., Malaurie, J., Brun, L., Kepanga, M., Hoang-Opermann, V.,... Hervé, C. (2017). A new definition of health? An open letter of autochthonous peoples and medical anthropologists to the WHO. *European Journal of Internal Medicine,* 37, 33–37.

Cooper, C. D., & Kurland, N. B. (2002). Telecommuting, professional isolation, and employee development in public and private organizations. *Journal of Organizational Behavior*, 23(4), 511–532.

Costa, G. (1996). The impact of shift and night work on health. *Applied Ergonomics*, 27(1), 9–16.

Croda, E., & Grossbard, S. (2021). Women pay the price of COVID-19 more than men. *Review of Economics of the Household*, 19(1), 1–9.

Crook, H., Raza, S., Nowell, J., Young, M., & Edison, P. (2021). Long covid – mechanisms, risk factors, and management. *BMJ*, 374.

Dextras-Gauthier, J., Marchand, A., & Haines III, V. (2012). Organizational culture, work organization conditions, and mental health: A proposed integration. *International Journal of Stress Management*, 19(2), 81.

Dong, X. S., West, G. H., Holloway-Beth, A., Wang, X., & Sokas, R. K. (2019). Heat-related deaths among construction workers in the United States. *American Journal of Industrial Medicine*, 62(12), 1047–1057.

Durie, M. H. (1985). A Maori perspective of health. *Social Science & Medicine*, 20(5), 483–486.

Felknor, S. A., Streit, J. M., McDaniel, M., Schulte, P. A., Chosewood, L. C., & Delclos, G. L. (2021). How will the future of work shape OSH research and practice? A workshop summary. *International Journal of Environmental Research and Public Health*, 18(11), 5696.

Felstead, A., & Henseke, G. (2017). Assessing the growth of remote working and its consequences for effort, well-being and work-life balance. *New Technology, Work and Employment*, 32(3), 195–212.

Frasquilho, D., Matos, M. G., Salonna, F., Guerreiro, D., Storti, C. C., Gaspar, T., & Caldas-de-Almeida, J. M. (2015). Mental health outcomes in times of economic recession: a systematic literature review. *BMC Public Health*, 16(1), 1–40.

Gajendran, R. S., & Harrison, D. A. (2007). The good, the bad, and the unknown about telecommuting: Meta-analysis of psychological mediators and individual consequences. *Journal of Applied Psychology*, 92(6), 1524.

Godeau, D., Petit, A., Richard, I., Roquelaure, Y., & Descatha, A. (2021). Return-to-work, disabilities and occupational health in the age of COVID-19. *Scandinavian Journal of Work, Environment & Health*, 47(5), 408.

Godderis, L., & Luyten, J. (2020). Challenges and opportunities for occupational health and safety after the COVID-19 lockdowns. *Occupational and Environmental Medicine*, 77(8), 511–512.

Green Building Council of Australia. (2022). Accessed 24 September 2022 from: https://new.gbca.org.au/

Gross, J. V., Fritschi, L., Mohren, J., Wild, U., & Erren, T. C. (2021). Contribution of Occupational Health to multidisciplinary team work for Covid-19 prevention and management. *La Medicina del Lavoro*, 112(2), 171.

The Guardian. (2019). *Revealed: hundreds of migrant workers dying of heat stress in Qatar each year.* Accessed 22 September 2022 from: www.theguardian.com/global-development/2019/oct/02/revealed-hundreds-of-migrant-workers-dying-of-heat-stress-in-qatar-each-year

Hallin, H. (2020). *Home-Based Telework During the Covid-19 Pandemic.* School of Health, Care and Social Welfare, Mälardarlen University Sweden.

Harrison, J., & Dawson, L. (2016). Occupational health: Meeting the challenges of the next 20 years. Safety and Health at Work, 7(2), 143–149.

Hayes, K., & Poland, B. (2018). Addressing mental health in a changing climate: Incorporating mental health indicators into climate change and health vulnerability and adaptation assessments. *International Journal of Environmental Research and Public Health*, 15(9), 1806.

International Labour Organization (ILO). (2019). *Safety and Health at the Heart of the Future of Work*, International Labour Organization.

International Labour Organization (ILO). (2021). *New Legislation in Qatar Provides Greater Protection To Workers From Heat Stress.* Accessed 23 September 2022 from: www.ilo.org/global/about-the-ilo/newsroom/news/WCMS_794475/lang--en/index.htm

ISO. (1989). ISO 7243:1989 Hot environments – Estimation of the heat stress on working man, based on the WBGT-index (wet bulb globe temperature). ISO.

Jacobs, J. A., & Gerson, K. (2001). Overworked individuals or overworked families? Explaining trends in work, leisure, and family time. *Work and Occupations*, 28(1), 40–63.

Johansen, M. D., Mahbub, R. M., Idrees, S., Nguyen, D. H., Miemczyk, S., Pathinayake, P.,... & Hansbro, P. M. (2022). Increased SARS-CoV-2 Infection, Protease and Inflammatory Responses in COPD Primary Bronchial Epithelial Cells Defined with Single Cell RNA-Sequencing. *American Journal of Respiratory and Critical Care Medicine* (ja).

Jones, W., Gibb, A. G., & Chow, V. (2021). Adapting to COVID-19 on construction sites: what are the lessons for long-term improvements in safety and worker effectiveness? *Journal of Engineering, Design and Technology*, 20(1), 66–85.

Karanikolos, M., Heino, P., McKee, M., Stuckler, D., & Legido-Quigley, H. (2016). Effects of the global financial crisis on health in high-income OECD countries: A narrative review. *International Journal of Health Services*, 46(2), 208–240.

Kjellstrom, T., Briggs, D., Freyberg, C., Lemke, B., Otto, M., & Hyatt, O. (2016). Heat, human performance, and occupational health: a key issue for the assessment of global climate change impacts. *Annual Review of Public Health*, 37, 97–112.

Kjellstrom, T., Holmer, I., & Lemke, B. (2009). Workplace heat stress, health and productivity–an increasing challenge for low and middle-income countries during climate change. *Global Health Action*, 2(1), 2047.

Knibb-Lamouche, J. (2012). *Culture as a Social Determinant of Health.* Accessed 24 September 2022 from: www.ncbi.nlm.nih.gov/books/NBK201298/

Koh, D. (2020). Migrant workers and COVID-19. *Occupational and Environmental Medicine*, 77(9), 634–636.

Kozlovska, M., Klosova, D., & Strukova, Z. (2021). Impact of industry 4.0 platform on the formation of construction 4.0 concept: A literature review. *Sustainability*, 13(5), 2683.

Leonardi, F. (2018). The definition of health: Towards new perspectives. *International Journal of Health Services*, 48(4), 735–748.

Lingard, H., & Turner, M. (2015). Improving the health of male, blue collar construction workers: a social ecological perspective. *Construction Management and Economics*, 33(1), 18–34.

Lingard, H., Raj, I. S., Lythgo, N., Troynikov, O., & Fitzgerald, C. (2019). The impact of tool selection on back and wrist injury risk in tying steel reinforcement bars: A single case experiment. *Construction Economics and Building*, 19(1), 1–19.

Ministry of Health. (2017). *Māori Health Models – Te Whare Tapa Whā.* Accessed 25 September 2022 from: www.health.govt.nz/our-work/populations/maori-health/maori-health-models/maori-health-models-te-whare-tapa-wha

Montreuil, S., & Lippel, K. (2003). Telework and occupational health: A Quebec empirical study and regulatory implications. *Safety Science*, 41(4), 339–358.

Newby, J. M., K. O'Moore, S. Tang, H. Christensen, & K. Faasse. (2020). Acute mental health responses during the COVID-19 pandemic in Australia. *PLoS One*, 15 (7): e0236562. https://doi.org/10.1371/journal.pone.0236562

Newman, F., & Humphrys, E. (2020). Construction workers in a climate precarious world. *Critical Sociology*, 46(4–5), 557–572.

Noble, S. M., Mende, M., Grewal, D., & Parasuraman, A. (2022). The Fifth Industrial Revolution: How Harmonious Human–Machine Collaboration is Triggering a Retail and Service [R]evolution. *Journal of Retailing*, 98(2), 199–208.

Office For National Statistics. (2021). *Coronavirus (COVID-19) related deaths by occupation, England and Wales,* www.ons.gov.uk/peoplepopulationandcommunity/healthandsoc ialcare/causesofdeath/datasets/coronaviruscovid19relateddeathsbyoccupationengl andandwales, accessed 18 September 2022.

Oleribe, O. O., Ukwedeh, O., Burstow, N. J., Gomaa, A. I., Sonderup, M. W., Cook, N.,... Taylor-Robinson, S. D. (2018). Health: redefined. *Pan African Medical Journal.* Accessed 25 September 2022 from: www.panafrican-med-journal.com/content/arti cle/30/292/full/

Pasco, R. F., Fox, S. J., Johnston, S. C., Pignone, M., & Meyers, L. A. (2020). Estimated association of construction work with risks of COVID-19 infection and hospitalization in Texas. *JAMA Network Open,* 3(10), e2026373–e2026373.

Peckham, T. K., Baker, M. G., Camp, J. E., Kaufman, J. D., & Seixas, N. S. (2017). Creating a future for occupational health. *Annals of Work Exposures and Health,* 61(1), 3–15.

Pirzadeh, P., & Lingard, H. (2021). Working from home during the COVID-19 pandemic: Health and well-being of project-based construction workers. *Journal of Construction Engineering and Management,* 147(6), 1–17.

Pradhan, B., Kjellstrom, T., Atar, D., Sharma, P., Kayastha, B., Bhandari, G., & Pradhan, P. K. (2019). Heat stress impacts on cardiac mortality in Nepali migrant workers in Qatar. *Cardiology,* 143(1), 37–48.

Ragan, K. R., Lunsford, N. B., Thomas, C. C., Tai, E. W., Sussell, A., & Holman, D. M. (2019). Peer Reviewed: Skin Cancer Prevention Behaviors Among Agricultural and Construction Workers in the United States, 2015. *Preventing Chronic Disease,* 16. http://dx.doi.org/10.5888/pcd16.180446external icon.

Rosen, J., Miller, A., Hughes Jr, J., & Remington, J. (2015). National Institute of Environmental Health Sciences Worker Training Program: perspectives on the health and safety of workers, volunteers, and residents involved in the cleanup and rebuilding of New York City housing damaged by Hurricane Sandy. *Environmental Justice,* 8(3), 105–109.

Schulte, P. A., & Chun, H. (2009). Climate change and occupational safety and health: establishing a preliminary framework. *Journal of Occupational and Environmental Hygiene,* 6(9), 542–554.

Schulte, P. A., Bhattacharya, A., Butler, C. R., Chun, H. K., Jacklitsch, B., Jacobs, T.,... & Wagner, G. R. (2016). Advancing the framework for considering the effects of climate change on worker safety and health. *Journal of Occupational and Environmental Hygiene,* 13(11), 847–865.

Schulte, P. A., Delclos, G., Felknor, S. A., & Chosewood, L. C. (2019). Toward an expanded focus for occupational safety and health: A commentary. *International Journal of Environmental Research and Public Health,* 16(24), 4946.

Schulte, P. A., Streit, J. M., Sheriff, F., Delclos, G., Felknor, S. A., Tamers, S. L.,... & Sala, R. (2020). Potential scenarios and hazards in the work of the future: A systematic review of the peer-reviewed and gray literatures. *Annals of Work Exposures and Health,* 64(8), 786–816.

Sevilla, A., & Smith, S. (2020). Baby steps: The gender division of childcare during the COVID-19 pandemic. *Oxford Review of Economic Policy,* 36(Supplement 1), S169–S186.

Sherratt, F., & Dainty, A. (2022). The power of a pandemic: How Covid-19 should transform UK construction worker health, safety and wellbeing. *Construction Management and Economics,* 1–8. https://doi.org/10.1080/01446193.2022.2104890

Sherratt, F., Dowsett, R., & Sherratt, S. (2020). Construction 4.0 and its potential impact on people working in the construction industry. *Proceedings of the Institution of Civil Engineers – Management, Procurement and Law,* 173(4), 145–152.

Sinclair, R. R., Allen, T., Barber, L., Bergman, M., Britt, T., Butler, A.,... & Yuan, Z. (2020). Occupational health science in the time of COVID-19: Now more than ever. *Occupational Health Science,* 4(1), 1–22.

Sinclair, R. R., Probst, T. M., Watson, G. P., & Bazzoli, A. (2021). Caught between Scylla and Charybdis: How economic stressors and occupational risk factors influence workers' occupational health reactions to COVID-19. *Applied Psychology,* 70(1), 85–119.

Sneller, T. N., Choi, S. D., & Ahn, K. (2018). Awareness and perceptions of ergonomic programs between workers and managers surveyed in the construction industry. *Work,* 61(1), 41–54.

Tamers, S. L., Streit, J., Pana-Cryan, R., Ray, T., Syron, L., Flynn, M. A.,... & Howard, J. (2020). Envisioning the future of work to safeguard the safety, health, and well-being of the workforce: A perspective from the CDC's National Institute for Occupational Safety and Health. *American Journal of Industrial Medicine,* 63(12), 1065–1084.

Torres, R., Heyman, R., Munoz, S., Apgar, L., Timm, E., Tzintzun, C.,... & Tang, E. (2013). Building Austin, building justice: Immigrant construction workers, precarious labor regimes and social citizenship. *Geoforum,* 45, 145–155.

Uddin, S. J., Ganapati, N. E., Pradhananga, N., Prajapati, J., & Albert, A. (2021). Is the workers' health and safety scenario different in post-disaster reconstruction from conventional construction? A case study in Bhaktapur, Nepal. *International Journal of Disaster Risk Reduction,* 64, 102529.

Wheatley, D. (2012). Good to be home? Time-use and satisfaction levels among home-based teleworkers. *New Technology, Work and Employment,* 27(3), 224–241.

World Health Organization. (2010). *A Conceptual Framework for Action on the Social Determinants of Health.* World Health Organization.

Xiang, J., Hansen, A., Pisaniello, D., & Bi, P. (2016). Workers' perceptions of climate change related extreme heat exposure in South Australia: A cross-sectional survey. *BMC Public Health,* 16(1), 1–12.

Yavorsky, J. E., Qian, Y., & Sargent, A. C. (2021). The gendered pandemic: The implications of COVID-19 for work and family. *Sociology Compass,* 15(6), e12881.

Zamarro, G., & Prados, M. J. (2021). Gender differences in couples' division of childcare, work and mental health during COVID-19. *Review of Economics of the Household,* 19(1), 11–40.

INDEX

absenteeism 10, 61, 64, 104, 185–6
abusive leadership 211–13
Ackerman, P. L. 239
acrylic sealants 47
Adam, B., 93
administrative controls 32–3, 42, 46, 71, 80
aerobic capacity 6, 223
age factors: ageing population 223; ageing process 223–5; cognitive decline 226–7; discrimination 240–1; healthy ageing 222–45; injuries 231–2; interventions 242–5; lifespan perspective 238–40; lifestyle 228–9; mortality 198, 231–2; pain 225–6; physical health 229–31; psychological health 232–8; retirement, early 3, 48–9, 227–8; social context of work 240–1; South Africa 186; stereotyping 240, 243; work ability 227–8; work capacity 223–4; work-life balance 244; *see also* young construction workers
age management 241–2
airborne pollutants 29, 31, 35, 41–2, 199, 282–3
Alavinia S. M. 229
alcohol consumption: gender based violence 131; HIV/AIDS 183; lifestyle interventions 6; mental ill health 66; sexual harassment 120; Sub Saharan Africa 180, 185, 189; young workers 204
Allis, P. 260
Alzheimer's disease 114

American Conference of Governmental Industrial Hygienists 38
Andersson, L. M. 261
Angola 171
anxiety: discrimination and 125; gender based violence 131; job control 6; long hours 89; psychological hazards 67; subcontracting 65; United Kingdom 2020 28; work-family conflict 91; young workers 206
ANZSCO classification code 233, 235
ANZSIC classification code 233, 235
apprenticeships 194–7, 200–13
Arndt, V. 225, 229
arthritis 49, 114, 225
asbestos 3, 30–1, 34–7, 42, 199
AS/NZS 1716–Respiratory protective devices 41
asphalt 47
Attitude to Work programme (Finland) 214–15
Australian and New Zealand Society of Occupational Medicine 40
Australian Bureau of Statistics 229
Australian Constructors Association 286
Australian Human Rights and Equal Opportunity Commission 120
Australian Human Rights Commission 18, 131–2
Australian Institute of Health and Safety 40

Australian Institute of Occupational
  Hygienists 32–3
*Australian National Health Survey
  2017–2018* 2
Australian National Standard for
  Occupational Noise 44
Australian Workplace Exposure Survey 47
autoimmune diseases 37, 114

back pain 3, 224–5, 230–1, 242
Baicker, K. 11
Baltes, M. M. 239
Baltes, P. B. 239
Bambra, C. 98
Bardoel, E. A. 260
Barnett, T. 185
Barton, C. J. 291
Beaumont, David 288
Bednarz, A. 196
Belgium 175, 206
Betta Stone 40
Bies, R. J. 261
bitumen 47
Black Asian or Minority Ethnic (BAME)
  background 6
Blewett, V. 210
Bonanno, G. A. 151
Booysen, F. 182
Borsting Jacobsen, H. 231
Boschman, J. S. 65
Botswana 181–2
Bowen, P. 184, 187
Brauner, C. 97
Breslin, F. C. 197–202
bricklayers 65
Bridges, D. 123, 129
Brief Resilience Scale 157
Brief Sense of Community Scale 263
Britt, T. W. 150
Brough, P. 258
Bryan, C. 160
bullying 66, 68, 72–4, 81, 122, 127,
  206–7
Bureau for Economic Research (S. Africa)
  184
Burke, Tarana 130
Burkina Faso 181
burnout: dimensions 260; long hours
  89; mental ill health 78, 81; older
  workers 232; organisational culture
  255, 259, 286; recovery 104; resilience
  153; respect and civility 262; work-
  family conflict 260; work-to-home
  interference 106

Burrowes, K. 114
business case for occupational health
  measures 10–11
Butterworth, P. 62, 232
Buyens, D. 244
"Buy Quiet" 46

cable-pulling 49
cadmium 31
Campion, M. A. 240
Canada 156, 197, 201
cancer: breast 125; construction
  industry 3, 34–7; diesel exhaust
  exposure 32; latency 30, 34; mortality
  3, 31–2, 35; older workers 230;
  ultraviolet radiation 283; United
  Kingdom 29, 34
Cancer Council 40–1
cannabis 204
Caplan, R. D. 263
Caponecchia, C. 275
carcinogens 34, 37
cardiovascular disease 31–2, 68, 89, 104,
  114, 229
career development 63, 68, 72, 153, 155,
  160, 242
Caribbean 282
Carmody, M. 48
carpal tunnel syndrome 49
carpenters 35, 132
Cattell, K. 170
cement 35, 47–9
cement workers 48
Census of Fatal Occupational Injuries
  (US) 232
Center for Construction Research and
  Training 134
Central Africa 282
Central African Republic 182
Central America 282
Chan, A. P. C. 66, 254
Chapman, J. 204
Chapman, M. T. 149
Chartered Institute of Building (UK) 65,
  90, 223, 254
Chau, N. 197–8
Chavis, D. M. 260
Chen, Y. 156
Chin, P. 213
China 156, 159, 174
Choi, S. 115
chromate 48–9
chromium III 48
chronic fatigue syndrome 114

chronic obstructive pulmonary disease 2, 29–31; *see also* lung disease
chronic toxic encephalopathy 29
Churchyard, G. J. 178
Cicmil, S. 254
Civil Contractors Federation (CCF) of Victoria 81–2
civility 261–2
Civility Norms Questionnaire-Brief 263
Claessen, H. 228
climate change 280–4
coal tar 35
cocaine 204
community, sense of 259–60, 263, 265
competitive tendering 17, 65
conceptual model of sense of place 258
Connor-Davidson Resilience Scale 156
Conrad, P. 8
"Construction 4.0" 291
Construction by Constructible 132
Construction Concrete 132
contact dermatitis 3, 29, 230
Cooklin, A. R. 91
Cooper, C. L. 150
Costa, G. 227, 244
COVID-19: economic effects 276; health inequality 5–6; long COVID 276; mortality 274; responses 273–6; Singapore 273; Sub Saharan Africa 171, 174, 176–7; suicide 4; teleworking 106; working from home 277–9
Cropanzano, R. 262
cryptococcal meningitis 179
crystallised intelligence 227
Csikszentmihalyi, M. 256
Curtis, H. M. 121
cytomegalovirus 179

Dahlgren and Whitehead model 4–5
Dahlgren, G. 4, 6
Dainty, A. 291
DALYs (disability-adjusted life years) 2, 22
Daniell, W. E. 45
De Cremer, D. 261
De Witte, H. D. 206
deadlines 65, 68, 72–3, 80, 88, 90
Decent Work Agenda (UN) 64
degreasers 47
Del Castillo, A. P. 133
Dement, J. M. 30, 35, 45
Demerouti, E. 263
Denmark 48, 231

depression: clinical assessment 77; discrimination and 125; gender based violence 131; long hours 89; organisational culture 78; psychological hazards 67; recovery time 104; subcontracting 65; supervisors 65; United Kingdom 2020 28; women 18, 116; work hours 94; work speed 65; work-family conflict 91; young workers 206
dermatitis 3
descalers 48
detergents 48
developing countries 169–90
Dextras-Gauthier, J. 78, 255, 286
diabetes 31, 68, 89
diesel 47
diesel engine exhaust exposure 3, 32–5
diet 6, 12, 90, 154; lifestyle interventions 6
digitisation 290–1
Dinh, H. 91–2
disability-adjusted life years 2
Dong, X. S. 232
Dowling, N. 204
Drake, C. 241

early school leavers 200
Echloff, T. 261
economic impact 30
effort-reward fairness 72, 233, 236–8
effort-reward imbalance (ERI) model 61–4
XVIII World Congress on Safety and Health at Work 10
Einarsen, S. 127
electricians 35
elimination of risk/stress 32–3, 42, 71, 80–1
Else-Quest, N. 130
Employee Assistance Programmes 79–80
employee resilience 150–3, 156–7
Employee Resilience Scale 157–8, 263
employee surveys 70, 77
employment, precarious 16–18, 73, 176, 199, 237, 241, 276, 281–2; *see also* job security
engagement 260–1, 263, 265
engineered stone 38–41
engineering controls 32–3, 42, 46, 71, 80
Engineering News Record 131
enterprise community involvement 14
epoxy resins 47
ergonomics 49, 51, 132–3, 213, 244–5, 279–80

Eritrea 181
ethics 10, 289, 291
Ethiopia 158, 180–1
European Agency for Safety and Health at
    Work 114, 133, 197–8
European Union: Directive 2003/53/
    EC 48; European Union Framework
    Directive 339/89/EEC 69; "right to
    disconnect" 106; young workers 197
exercise 3, 6–7, 12, 90, 242–4

Farrell, P. 132
Farrow, A. 230
fatigue 18, 65, 68, 89–90, 103–6, 179
Feldman, C. 226, 229, 240
fibromyalgia 114
FIFA World Cup 281
Fifth Industrial Revolution 291
Fine, C. 130
Finland 48, 214
Fisher, R. 133
flexible work arrangements 65, 92, 97,
    243–4, 278, 286
fluid intelligence 227
Flynn, M. A. 134
focus groups 77
Foley, S. 253
Fourth Industrial Revolution 290–1
France 175
Francis, V. 93
Fritschi, L. 40

Galea, N. 117–18, 130
Gambelunghe, A. 31
gambling 204
gases and fumes 31–2; lung disease 3;
    mortality 2
gastrointestinal disorders 284
Gee, G. C. 126
gender 113–36; apprenticeships 195–6;
    bullying 127; discrimination 116–17,
    120–2, 124–6, 132; equity initiatives
    117–18; gender roles 18, 92, 116, 118;
    health differences 114; homicides
    115; injuries 115, 122; intimidation
    of women 118–19, 123–4, 127–9;
    isolation 127–8; mental ill health 121;
    misdiagnoses 114; neurosexism 130;
    objectification of women 118–20; pay
    gap 93; personal protective equipment
    133–5; research bias 115–16; resilience
    157–60; safety voice behaviour 200; sex
    and 115–16; as social determinant of
    health 116–22; survival strategies 121;

vocational education 122–4; women's
    participation in construction 18, 115,
    127–8; work hours 117; working from
    home 277–80; work-life balance 18,
    122; workplace violence 18, 115, 119,
    130–2; World Health Organization 18;
    see also sexual harassment
Germany 48, 97, 175, 229
Geurts, S. A. 105
Gherardi, S. 195
Glimskär, B. 245
Godeau, D. 276
graffiti 132
Grandy, G. 213
Grant, L. 157
greases 47
"green" technologies 283
Griffiths, A. 239
Gucciardi, D. F. 149

Haar, J. 99, 263
Haar, J. M. 260
Habib, R. R. 132
Hakanen, J. J. 255, 261
Hall, E. M. 259
Hallberg, D. 93
Hanvold, T. N. 214
harassment 66, 73, 81, 119, 127
Härmä, M. 94
Hartmann, S. 148, 153–4, 157
Hartwig, A. 148
He, C. 156
Health and Safety Executive (UK) 30,
    65, 70
health definitions 12, 288–90
health promotion programmes:
    legal requirements 11–12; lifestyle
    interventions 3; organisational
    motivations 10–12; *see also* interventions
hearing loss, occupational 41, 43–7, 230;
    see also noise exposure
hearing protection devices 45–6
heart disease 2, 89, 114, 116; *see also*
    cardiovascular disease
heat stress 280–2
Henry, J. 257
hepatitis 189
Herzog, A. 244
hexavalent chromium 48
hierarchy of control 15–16, 27, 32–3, 42,
    46, 70–1, 79–80
"Hierarchy of Controls Applied to
    NIOSH Total Worker Health" 15–16
HILDA 232–7

HIV/AIDS: pathology and treatment 179–80; South Africa 182–9; Sub Saharan Africa 172, 178–90
Holmqvist, M. 8
home-work interface 68, 73; *see also* work-life balance
Hon, A. H. Y. 158
Hong, O. 46
Hoonakker, P. 224, 230
Hopkins, K. 259
Household, Income and Labour Dynamics in Australia 62, 232–7
households 182, 236, 285
Human Sciences Research Council 178
humour 129, 207–9
hypertension 125, 186, 284

Ijntema, R. C. 160–2
Ilmarinen, J. 94, 223
Indigenous workers 175, 287
inequality in health 4, 6, 20, 91, 113–16
Innstrand, S. T. 260–1
Institute of Medicine (US) 182
insulation workers 44
interactionist model of resilience 21, 145, 149, 151, 161
International Agency for Research on Cancer 32, 34, 37
International Labour Conference 2022 9
International Labour Office 67, 114
International Labour Organization: asbestos risks 36; broadening occupational health 284–5; Convention no 162 36; Fundamental Principles and Rights at Work 9–10; global monitoring study 2; Global Program for the Elimination of Silicosis (WHO/ILO) 38; "green" technologies 283; occupational health 134; silica risks 37; WHO/ILO Global Monitoring Report 2; work hours 93; working hours 89
interpersonal relationships 68, 72, 75, 81, 156, 196
interventions: changing job conditions 6; culture change 286–7; ethical aspects 205; lifestyle programs 6–8; mental health programmes 78–83; mental ill health 6; nutrition 6; for older workers 242–5; positive psychology 256–8; primary 6, 38, 76, 79–80, 151–2; secondary 38, 76, 79–80, 151–2; tertiary 38, 79–80, 152; worker participation in decision making 6; for

young workers 213–15; *see also* health promotion programmes
ironworkers 44, 46
ischaemic heart disease 2
ischaemic strokes 186
ISO 45003, *Occupational health and safety management–Psychological health and safety at work–Guidelines for managing psychosocial risks* 20, 71–8, 83
isocyanates 31
isolated work 72
Italy 227

jackhammering 49
Jain, A. 117
Jarvholm, B. 231
job control: low 61, 65–8, 96, 254; older workers 231, 233, 236–9, 244; psychological health 63, 72, 94; stress reduction 6; sustainable schedules 97; young workers 206
job demand-control (JD-C) model 62–3, 65, 259
job demands: high 157; job quality 61–3; older workers 233, 235–9, 244; psychological health 67, 72–3, 80, 99, 116, 199; recovery 104; as risk factor 66; young workers 206
job demands-resources (JD-R) model 62–3
job quality 61–2, 232–8
job security: construction industry 16; effort-reward imbalance 63–4; low 4, 61–2; older workers 233, 236–7, 241; psychological health 65, 73; Sub Saharan Africa 174, 176; subcontractors 74; young workers 4, 199
job support 65–7, 72
Johansson, J. 122
Johnson, J. V. 259
Johnson, R. W. 240
Johnstone, R. 69
joint pain 224–5
Jones, A. 196

Kanfer, R. 239
Karasek, R. A. 63
Karim, Q. A. 178, 180
Kenny, G. P. 242
Kenya 180–1
Kharsany, A. B. M. 178, 180
kidney disease 37, 280
King, T. L. 4
Kinman, G. 157

Kjellstrom, T. 282
Knies, E. 244
Kooij, D. T. 239
Kossek, E. E. 91, 155, 157, 259
Kristensen, T. S. 94
Kudryavtsev, A. 252
Kuntz, J. R. C. 161

Laberge, M. 115, 201–2
labour hire agencies 17
Lambert, S. J. 259
Lamontagne, A. D. 4
Landwehr, K. R. 33
Leensen, M. C. J. 44–6
Leisink, P. L. 244
Leiter, M. P. 260
Leka, S. 68
Leonardi, F. 289
León-Jiménez, A. 39
Leso, V. 39
Leung, M-Y. 169
LEV *see* local exhaust ventilation systems
Lewkowski, K. 44, 47
LGBTI+ 207
Li, W. 159
Liao, Y. 158–9
Lin, T. T. 158–9
Lingard, H. 9–10, 90, 93, 224
local exhaust ventilation systems 38, 40–2
Loudoun, R. J. 199
Lundberg, S. 245
lung disease 3, 31, 37, 39, 230
Lung Foundation Australia 40
Luthans, F. 157
Lyme disease 114

malaria 177–8
Malawi 180–2
Managing Psychosocial Hazards at Work: Code of Practice (SafeWork Australia) 80
Manual Handling Code of Practice (WorkSafe Victoria) 50–1
manual handling practices 50–1, 230
Māori 287–8
Maslach, C. 260
masons 29, 39–40, 213
Masten, A. S. 146
Mates in Construction 78
Mayhew, C. 65
Mayland, E. C. 275
McCormack, D. 206
McEwan, K. 150
McMahan, S. 244
McMillan, D. W. 259–60

Mealer, M. 157
Meding, B. 48
Melchior, M. 206
mental health programmes 78–83
mental ill health 60–83; age factors 62, 232–8; COVID-19 275–6, 278–80; incidence 3; interventions 6; job quality 61–2; levels of reward 6; mental health action plans 81–2; mental health programmes 78–83; return-to-work monitoring 77; risk factors 66, 254–5; social support 209–13; subsidised clinical assessments 77; women 121; work hours 92; young workers 205–7
mental wellbeing 22, 61, 65, 78, 244, 260, 263–5, 267, 278, 286
mesothelioma 3, 35, 230
Messing, K. 116, 132
meth/amphetamine 204
#MeToo movement 130–2
Mexico 37, 281
Meyer, I. H. 125
Meyers, M. C. 256–7
migrant workers 6, 40, 174, 185, 189, 273, 276, 281–2
Milano, Alyssa 130
Miller, N. G. 253
Milner, A. 62, 66, 89, 206
minority stress 124–6
Moag, J. F. 261
Model Work Health and Safety Act 11–12
Model Work Health and Safety Regulations 12
morality 10, 289
mortality: cancer 3, 31–2, 35; gases and fumes 2; heart disease 2; heat stress 281; incidence 281; long work hours 2; non-communicable diseases 2016 2; occupational particulate matter 2; older workers 231–2; stroke 2; work related diseases 2016 2; young workers 198
Mowday, R. T. 259
Mozambique 180
MSD *see* musculoskeletal disorders
multiple sclerosis 114
Murgia, N. 31
musculoskeletal disorders 3, 28, 49–51, 68, 229–31, 280
Myers, D. J. 198

Näswall, K. 158, 263
National Centre for Vocational Education Research 195

National Institute for Occupational Safety and Health (USA) 13–14, 44–6, 133, 280
Neitzel, R. 46
Netherlands 29, 43–4, 175, 229–30, 232
neurological damage 30, 32
neurosexism 130
New York Committee for Occupational Safety & Health 132
New Zealand 158–9, 206, 264, 287–8
Ng, T. W. 226, 229, 240
Nguyen, Q. 159
Nicolini, D. 195
Nielsen, M. B. 127
Nielsen, M. L. 199, 201
Nigeria 156, 180, 182
NIHL *see* noise-induced hearing loss
NIOSH *see* National Institute for Occupational Safety and Health
Noble, S. M. 291
noise exposure 3, 29–30; *see also* hearing loss, occupational
noise-induced hearing loss 43–7
non-malignant pleural disease 3
nutrition 2–3
Nwaogu, J. M. 122, 157
Nykänen, M. 214

OACD *see* occupational allergic contact dermatitis
obesity 2, 229
obsessive-compulsive disorder 131
occupational allergic contact dermatitis 48–9
occupational exposure limits 37–8
occupational health: challenges 30–1; distinction from safety 28, 30; risk controls 32–3
Occupational Health and Safety Act (S. Africa) 188
occupational particulate matter 2
Occupational Safety and Health Administration (US) 44, 128, 133, 135
Oceania 282
O'Driscoll, M. 260
OEL *see* occupational exposure limits
Office for Total Worker Health 15
oils 47
Okun, A. H. 198
Oldenburg Burnout Inventory 263
Olsson, C. 163
O'Neil, A. 131
O'Neill, R. 31
O'Neill, T. 223

Oo, B. L. 122–3
oral thrush 179
organic solvents 29, 47
Organisation for Economic Co-operation and Development 131
organisational change management 68, 72, 76, 79, 152–3
organisational culture 68, 70, 72, 106, 127, 255, 286
organisational justice 262
osteoarthritis 229
ototoxic chemicals 47
Ottawa system 98
Oude Hengel, K. M. 229
overtime 77, 90, 94–5, 97, 101–2, 105–6, 239

painters: cancer 3, 34–5; organic solvent exposure 29
"painter's syndrome" 29
Park Health 103
Pascoe, E. A. 125–6
paviors 35
Pears, J. 258
Pearson, C. M. 261
Pek, S. 201
performance monitoring 77
"period dignity" 135
PERMA 257
Perpetual Guardian 99
Perrigino, M. B. 155
personal health resources 13–14
personal protective equipment 32–3, 41–3, 46, 80, 122, 132–5
Petersen, J. S. 3
Peterson, N. A. 263
petrol 33, 47
Phillips, K. 245
physical work environment 13–14, 71
Pidd, K. 206
Pietrangelo, A. 179
place attachment 252
place meaning 252
pleural disease 230
plumbers 35, 48
pneumonia 179
polycyclic 1 aromatic hydrocarbons 31
population ageing 222
Portugal 175
Positive Plans–Positive Futures Program 81–2
positive psychology 255–7
Posthuma, R. A. 240
post-traumatic stress disorder 67, 131

PPE *see* personal protective equipment
Pradhan, P. K. 281
presenteeism 11, 95, 104, 255
productivity: decrease 11, 64, 90, 100, 170, 172, 177, 182, 186; increase 6, 8, 99, 152–3, 172, 175, 276, 290–1
Productivity Commission 152
progressive massive fibrosis 39
project-based work: COVID-19 278; job security 237; long hours 2, 20, 65, 88–90, 92, 94–7; positive psychology 256; psychological conditions 232; rigid hours 117; sense of place 253–4; work-life balance 99
psychological health *see* mental ill health
psychosocial hazards 67–78
psychosocial risks 67–78
psychosocial work environment 14, 67–71
public health approach 273–5, 284–5
Public Health Association of Australia 40

Qatar 281
Quinlan, M. 65

Rampen, J. 135
Rauscher, K. J. 198
RAW framework 154
Rawlinson, F. 132
recommended exposure limit 44
rehabilitation 36, 77, 79–80
Reid, A. 40
REL 44
remote work 72
reproductive hazards 135
resilience 145–63; definitions 145–8, 262; employee resilience 150–3, 156–7; interactionist framework 21, 145, 149, 151, 161; measurement scales 157, 263; mental wellbeing 266; protective factors 153–4; risk-reduction approach 163; systems framework 146; team resilience 148–50; training 160–3
Resilience at Work (RAW) framework 154
respect 261–3, 265
Respect Code (Victoria) 81
respiratory protective equipment 38, 41, 43
respiratory system 32, 43, 223; *see also* chronic obstructive pulmonary disease; lung disease; pneumonia; tuberculosis
Responsible Construction Practices credits 283–4
retirement, early 3, 48–9, 227–8, 231–2

Reynolds, F. 230
rheumatoid arthritis 114
"right to disconnect" 106
Ringen, K. 29
risk controls 32–3
risk-reduction approach 163
road surfacers 35
roadmen 35
Robens-style model 32, 69
Robertson, I. T., 152–3, 157, 160–1
Roche, A. M. 78, 254
role play 75
roof plumbers 225–6
roofers 35, 232
Rose, C. 40
Royal Australian College of General Practitioners 113–14
Rwanda 181

safety compliance 156, 200
safety voice behaviour 200–2
Safety Voice for Ergonomics programme 213
SafeWork Australia 39, 71, 78, 80, 119, 199, 231; Code of Practice 69–70
Saleh, S. 46–7
Sámano-Ríos, M. L. 214
Sang, K. 135
sanitary facilities 135–6
Sartori. S. 227, 244
Schaufeli, W. B. 255, 260–1
SDGs *see* Sustainable Development Goals
Seixas, N. 46
self-employed workers 17, 40, 170, 274
Seligman, M. 256–7
Senbeto, D. L. 158
sense of place 252–67
sense of place scales 262–3
sex: transactional 189; unsafe practices 185, 189
sexual harassment 18, 73, 81, 120, 122, 131–2
Shatté, A. 157
Shaw, D. S. 150
Sherratt, F. 7–9, 12, 18, 28, 291
shift work 34–5, 68, 73, 97–8, 103–4
shotcreting 49
shoulder pain 6, 224–5, 230
shovelling 49
Siegrist, J. 64
silica 3, 31, 34–5, 37–42
silicosis 37, 39–40
Sinclair, R. R. 274
Singapore 6, 273

Sinyai, C. 115
skin disease, occupational 47–8
skin neoplasma 3
sleep disorders 67, 91, 104, 121
sleep quality 31
Smallwood, J. 9–10
Smart Richman, L. 125–6
Smith, J. 181
Smith, P. 197
smoking 2–3, 6, 31
Snashall, D. 29
social determinants of health 4–9
social support 148, 201, 209–13, 258–9, 263
Social Support from Coworkers Index 263
Social Support from Supervisor Index 263
Soderlund, J. 88–9
"soft skills" 75, 213
solar radiation 35
solvents 29, 47, 122
Sonnentag, S. 105
South Africa 172–6, 178, 180–8
South African Business Coalition on HIV/AIDS 184
South Asia 282
Southeast Asia 282
Starratt, A. 213
Statistics South Africa 185
Stattin, M. 231
steel-fixing 49–51, 279–80
Stellman, J. M. 116
Stocks, S. J. 229
stonemasons 29, 39–40, 213
Strazdins, L. 62
stress: co-factors 31; conservation of resources 105; construction industry 64–7; discrimination and 125–6; gender differences 121–2; lifestyle 3; long hours 90; minority stress 124, 126; psychosocial work environment 14; recovery time 104–6; reduction interventions 6; United Kingdom 2020 28; work hours 99; *see also* mental ill health
stroke 2, 89, 186, 280
Sub Saharan Africa 169–90; carbon dioxide emissions 172; colonialism 175; construction industry 173–6, 184–90; COVID-19 171, 174, 176–7; gross domestic fixed investment 173; gross national income 172; HIV/AIDS 172, 178–90; job security 174, 176; malaria 177–8; personal protective equipment 177; population 172; public-private partnerships 174–5; social issues 175–6; tuberculosis 178
subcontracting 17, 65, 71
substance misuse 91, 125, 176, 181, 189, 194, 204, 276
substitution of hazards 32–3, 42, 71, 80
suicide: gender based violence 131; lack of job control 65; rates 3–4; risk factors 66; work hours 89; young workers 206–7
Sun, C. 66–7
supervisors: of apprentices 196, 202, 205–6, 209; depression 65; harassment from 131, 150; harmful practices 15; hostility from 128, 156, 212–13; musculoskeletal disorders 49; support from 21, 65, 72, 75, 99, 122, 194–5, 201–4, 209–11, 259, 263, 265; of young women 200; young workers 202
Sustainable Development Goals 1, 9
Sweden 31, 45, 48, 231
SWEMWBS 264
systems framework 146
systems level conceptual model of work, safety, health and wellbeing 16

Taiwan 158–9
Tanzania 180–1
team resilience 148–50
technology: growth of 290–1; job displacement 290–1; overload 65, 90, 254; risks 290
teleworking 106
Thames Tideway Tunnel 102–4
Theorell, T. 63
Thoracic Society of Australia & New Zealand 40
time management 80
time performance 88–9
time poverty 7–8
toilets 132, 135
Tonkin, K. 159
Total Worker Health model 13–16
Townsend, K. 100–1
trade unions 36, 98
training for resilience 160–3
truck drivers 32
Truxillo, D. M. 227, 239, 242
tuberculosis 37, 176, 178–9, 183, 188–9
Tucker, S. 201
tunnel workers 29, 32, 102–4
Turner, M. 90, 123, 130, 154, 157–9, 224
Turner, N. 200–1

turnover, employee 10–11, 64, 70, 91, 211, 242, 260
Tyler, T. R. 261

Uganda 180–1
UK Health and Safety Executive 3
UNAIDS 178, 181
unemployment 61, 162, 185, 276, 291
United Kingdom: Chartered Institute of Building 90, 223; COVID-19 274, 277; Health and Safety Executive 70; ill health rates 28, 229; mental health 62, 121, 264; occupational allergic contact dermatitis 48; occupational cancer 35; older workers 241; Robens-style model 69; shift work 102; socioeconomic inequalities 5; suicide 4; women in construction 115, 117
United Nations: Agenda for Sustainable Development 64; Department of Economic and Social Affairs–Population Division 185; General Assembly 64, 130; Human Development Index 171; population ageing 222; 2030 Agenda of Sustainable Development Goals 1; working age 224
United Nations Development Programme 171
United States: asbestos 37; back pain 3; Center for Construction Research and Training 134; climate change 280–1; COVID-19 274; illness rates 29; long hours 89; lung cancer 35; mental health 275; National Institute for Occupational Safety and Health 13; noise-induced hearing loss 43–7, 230; older workers 223, 229, 232; sexist graffiti 132; sexual harassment 131; silicosis 40; suicide 3–4; wellness programmes 11; women in construction 115, 135; young workers 198, 232
urinary tract infection 135

value statements 8–9
van der Molen, H. F. 29, 51, 245
van Duivenbooden, C. 224, 230
Van Hooff, M. L. 105–6
van Quaquebeke, N. 261
van Steenbergen, E. F. 260
vanadium 31
Vanderbilt-Adriance, E. 150
Vanhove, A. J. 160
Varianou-Mikellidou, C. 241–2
Venkatesh, K. K. 183

vibration effects 3, 29–30
Victorian Trades Hall Council 131
Victorian Women in Construction Strategy 2019–2022: Building Gender Equity 117
violence, workplace 67, 73, 81, 115, 119, 130–2
vitreous fibres 31
Volkswagen 98

Wagner, H. 134
Walsh, B. M. 263
Walsh, D. C. 8
Warwick-Edinburgh Mental Wellbeing Short-Form 263–4
Watts, J. 129
West Africa 282
wet dust suppression 38, 40–2
Whitehead, M. 4, 7
Whiteside, A. 185
Widjaja, E. C. 122–3
wind turbine construction 283
Winder, C. 48, 153
Windle, G. 150, 157, 262
Winwood, P. C. 154
women see gender
wood dust, 31
work ability 94–6, 224, 227–8, 239, 241–2, 244–5
work conditions: psychosocial hazards 72; significance for health 16
worker participation in decision making 6, 13; see also job control
work-family conflict 91, 101
workforce casualisation 65, 174, 176, 185
work hours 88–107; compressed hours 98; culture change 286–7; gender 91–3, 117; irregular 16–17; job control 94; job demand 66; long 2, 17, 66, 89–90, 94–6, 105; modifying 98–104; mortality 2; psychosocial risk 77; recovery time 104–6; timing 93; weekend work 94–5, 97, 101–2, 105–6; WHO/ILO Global Monitoring Report 2; working from home 277–80; young construction workers 199; see also overtime; shift work
working days lost 9, 30
working from home 277–9
work-life balance 73, 89–96, 99–102, 122, 260, 263, 265
workload see job demand
work pace 68, 73, 79–80, 93–4

workplace wellness programmes 8–9, 11; *see also* interventions
work related diseases: construction industry 27; economic costs 30; global statistics 2; United Kingdom 2020 28; United States 29
work related injuries: gender differences 115; global statistics 2; young workers 194, 197–202
Work-Related Stress Indicator Tool 70
WorkSafe Victoria 50–1, 81–2
WorkWell Mental Health Improvement Fund 81
World Bank 171–2
World Health Organization: alcohol and drug use Sub Saharan Africa 189; asbestos risks 35–7; definition of health 12, 288; gender based approach 18; gender based violence 131; Global Burden of Disease 37; global monitoring study 2; Global Program for the Elimination of Silicosis (WHO/ILO) 38; health promotion by organisations 10–12; healthy workplaces 13, 15; HIV/AIDS 178; occupational health 134; Sustainable Development Goals 9; WHO/ILO Global Monitoring Report 2; working hours 89

young construction workers 194–215; alcohol consumption 204; apprenticeships 194–7, 200–4, 206–13; bullying 206–7; gambling 204; health promotion 213–15; injuries 197–202; job control 206; job demands 206; mental health 205–7; safety voice behaviour 200–2; social support 209–13; substance misuse 204; suicide 206–7; work hours 199; *see also* age factors

Zacher, H. 239
Zambia 180, 182
Zapf, D. 127
Zhu, Y. 159
Zierold, K. M. 202
Zimbabwe 171, 180–2
Zoller, H. M. 7
Zwerling, C. 3